Cerebral Vascular Smooth Muscle and its Control

The Ciba Foundation for the promotion of international cooperation in medical and chemical research is a scientific and educational charity established by CIBA Limited – now CIBA-GEIGY Limited – of Basle. The Foundation operates independently in London under English trust law.

Ciba Foundation Symposia are published in collaboration with Elsevier Scientific Publishing Company / Excerpta Medica / North-Holland Publishing Company in Amsterdam

Elsevier / Excerpta Medica / North-Holland, P.O. Box 211, Amsterdam

Cerebral Vascular Smooth Muscle and its Control

Ciba Foundation Symposium 56 (new series)

1979

Excerpta Medica

Amsterdam · Oxford · New York

Second printing March 1979

ISBN Excerpta Medica 90-219-4062-0
ISBN Elsevier/North-Holland Inc., 0-444-90026-8

Published in March 1978 by Elsevier/Excerpta Medica/North-Holland, P.O. Box 211, Amsterdam and Elsevier/North-Holland Inc., 52 Vanderbilt Avenue, New York, N.Y. 10017.

Suggested series entry for library catalogues: Ciba Foundation Symposia.
Suggested publisher's entry for library catalogues: Elsevier/Excerpta Medica/North-Holland

Ciba Foundation Symposium 56 (new series)

408 pages, 87 figures, 22 tables

Library of Congress Cataloging in Publication Data

Symposium on the Control of Cerebral Vascular Smooth Muscle, London, Eng., 1977.
Cerebral vascular smooth muscle and its control.

(Ciba Foundation symposium; 56 (new series)).
Bibliography: p. Includes index.
1. Brain–Blood-vessels–Congresses. 2. Vascular smooth muscle–Congresses.
I. Title. II. Series: Ciba Foundation. Symposium; new ser., 56.
QP108.5.C4S95 1977 612′.824 77–28855
ISBN 0-444-90026-8.

Printed in The Netherlands by Casparie, Alkmaar

Contents

Participants

Symposium on The Control of Cerebral Vascular Smooth Muscle *held at the Ciba Foundation, London, 11th–13th July 1977*

Chairman: M. J. PURVES Department of Physiology, School of Veterinary Science, University of Bristol, Park Row, Bristol BS1 5LS, UK

J. ASTRUP Department of Clinical Physiology, Bispebjerg Hospital, 2400 Copenhagen NV, Denmark

L. EDVINSSON Department of Histology, University of Lund, Biskopsgatan 5, S-223 62 Lund, Sweden

D. D. HEISTAD Department of Internal Medicine, University Hospitals and Clinics, Iowa City, Iowa 52242, USA

D. HEUSER Physiologisches Institut (1), University of Tübingen, Gmelinstr. 5, 74 Tübingen, West Germany

F. F. JÖBSIS Department of Physiology, Duke University Medical School, Durham, North Carolina 27710, USA

W. R. KEATINGE Department of Physiology, The London Hospital Medical College, Turner Street, London E1 2AD, UK

D. W. LÜBBERS Max-Planck-Institut für Systemphysiologie, Rheinlanddamm 201, D-4600 Dortmund, West Germany

D. G. MCDOWALL Department of Anaesthesia, University of Leeds Medical School, 24 Hyde Terrace, Leeds LS2 9LN, UK

B. S. MELDRUM Department of Neurology, Institute of Psychiatry, De Crespigny Park, Denmark Hill, London SE5 8AF, UK

M. A. MOSKOWITZ Department of Neurology, Peter Bent Brigham Hospital, Huntington Avenue, Boston, Massachusetts 02115, USA

B. NILSSON Brain Research Laboratory, E-Blocket, University Hospital, S-221 85 Lund, Sweden

C. OWMAN Department of Histology, University of Lund, Biskopsgatan 5, S-223 62 Lund, Sweden

SIR GEORGE PICKERING 5 Horwood Close, Headington, Oxford OX3 7RF, UK

F. PLUM Department of Neurology, The New York Hospital, Cornell Medical Center, 525 East 68th Street, New York, NY 10021, USA

M. E. RAICHLE Division of Radiation Sciences, The Edward Mallinckrodt Institute of Radiology, Washington University, 510 South Kingshighway, St Louis, Missouri 63110, USA

S. I. RAPOPORT Laboratory of Neurophysiology, National Institute of Mental Health, 9000 Rockville Pike, Bethesda, Maryland 20014, USA

D. REIS Laboratory of Neurobiology, Department of Neurology, Cornell University Medical College, 1300 York Avenue, New York, NY 10021, USA

C. ROSENDORFF Department of Physiology, University of the Witwatersrand, Medical School, Hospital Street, Johannesburg, Republic of South Africa

R. RUBIO Department of Physiology, University of Virginia, School of Medicine, Charlottesville, Virginia, USA

M. SANDLER Bernard Baron Memorial Research Laboratories, Department of Chemical Pathology, Queen Charlotte's Hospital for Women, Goldhawk Road, London W6 OXG, UK

B. K. SIESJÖ Research Department 4, E-Blocket, University Hospital, S-211 85 Lund, Sweden

I. A. SILVER Department of Pathology, University of Bristol Medical School, University Walk, Bristol BS8 1TD, UK

L. SOKOLOFF Laboratory of Cerebral Metabolism, Building 36, Room 1A-27, National Institute of Mental Health, 9000 Rockville Pike, Bethesda, Maryland 20014, USA

Editors KATHERINE ELLIOTT (*Organizer*) and MAEVE O'CONNOR

Chairman's opening remarks

M. J. PURVES

Department of Physiology, University of Bristol

The purpose of this symposium is to consider some aspects of the regulation of cerebral vascular smooth muscle. In particular, we wish to consider the evidence which suggests that if the metabolism of part of the brain alters, there is a compensatory change in local blood flow; and if this compensation occurs, we should consider what coupling factors might be involved. We think that this is an opportune time to hold such a meeting because during the past year or two there have been a number of important advances in techniques for measuring local cerebral blood flow and metabolism. At the same time, since a number of ions have been proposed as coupling factors, it is appropriate to consider how the level of these ions actually changes in interstitial fluid of the brain, so exploiting recent advances in the use of ion-selective microelectrodes.

Although one meeting never solves any problems, meetings often highlight areas of ignorance and problems which are ripe for solving. And with the possibility of a more leisurely and informed discussion here than at most large international meetings, it should become clearer which questions can be temporarily laid aside and which ought to be pursued energetically over the next year or two.

We felt that it would be useful to have, right at the beginning of this meeting, a review of the field which would place our present preoccupation in some sort of historical context. Professor Plum has responded to some gentle persuasion and has agreed to do this for us. His qualifications are apt. As a neurologist and editor of distinction, he has both contributed to and followed the developments in this field, and because he has studiously avoided the in-fighting we are assured of an objective viewpoint.

Introduction: a multiple factor theory for control of cerebral vascular smooth muscle?

FRED PLUM

Cerebral Vascular Disease Research Center and Department of Neurology, The New York Hospital-Cornell University Medical College, New York

It seems remarkably appropriate to meet in London to discuss the circulation of the brain just nine months shy of the 400th anniversary of Harvey's birth. It comes as a less enchanting reflection to realize that it is now 87 years since another celebrated British team, Roy and Sherrington, first described in 1890 the powerful effect of CO_2 on the cerebral circulation. Yet we still haven't determined the mechanism of how that major product of cerebral metabolism exerts its effect, nor are we certain what part, if any, the CO_2 response plays in regulating the normal coupling that tightly links blood flow to metabolism in the brain.

The last few years have seen a spate of short-paper conferences on various aspects of the cerebral circulation. Many of these have left the impression of having transmitted messages that were fragmented, inconclusive and as often as not either contradictory or repetitious. To avoid these pitfalls would seem to require that we depart here from the usual form of safe presentations and focus more on the questions than on producing comfortable but limited answers. Almost all of us have heard or read much of each others' data before. What we have done less of is to discuss how to integrate the various pieces of information so that we can grasp the relative biological importance of any given experimental finding in relation to health and disease.

Until now, knowledge of cerebral circulatory physiology has advanced in a series of more or less clearly defined epochs (Table 1). The first lasted from Roy and Sherrington until the late 1940s. It collected and consolidated most of the major anatomical facts about the cerebral vasculature and provided the initial leads to many important physiological considerations, but failed to integrate these fragments into a satisfactory synthesis of how the cerebral circulation worked. Kety & Schmidt's nitrous oxide method (1948) solved that impasse and the next decade saw the rapid accumulation of observations

TABLE 1

Methodological epochs in cerebral vascular physiology

1890–1948	Classical period
1948–1960	N_2O method measures global CBF and CMR_{O_2} *in vivo*
1961–1974	Isotope injection method measures regional CBF *in vivo*
1970– →	Short-life isotopes measure regional cerebral metabolism *in vivo*
1975– →	Quantitative 2-DG method measures cerebral micro-metabolism

CBF: cerebral blood flow; CMR_{O_2}: cerebral metabolic rate of oxygen.

which disclosed how over-all cerebral vascular physiology adjusted or changed in health and disease. In 1961 Lassen & Ingvar opened the next epoch with a practical and accurate method for measuring regional cerebral blood flow in animals and man. The decade following that technical development provided, first, an understanding of how regional cerebral flow changed in health, then of how it was altered by disease, and, most recently, demonstrated that regional flow increased or decreased during altered states of physiological function. This last development directly presaged Ter-Pogossian's and Sokoloff's pioneering methods for measuring regional cerebral metabolism (Ter-Pogossian *et al.* 1970; Sokoloff *et al.* 1977). Sokoloff's 2-deoxyglucose (2-DG) method, of course, when combined with other autoradiographic tracers, will for the first time allow flow and metabolism to be quantified simultaneously in even microscopically small regions of brain. The exploration of the 2-DG method is just beginning, as is the exploration, by Raichle (1975), Reivich (1977) and their co-workers, of new techniques that can measure regional cerebral metabolism in awake man by radionuclide emission scanning.

These epochal, method-based, advances in understanding cerebral vascular physiology and metabolism have left several major questions unanswered, however, which perhaps implies that their solution requires different approaches (Table 2). An example is the mystery that still surrounds the function of the perivascular nerve plexuses of the brain.

Dr Purves in his monograph (1972) nicely reviews the classic anatomy of the rich plexus of nerves that invest the intracranial vessels, and Edvinsson (1975) has clearly described the pharmacological subdivisions of this network as outlined by the beautiful histochemical techniques of Professor Owman and his co-workers of the Lund school. Several physiological and pharmacological

TABLE 2

Major questions unsolved by present methods

1.	What is physiological function of perivascular innervations?
2.	Is cerebral vascular resistance (CVR) inhibited by specific or non-specific (multiple?) receptors?
3.	What messenger(s) couple(s) local metabolism to local CVR?
4.	Does alteration of CVR have clinical significance?

studies have demonstrated the unequivocal alterations in cerebral vascular smooth muscle function that occur when these nerves or their transmitters have been cut, stimulated or blocked. What has been less clear is (1) whether neurogenic influences importantly and normally regulate cerebral vascular adjustments to physiological demands by the organism, or (2) whether they function as an emergency mechanism designed to prevent extreme perturbation in the system, or (3) whether they are physiologically superfluous, with little or no biological importance in regulating mammalian cerebral circulation.

The lessons of human diseases suggest to us that these autonomic nerves do in fact make a physiological contribution. The disease idiopathic autonomic insufficiency varies widely in its anatomical severity as well as in the quality and quantity of autonomic functional loss it produces (Black & Petito 1978). Probably all patients with this disease have abnormalities of peripheral sympathetic ganglia, but not all have morphological abnormalities of central autonomic structures. When central structures are involved, however, the impairment can include the solitary complex of the medulla as well as the locus coeruleus, both of which have been regarded as possessing autonomic functions. Several investigators, including Caronna and myself (1973), have studied cerebral vascular resistance in idiopathic autonomic insufficiency. All of the patients so studied retained CO_2 responsiveness in the cerebral vascular bed. Some, especially those with milder forms of the disease, retained cerebral autoregulatory responses to altered blood pressure. The more severely involved patients, however, were found to have pressure-passive cerebral vascular beds during either increases or decreases in systemic blood pressure. Although these subjects with loss of cerebral autoregulation all had advanced disease, with signs of severe peripheral autonomic denervation, they were not systemically ill or hypovolaemic when studied. Since no autopsies were available, one cannot accurately correlate the loss of cerebral vascular pressure regulation with a predominance of either peripheral or central autonomic denervation.

What is inescapable, however, is that the only human condition known to produce nearly complete peripheral autonomic denervation and sometimes extensive central adrenergic denervation removes the normal capacity of the cerebral vascular smooth muscle to adjust to either increases or reductions in the systemic blood pressure. To the clinical investigator, these findings imply that the autonomic innervation of the cerebral vessels *must* be of physiological importance.

A striking and disconcerting aspect of physiological studies on the cerebral circulation has been that the more we have learned, the harder it has become to regard carbon dioxide or the hydrogen ion as the universal messenger that links increased tissue metabolism to the relaxation of cerebral vascular smooth muscle. Brennan and I (see Plum 1971) and Howse *et al.* (1974) tried to measure a change in brain surface pH during the sudden increase in blood flow that accompanies seizures. In those experiments surface pH readings as often turned alkaline as they did acid. Biochemical changes in the tissue, however, demonstrated an increased lactic acid production and we rather unsatisfactorily concluded that impermeability of pia arachnoid membranes to the hydrogen ion might have prevented us from recording the early release of acid. As Astrup and Siesjö will tell us at this meeting, we probably should have believed our electrodes and not our calculated chemistry values. Astrup's and Siesjö's abstracts indicate, however, that while H^+ itself is not the messenger that keeps the brain acid–base balance within such narrow confines, they are unable to propose a specific alternative. Nor do other reported studies identify a satisfactory candidate for the universal messenger.

Perhaps there is no single messenger, and perhaps we should not expect one in a system with several metabolic end-products. It is difficult, for example, to postulate a single molecular messenger that could act as the common intermediary to the cerebral smooth muscle from all the different drugs that affect the cerebral circulation. It may be that many products of cerebral metabolism can inhibit the contraction of cerebral vascular smooth muscle. Hydrogen ions, CO_2, calcium, potassium, adenosine and prostaglandins have all been shown to alter cerebral vascular resistance but none of them qualify as the universal messenger. Such a multiple factor theory for the regulation of cerebral vascular resistance would be analogous to that believed to explain the regulation of pulmonary ventilation.

The cerebral vascular smooth muscle provides one of the major regulators that rapidly adjust the metabolic supply and excretion of the brain. It shares this function with the cerebral vascular endothelium whose enzymes ensure the movement of crucial stuffs between blood and brain, with the astrocytes that control the concentrations of at least H^+, K^+, and NH_4 in the extracellular space of the brain, and with the systemic blood pressure and respiratory apparatus. One would anticipate that biological stimuli that importantly alter one of these systems might turn out to affect others as well. At least I hope that may be one of the ideas this conference will discuss.

References

BLACK, I. B. & PETITO, C. K. (1978) Transsynaptic regulation in idiopathic autonomic insufficiency. *Ann. Neurol.*, in press

CARONNA, J. J. & PLUM, F. (1973) Cerebrovascular regulation in preganglionic and postganglionic autonomic insufficiency. *Stroke 4*, 12–19

EDVINSSON, L. (1975) Neurogenic mechanisms in the cerebrovascular bed. *Acta Physiol. Scand. Suppl. 427*, 1–35

HOWSE, D. C., CARONNA, J. J., DUFFY, T. E. & PLUM, F. (1974) Cerebral energy metabolism, pH and blood flow during seizures in the cat. *Am. J. Physiol. 227*, 1444–1451

KETY, S. S. & SCHMIDT, C. F. (1948) The nitrous oxide method for the quantitative determination of cerebral blood flow in man: theory, procedure and normal values. *J. Clin. Invest. 27*, 476–483

LASSEN, N. A. & INGVAR, D. H. (1961) Blood flow of the cerebral cortex determined by radioactive krypton. *Experientia (Basel) 17*, 42–45

PLUM, F. (1971) The effect of epileptic seizures and comatose states on the oxidative metabolism of the brain, in *Ion Homeostasis of the Brain* (Siesjö, B. K. & Sörenson, S. C., eds.), pp. 439–453, Munksgaard, Copenhagen

PURVES, M. J. (1972) *The Physiology of thc Cerebral Circulation*, Cambridge University Press, London

RAICHLE, M. (1975) Cerebral blood flow and metabolism, in *Outcome of Severe Damage to the Central Nervous System (Ciba Found. Symp. 34)*, pp. 85–92, Elsevier/Excerpta Medica/North-Holland, Amsterdam

REIVICH, M., KUHL, D., WOLF, A., GREENBERG, J., PHELPS, M., IDO, T., CASELLA, V., FOWLER, J., GALLAGHER, B., HOFFMAN, E., ALAVI, A. & SOKOLOFF, L. (1977) Local cerebral glucose metabolism determination in man with ^{18}F-2-deoxy-2-fluoro-D-glucose. *Ann. Neurol. 1*, 495–496

ROY, C. S. & SHERRINGTON, C. S. (1890) The regulation of the blood supply of the brain. *J. Physiol. (Lond.) 11*, 85–108

SOKOLOFF, L., REIVICH, M., KENNEDY, C., DES ROSIERS, M. D., PATLAK, C. S., PETTIGREW, K. D., SAKURADA, O. & SHINOHARA, M. (1977) The (^{14}C) deoxyglucose method for the measurement of local cerebral glucose utilization: theory, procedure, and normal values in the conscious and anesthetized albino rat. *J. Neurochem. 28*, 897–917

TER-POGOSSIAN, M. D., EICHLING, J. O., DAVIS, D. & WELCH, M. J. (1970) The measurement *in vivo* of regional cerebral oxygen utilization by means of oxyhemoglobin labelled with radioactive oxygen-15. *J. Clin. Invest. 49*, 381–389

How vascular smooth muscle works

WILLIAM R. KEATINGE

The London Hospital Medical College, London

Abstract Electrical recordings made from vascular smooth muscle during the last 15 years make it clear that the role of electrical activity in controlling contraction is often important but varies greatly both between different vessels and for different responses of a given vessel. Only a few mammalian vessels have widely conducted electrical activity, but others can develop this activity, with consequent rhythmical contraction, when made anoxic and stimulated. Action potentials play a part in smooth non-rhythmical responses of arteries to nerves and hormones, while passive conduction of depolarization round the vessel wall is responsible for ring contractions of arteries after local injury. Ca and K cause vasodilatation largely by hyperpolarizing the smooth muscle cells. Electrical activity plays no part in some responses. In particular noradrenaline can contract arteries by directly promoting entry of extracellular Ca, and also by releasing Ca stores by non-electrical means. These processes are particularly important in the inner muscle of arteries, which is not directly innervated.

The extent to which activation of one point on a blood vessel is followed by conduction of electrical activity from cell to cell is probably the most important question to be settled in understanding the behaviour of any given blood vessel. The extent of such conduction varies in different vessels, and varies even in the same vessel under different circumstances. A few large vessels, particularly mammalian portal veins, and the aorta of turtles and newborn rats, have been known for some time to have spontaneous and widely conducted electrical discharges (Funaki & Bohr 1964; Roddie 1962; Biamino & Krukenberg 1969). These discharges are relatively easy to record, and they give rise to synchronized rhythmical contractions. At the other extreme some vessels such as rabbit pulmonary artery rarely seem to produce electrical discharges (Su *et al.* 1964). The electrical behaviour of intracerebral vessels is largely obscure, but electrical activity has proved to play an important role in certain reactions of the common carotid artery in sheep, the main artery supplying the brain.

Prolonged electrical and mechanical records can be made from this artery by the sucrose-gap method (Keatinge 1964). These records show that spontaneous activity is absent, but that electrical activity can be induced by vasoconstrictor agents such as noradrenaline and angiotensin. Similar results are obtained by microelectrode studies of the rabbit carotid (Mekata 1971). The electrical activity is often only of brief duration, with one or a short series of discharges. After these discharges activity may cease entirely even though the vasoconstrictor agent remains in high concentration. At this stage there is sustained, steady depolarization. This can in part account for the contraction, which continues, but the main cause of the sustained mechanical response to persistent high concentrations of noradrenaline is independent of electrical changes. The evidence for this is that noradrenaline and other constrictor agents produce much the same degree of sustained contraction when all electrical response has been eliminated by K-rich solutions as they do when electrical activity is present. The main role of electrical activity in the arteries' mechanical response to sustained high concentrations of constrictor hormones is therefore to accelerate the initial contraction when the hormones are first applied.

Although noradrenaline also mediates the arteries' constrictor response to sympathetic nerves, electrical activity in the smooth muscle plays a larger role in bringing about this particular response. One reason for this is the different pattern of stimulation, small packages of noradrenaline being released by individual neurons and acting locally in high concentration for only a short time before being taken up again by the nerve. There is therefore a brief but powerful stimulus to a succession of groups of smooth muscle cells, each group being activated by a single nerve fibre. This leads to a synchronized action potential in the group of smooth muscle cells stimulated (Keatinge 1966). The extent to which these discharges are conducted to adjacent cells is not known but recent microelectrode studies (C. Torrie & W. R. Keatinge, unpublished work) suggest that the distance of conduction is usually very short indeed. The conduction certainly involves cells in only a small part of the thickness of the vessel wall. Smooth muscle cells in the outermost part of the wall, though aligned circularly round the wall like inner cells, are separated into distinct bundles by connective tissue, and though it is likely that electrical activity spreads through the cells of a given bundle, it does not seem to spread to adjacent bundles.

In any event, it is unlikely that nerve-induced action potentials in cells of the outer part of the artery wall often spread to the inner muscle. Since the inner muscle has no direct nerve supply, this raises the question of how the inner muscle cells are activated. A major factor is that the inner cells are much more sensitive than the outer cells to both noradrenaline and other vasoconstrictor agents. This was shown first when either the inner or the outer region of strips of artery wall was damaged by heat, so that only outer or only inner cells, respectively, remained alive (Graham & Keatinge 1972). Such preparations showed that inner cells were 10- to 100-fold more sensitive than outer cells, responding with large contractions to concentrations of constrictor hormones that produced no response from outer tissue. The difference in sensitivity is a real difference in responsiveness by the cells of the two regions rather than a result of differential uptake of the hormones by nerves in the outer region, since the difference remained when nerve uptake was blocked. However, the difference was reduced by prolonged denervation, and is probably produced over a long period by the nerves in the outer region; it represents a reduced sensitivity that is the counterpart of the familiar non-specific type of denervation supersensitivity. It is interesting that the normal absence of nerves from the inner region of arteries in turn seems to be a result of the high pressure in the inner tissues which is sufficient to exclude nerves from the region (Keatinge & Torrie 1976). In any event the inner muscle is the only part of the artery wall that is sensitive enough to respond to common circulating concentrations of vasoconstrictor agents. The inner muscle also contributes to the vessel's response to vasoconstrictor nerves, probably because its high sensitivity enables it to respond to small amounts of transmitter that diffuse to it from the innervated outer region. Small arteries present considerable technical difficulties, but it is at least clear that some of them, such as those of rat mesentery (Trail 1963), fire action potentials in response to sympathetic nerve activity, while others (Von Loh & Bohr 1973) apparently do not.

The inner muscle of the sheep carotid, though it does not readily give persistent rhythmical discharges, can conduct depolarization passively over considerable distances from cell to cell. The direction of this conduction is almost entirely around the vessel wall, in the direction of the long axis of the smooth muscle cells; there is little conduction along the wall. The most important result of this conduction is that a ring contraction of the vessel is produced when one point is injured. It is interesting that action potentials normally play little or no part in this process. No action potentials could be recorded even within 1 mm of the site of injury unless procaine, which facilitated action potentials in vascular smooth muscle, was present. In the absence of procaine the depolarization decayed steadily, with a space constant of approximately 2.4 mm in the circular direction round the vessel wall (Graham & Keatinge 1975). These ring contractions are clearly important in the ability of the vessel to respond directly to injury and so to arrest haemorrhage caused by injury.

Another major factor in the arrest of arterial haemorrhage is the vessel's response to vasoconstrictor substances released by clotting blood. The role of these, the most important of which are 5-hydroxytryptamine, noradrenaline, histamine and vasoactive proteins (Kapp *et al.* 1968), has long been known. It has recently become clear that the outer muscle gives relatively little response to the concentrations of these substances produced by clotting blood (Graham & Keatinge 1975). The major part of the vessel's response to these is produced by its highly sensitive inner muscle, and it is clear that any injury or disease that results in the inner muscle coming into close contact with thrombus or its products will cause powerful contraction. This could clearly cause acute ischaemia by suddenly completing the occlusion of an artery that is already partly obstructed by thrombosis. The mechanism of an artery for closing an injury to its wall is therefore a moderately complex one. It is in general well adapted to halting leakage of blood through a traumatic lesion of the wall without unduly restricting flow through the lumen. The mechanism can, however, operate inappropriately to halt flow through an artery whose wall is physically intact if a sufficiently intense mechanical or chemical stimulus reaches the inner muscle.

The action potentials of sheep carotid smooth muscle, which usually last about a second, are at least partly Na-based, though they differ from Na-based action potentials of nerve and striated muscle in being insensitive to tetrodotoxin. The evidence is that they are readily obtained in Ca-free saline but cannot be elicited when Na is also removed, and that they are accompanied by influx of Na into the cells (Keatinge 1968*a*, *b*). However, action potentials could sometimes be elicited from the arteries in Ca-containing solution free of Na. This was so particularly when tetraethylammonium or procaine was present to block stabilizing K channels (Jacobs & Keatinge 1974). The channels carrying the inward current therefore seem to be able to admit Ca as well as Na. The arteries can also produce slow discharges lasting many seconds. These occur particularly during anoxia with Ca present or in the presence of high concentrations of Mg or Mn (Keatinge 1976). Recent evidence (unpublished) indicates that these discharges are associated with an increase in membrane conductance and are due to a slowly inactivated inward current that can be carried by any of these three ions. Neither these nor spike discharges are easily elicited by simple electrical stimulation in physiological solutions, either in rabbit (Mekata 1971) or sheep carotid arteries (Mekata & Keatinge 1975). This stability is due to the opening of K channels on depolarization, which produces powerful outward-going rectification which resists further depolarization. The slow discharges are readily produced only after the K channels are closed by Mn, Mg or some other agent. Both the spike discharges and the slow discharges are remarkably resistant to conventional blocking agents such as local anaesthetics and verapamil. Discovery of an agent that would act specifically on these channels, and allow the responses that they mediate to be controlled specifically, would clearly be of considerable value.

It might be expected that the mechanical response of arteries to depolarization would be produced by electrically mediated release of Ca from the endoplasmic reticulum, as is the response of striated muscle. Arterial smooth muscle cells contain large amounts of such reticulum, which often makes close contact with the surface membrane (Devine *et al.* 1972; Keatinge 1972*a*). Although it remains possible that some Ca can be released in this way after surface depolarization, clear evidence of such release has not been obtained. Mechanical responses of arteries to K depolarization cease rather quickly when external Ca is removed, and in the sheep carotid the time of cessation matches the time needed for extracellular Ca to fall to threshold level (Keatinge 1976). If depolarization does act by releasing Ca stores in arteries it must utilize some store that equilibrates rather rapidly with extracellular Ca. There is in fact no clear evidence at present that depolarization does not act simply by opening Ca channels in the cell membrane and allowing free extracellular Ca ions to enter.

The effect of small increases in external K and Ca on blood vessels is puzzling at first sight. Since an increase in K usually depolarizes cells, while an increase in Ca tends to increase Ca entry directly and so to cause contraction, it might be supposed that either K or Ca would increase the mechanical tone of arteries. In practice, small external increases in either ion usually cause vasodilatation. Small increases in K in fact hyperpolarize arteries by stimulating an electrogenic Na pump. At low external Ca concentrations, an increase in Ca also hyperpolarizes arteries, presumably because Ca binds to the outer surface of the cell membrane just as it does in nerves with Na-based action potentials.

Noradrenaline, unlike depolarization, can utilize a resistant Ca store from cells in arteries. A number of arteries have been shown to respond to noradrenaline after long periods in Ca-free solutions, or after the addition of lanthanum to block Ca entry (Van Breemen *et al.* 1972). Sheep carotid arteries respond, after exposure to Ca-free solution containing EDTA, for long enough to lower extracellular Ca throughout the tissue to well below the threshold level for contraction (Keatinge 1972*a*, *b*). Direct evidence of Ca release in the form of increased efflux of ^{45}Ca after noradrenaline has been added was first reported in rabbit aorta by Hudgins (1969). A feature of this response to noradrenaline, at least in sheep carotid arteries, is that it can be obtained in Ca-free saline when the normal depolarizing response to noradrenaline is not only depressed but also reversed in direction. It seems clear that the mechanism by which noradrenaline activates the arteries in Ca-free solution is chemical and does not depend on the electrical depolarization of the cell membrane. It should be mentioned that noradrenaline also seems to allow entry of Ca from the extracellular space, and that the slow, sustained phase of mechanical response to noradrenaline is due to this Ca entry. With the electrically mediated response there are therefore three routes by which noradrenaline can produce vascular contraction.

The local organization of arterial contraction is therefore complex. How many of the mechanisms present in the common carotid are shared by the cerebral arteries remains to be seen. It is at least known that the pattern of innervation of the larger intracranial vessels is not very different from that of the common carotid. It would be surprising if the intracranial arteries did not also share many of its mechanisms of response.

References

BIAMINO, G. & KRUKENBERG, P. (1969) Synchronization and conduction of excitation in the rat aorta. *Am. J. Physiol. 217*, 376–382

DEVINE, C. E., SOMLYO, A. V. & SOMLYO, A. P. (1972) Sarcoplasmic reticulum and excitation contraction coupling in mammalian smooth muscle. *J. Cell Biol. 52*, 690–718

FUNAKI, S. & BOHR, D. R. (1964) Electrical and mechanical activity of a mammalian vein. *Nature (Lond.) 203*, 192–194

GRAHAM, J. M. & KEATINGE, W. R. (1972) Differences in sensitivity to vasoconstrictor drugs within the wall of the sheep carotid artery. *J. Physiol. (Lond.) 221*, 477–492

GRAHAM, J. M. & KEATINGE, W. R. (1975) Responses of inner and outer muscle of the sheep carotid artery to injury. *J. Physiol. (Lond.) 247*, 473–482

HUDGINS, P. M. (1969) Some drug effects on calcium movements in aortic strips. *J. Pharmacol. Exp. Ther. 170*, 303–310

JACOBS, A. & KEATINGE, W. R. (1974) Effects of procaine and lignocaine on electrical and mechanical activity of smooth muscle of sheep carotid arteries. *Br. J. Pharmacol. 51*, 405–411

KAPP, J., MAHALEY, M. S. & ODOM, G. L. (1968) Cerebral artery spasm. Part 2. Experimental evaluation of mechanical and humoral factors in pathogenesis. *J. Neurosurg. 29*, 339–349.

KEATINGE, W. R. (1964) Mechanism of adrenergic stimulation of mammalian arteries and its failure at low temperatures. *J. Physiol. (Lond.) 174*, 184–205

KEATINGE, W. R. (1966) Electrical and mechanical response of arteries to stimulation of sympathetic nerves. *J. Physiol. (Lond.) 185*, 701–715

KEATINGE, W. R. (1968*a*) Ionic requirements for arterial action potential. *J. Physiol. (Lond.) 194*, 169–182

KEATINGE, W. R. (1968*b*) Sodium flux and electrical activity of arterial smooth muscle. *J. Physiol. (Lond.) 194*, 183–200

KEATINGE, W. R. (1972*a*) Mechanical response with reversed electrical reference to nor-adrenaline by Ca-deprived arterial smooth muscle. *J. Physiol. (Lond.) 224*, 21–34
KEATINGE, W. R. (1972*b*) Ca concentration and flux in Ca-deprived arteries. *J. Physiol. (Lond.) 224*, 35–59
KEATINGE, W. R. (1976) Calcium in the arterial smooth muscle cell in *Ionic Action in Vascular Smooth Muscle* (Betz, E., ed.), pp. 67–70, Springer-Verlag, Berlin
KEATINGE, W. R. & TORRIE, C. (1976) Action of sympathetic nerves on inner and outer muscle of sheep carotid artery, and effect of pressure on nerve distribution. *J. Physiol. (Lond.) 257*, 699–712
MEKATA, F. (1971) Electrophysiological studies of the smooth muscle cell membrane of the rabbit common carotid artery. *J. Gen. Physiol. 57*, 738–751
MEKATA, F. & KEATINGE, W. R. (1975) Electrical behaviour of inner and outer muscle of sheep carotid artery. *Nature (Lond.) 258*, 534–535
RODDIE, I. C. (1962) The transmembrane potentials associated with smooth muscle activity in turtle arteries and veins. *J. Physiol. (Lond.) 163*, 138–150
SU, C., BEVAN, J. A. & URSILLO, R. C. (1964) Electrical quiescence of pulmonary artery smooth muscle during sympathomimetic stimulation. *Circ. Res. 15*, 20–27
TRAIL, W. M. (1963) Intracellular studies on vascular smooth muscle. *J. Physiol. (Lond.) 167*, 17–18
VAN BREEMEN, C., FARINAS, B. R., GERBA, P. & MCNAUGHTON, E. D. (1972) Excitation contraction coupling in rabbit aorta studied by the lanthanum method for measuring cellular calcium influx. *Circ. Res. 30*, 44–55
VON LOH, D. & BOHR, D. R. (1973) Membrane potentials of smooth muscle cells of isolated resistance vessels. *Proc. Soc. Exp. Biol. Med. 144*, 513–516

Discussion

Purves: Professor Plum made the point that intracranial arteries characteristically respond physiologically to hyperpolarization by dilatation. Is anything known about the junctions between smooth muscle cells comparable to what is known for skeletal muscle cells about the way that current flows between cells, perhaps producing an overall hyperpolarization, particularly in the inner part? What sort of resistances might be involved?

Keatinge: The longitudinal resistance is high, but the basic membrane resistance is also high, with the net result that the space constant is long, often 3 mm, allowing widespread passive conduction around the vessel wall in sheep carotid arteries. There are large differences between arteries in this respect. I would hesitate to extrapolate to the cerebral vessels, but the segmental contractions of cerebral arteries seen in a number of conditions might be mediated electrically to some extent. The cell-to-cell connections responsible are the classical smooth muscle junctions which used to be described as tight junctions and are now generally called gap junctions or nexuses.

Siesjö: I have three simple questions. First, what is the arrangement of the muscle fibres in small resistance vessels? In other words, is dilatation always caused by relaxation of circularly arranged smooth muscle fibres?

Second, what sort of electrical activity in the cells is needed for dilatation to be induced? Third, would the cells always react to a restriction of their own oxygen or substrate supply by dilatation?

Keatinge: Speden (1964) and Steedman (1966) showed that mesenteric arterioles of rat and guinea-pig were electrically quiescent in the absence of stimulation but if the sympathetic nerve supply was naturally or artificially stimulated the cells fired action potentials. Other people have failed to find action potentials in other small arteries. Some of these negative results may reflect damage to cells, but there are enough negative findings to suggest that some arterioles rarely fire action potentials even when stimulated. They usually undergo depolarization when stimulated.

Purves: Professor Siesjö's question is, effectively, what is the mechanism of dilatation, even in the absence of action potentials? Is it some peculiar arrangement of smooth muscle, or changes in resting membrane potential, or what?

Keatinge: Potassium relaxation is seen in a lot of vessels, and seems to result from hyperpolarization brought about by direct activation of the sodium pump by external potassium. Our information about other physiological dilator agents is limited. The sheep carotid artery, like many others, is not very sensitive to vasodilators *in vitro*. Vasodilators however, like constrictors, act partly by hyperpolarization and partly by other means. Their effects are only seen after stimulation, for example by noradrenaline.

Reis: Could you dilate a little on the gradient of innervation across the carotid and its relationship to the arterial pressure? Sympathetic nerves are capable of great plasticity and under certain conditions the innervation may extend into the interior of the vessel. Bevan *et al.* (1975, 1976) have observed that, if intra-arterial pressure is increased by aortic ligation in the rabbit, there is an increase in the sympathetic innervation of the artery. The relationship to pressure gradients within arteries in the head would predict that there would be a denser innervation along the media.

Keatinge: There is in general quite good negative correlation between the intraluminal pressure in different arteries and the extent to which nerves penetrate the muscle layer. Some intracranial vessels, for example, have rather dense sympathetic innervation which penetrates quite a long way.

Purves: Are all these recordings made at what might be regarded as normal transmural pressure?

Keatinge: We mostly use helical strips of artery and the tension applied is enough to simulate the normal pressure.

Owman: I know that a relationship between pressure and innervation can be shown experimentally. I would not think that this is a decisive factor for the normal pattern of innervation of a blood vessel. For example, if one makes a lesion in the brain to stimulate sprouting or regeneration of central neurons, these newly forming fibres grow out also on the surface of the brain to innervate or reinnervate the vessels at the base of the brain (Katzman *et al.* 1971). In these circumstances the nerves penetrate throughout the entire media of that vessel, although the vessel is probably under the same luminal pressure as normally. Thus in general terms the nerve fibres appear to penetrate the entire vessel wall in certain parts of the circulation, or they are located on the surface of the vessel, irrespective of luminal pressure. Other conditions than pressure may govern a given pattern of vascular innervation.

Keatinge: Is this in vessels that are completely canalized? During repair of a vessel there is a period in which it is thrombosed.

Owman: The vessel itself is not at all involved in the lesion. The lesion is made in the brain parenchyma, for example in the region of the nigro-neostriatal tract. The tract of the lesion probe tends to lead the regenerating nerve fibres out to the surface of the brain. These fibres also supply the vessels with extremely dense networks of nerve fibres, for example from the substantia nigra in the case of dopamine fibres. Such vessels then achieve an abnormal pattern of innervation; the fibres innervate the entire vessel wall whereas under normal conditions that vessel is innervated only on the surface, with the nerves running in the adventitia.

Keatinge: It would be interesting to have some detailed histological accounts of how the nerves run. If nerves enter a vessel wall at a very low angle they might be able to penetrate without encountering a critical pressure gradient.

Edvinsson: The pial vessels are densely innervated by sympathetic adrenergic nerves and the medial layer is rather thin. In cat pial arteries at the base of the brain there are only six to eight layers of smooth muscle cells in the vessel wall. Furthermore, the response to noradrenaline in terms of ED_{50} values (concentration of the agonist resulting in half maximum effect) is obtained in cerebral vessels at relatively higher molar concentrations than in extracranial vessels. Could this be comparable with the responsiveness of the inner layer of the sheep carotid artery?

Keatinge: That is possible.

Lübbers: You spoke about the effect of anoxia on electrical activity. Is anything known about the effect of high oxygen tension?

Keatinge: I do not know of work in blood vessels with O_2 tensions greater than atmospheric pressure.

Lübbers: In your preparations you get electrical activity from the outer layer of the muscle. Does this still happen in denervation experiments?

Keatinge: We haven't looked at that yet.

Rosendorff: The differential sensitivity to noradrenaline of the inner and outer layers of arterial smooth muscle is interesting. The explanation may be more complex than has been suggested here, and may have something to do with the very potent inactivation mechanisms for noradrenaline and the distribution of these mechanisms through the thickness of the media. When noradrenaline is infused intravascularly, that is, applied to the media from the lumen side, it has very little effect on cerebral blood flow. We think that this is because of the very formidable barriers to ingress of the noradrenaline from blood to receptors in the media; these barriers include the uptake of noradrenaline into vascular smooth muscle cells ('uptake-2'), a variety of catabolic enzymes like monoamine oxidase (MAO; EC 1.4.3.4) and catechol-*O*-methyltransferase (COMT; EC 2.1.1.6), and, towards the adventitial side of the media where innervation density is highest, uptake into nerve terminals. By inhibiting any one or a combination of these inactivation mechanisms, one can increase the local concentration of noradrenaline available to receptors, and therefore increase the responsiveness of vascular smooth muscle to the amine. Have you any thoughts about the possibility that the differential sensitivity which you describe can be explained by differences in smooth muscle uptake of noradrenaline in the inner and outer layers, or by differences in MAO or COMT activity between these two regions?

Keatinge: I do not know, but we minimized the effect of such factors by doing our experiments with sustained concentrations of the hormone and using denervated arteries in some cases.

Owman: There is no information on differential levels of enzymes in the wall of arteries and arterioles. What we know is that the endothelial cells are rich in certain enzymes. I am thinking particularly of the information available on the capillary endothelium (Hardebo *et al.* 1976).

Rubio: The idea that the innervation of the deep layers can disappear because of an increase in the interstitial pressure surrounding the nerves doesn't fit too well with what happens in the heart. In the left ventricle there are high pressures in the endocardial layers. Both light microscopy and electron microscopy show that vessels in the endocardium, where the nerves are exposed to very high pressures, are all almost equally innervated.

Keatinge: Pressures in the arteries of the heart and in the cardiac muscle itself are of course intermittent. When the ventricle relaxes the pressure drops to near atmospheric. Perhaps nerves may tolerate intermittent spells of high pressure that they wouldn't tolerate if sustained. We certainly need more information on this.

References

BEVAN, R. D., PURDY, R. E., SU, C. & BEVAN, J. A. (1975) Evidence for an increase in adrenergic nerve function in blood vessels from experimental hypertensive rabbits. *Circ. Res. 37*, 503–508

BEVAN, R. D., VAN MARTHANS, E. & BEVAN, J. A. (1976) Hyperplasia of vascular smooth muscle in experimental hypertension. *Circ. Res. Suppl. 38*, 58–62

HARDEBO, J. E., EDVINSSON, L., FALCK, B. LINDVALL, M., OWMAN, CH., ROSENGREN, E. & SVENGAARD, N.-AA. (1976) Experimental models for histochemical and chemical studies of the enzymatic blood-brain barrier for amine precursors, in *The Cerebral Vessel Wall* (Cervós-Navarro, J. *et al.*, eds.), pp. 233–244, Raven Press, New York

KATZMAN, R., BJÖRKLUND, A., OWMAN, CH., STENEVI, U. & WEST, K. A. (1971) Evidence for regenerative axon sprouting of central catecholamine neurons in the rat mesencephalon following electrolytic lesions. *Brain Res. 25*, 579–596

SPEDEN, R. N. (1964) Electrical activity of single smooth muscle cells of the mesenteric artery produced by splanchnic nerve stimulation in the guinea-pig. *Nature (Lond.) 202*, 193–194

STEEDMAN, W. M. (1966) Microelectrode studies on vascular smooth muscle. *J. Physiol (Lond.) 186*, 382–400

Capillary flow in the brain cortex during changes in oxygen supply and state of activation

D. W. LÜBBERS and E. LENIGER-FOLLERT

Max-Planck-Institut für Systemphysiologie, Dortmund

Abstract Changes in regional blood flow do not always correspond to changes in capillary flow (microflow) at all sites in the brain cortex. Changes in microflow during activation of the brain tissue and the relationship of changes in P_{O_2}, pH and pK to changes in microflow were therefore studied.

Microflow was recorded continuously and simultaneously at several measuring sites by the local hydrogen clearance method. Additionally, local tissue P_{O_2} was measured in the same capillary area. When the tissue was locally activated by direct electrical stimulation, microflow increased within 1 to 2 s of the beginning of stimulation, and the increase was uniform at all measuring sites.

As local tissue P_{O_2} did not decrease but increased immediately after the beginning of stimulation in parallel with the increased microflow, the hyperaemia could not be triggered by local hypoxia. Local H^+ and K^+ activities were therefore studied with microelectrodes. The H^+ activity at first decreased and later increased, whereas the local K^+ activity increased very rapidly, within a few milliseconds. According to the time course of the activities, therefore, only K^+ could be the trigger for the initial rapid increase in microflow. Later, H^+ activity could play a role in the maintenance of functional hyperaemia. The increase in microflow also occurs when the cortex is activated in a more physiological way by indirect stimulation (evoked potentials).

It has been known for a long time that cerebral blood flow increases with an increase in arterial P_{CO_2} (Pa_{CO_2}) or a decrease in arterial P_{O_2} (Pa_{O_2}); vice versa, it decreases when Pa_{CO_2} decreases and Pa_{O_2} increases. Since an increased P_{CO_2} is produced by an increase in metabolism and a decreased Pa_{O_2} means a decrease in oxygen supply to the tissue, both situations indicate that a higher blood flow is needed to normalize the oxygen supply to the tissue. Both CO_2 and O_2 have an effect of their own. These effects, and the easy diffusibility of O_2 and CO_2, make them very suitable for playing a part in the overall metabolic regulation of tissue blood flow, and they could perhaps act as the main stimulus for the basic mechanisms of flow regulation: dilatation and

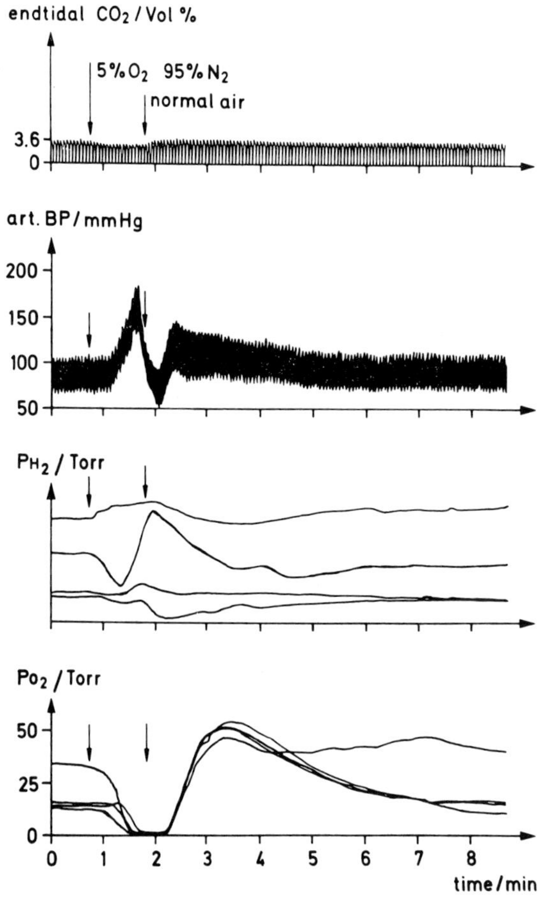

FIG. 1. Changes in microflow, P_{H_2} and tissue P_{O_2} during reduced arterial P_{O_2}. art BP: arterial blood pressure; P_{H_2}: tissue hydrogen pressure (an increase in P_{H_2} means a decrease in microflow); P_{O_2}: oxygen pressure measured on the brain surface (gyrus suprasylvius, cat; barbiturate anaesthesia). (Reproduced from Leniger-Follert *et al.* 1976, with permission.)

contraction of the vascular smooth muscle. Measurements of regional flow, as performed by local clearance with a radioactive tracer, have demonstrated that the same results can be found with regional flow through the grey and white matter (for review see Purves 1972; Lübbers 1972; Betz 1972). The distribution of O_2 and CO_2 in the tissue would imply a relatively homogeneous flow reaction in brain areas with changing metabolism. In animals breathing 5% O_2 in N_2, both total and regional blood flow always increase. Fig. 1

however, shows that, in spite of this well-known homogeneous reaction of regional flow, local flow through such a region can vary considerably (Leniger-Follert *et al.* 1976; Leniger-Follert & Lübbers 1977*a*). The figure shows four traces of local flow, that is flow at the capillary level, measured simultaneously in the cat. One trace follows the changes in blood pressure passively. Two traces show an increase and one—unexpectedly—shows a marked decrease in microflow. Since regional flow always increases under the same conditions local factors must exist which play an important role and modify the over-all reaction.

Aside from direct observations, two methods are available by which local flow can be monitored at the capillary level: (1) hydrogen clearance with hydrogen applied locally as a direct method; (2) measurement of local tissue Po_2 as an indirect method.

Local hydrogen clearance is a new method by which the flow is measured by generating hydrogen by an electrical current and measuring it polarographically (Lübbers & Stosseck 1970; Stosseck *et al.* 1974). We have mostly used multiwire surface elements (Leniger-Follert & Lübbers 1976). The distance between the H_2-producing and measuring wires was about 300 μm. Such an H_2–PH_2 element measures the flow in a tissue volume of about 0.05 to 0.2 mm^3 (Skolasinska *et al.* 1977). Acker *et al.* (1977) constructed a microneedle H_2–PH_2 element containing two 1 μm platinum microelectrodes. This element monitors the flow in a sphere of only about 80 μm in diameter.

Wodick (1976) was able to analyse quantitatively the transport of hydrogen in blood-perfused tissue with local generation of hydrogen. If hydrogen is supplied by a pulse, the time course of hydrogen, $p(t)$, is described by

$$p(t) = \frac{Q}{(D^*t)^{3/2}} \exp \frac{-r^2}{4D^*t} + \frac{x\bar{v}}{2D^*} - \frac{\bar{v}^2 t}{4D^*} \qquad (1)$$

where Q is a constant.

Equation (1) shows that microflow is characterized by three parameters: (1) mean flow per area, $\bar{v}$, which takes into account only the amount of indicator which leaves a plane perpendicular to the flow direction, (2) an apparent diffusion coefficient, D^*, being $D + \gamma v_w{}^2$, where v_w is the absolute flow per area, (3) x, where x is a projection of the direction of mean flow on the connecting line, r, between H_2 source and H_2 measuring site.

This analysis shows that, by local application of the indicator directly into the tissue, flow per area and not flow per volume is measured. Flow per area has the same dimension as flow velocity.

Recently we (R. Wodick, U. Grossmann & D. W. Lübbers, unpublished work) have developed equations which describe the continuous flow measurement. For the continuously measured hydrogen pressure, Ps, the following equation holds:

$$\text{ks} = \frac{2}{r}\,\frac{Q}{D^*}\,\exp\left[\frac{-\bar{v}(r-x)}{2D^*}\right] \tag{2}$$

The equation shows that the continuous flow depends on the same set of parameters as *p(t)* in Eq. (1). A change in Ps can mean: (1) a change in absolute flow per area, (2) a change in mean flow per area (for example, by a change in the fraction of countercurrent flow), (3) a change in the direction of mean flow. We call the P_{H_2} signal, Ps, produced by these flow parameters, 'microflow'.

We can easily compare the data on flow per area with the values of flow per volume of this area by an additional arterial injection of hydrogen (or, if possible, by hydrogen inhalation). Then the element is used to register the usual clearance curve; but, since the tissue is saturated with hydrogen from the arterial inflow of the capillary, this kind of clearance covers a larger tissue sample than does the microflow.

We also investigated microflow during changes in blood pressure. In spite of a well-defined autoregulatory reaction of regional flow, microflow showed only partial flow regulation. At other measuring sites, microflow increased with increased blood pressure and decreased as blood pressure decreased (Leniger-Follert & Lübbers 1975).

Before we discuss the possible meaning and importance of these inhomogeneous reactions of microflow, we shall demonstrate another example of indirect measurements of local flow reactions. Fig. 2 shows the change in tissue P_{O_2} in the cat when arterial P_{O_2} changes from about 90 to 180 mmHg (Leniger-Follert *et al.* 1975). P_{O_2} is measured with a multiwire surface element (Kessler & Lübbers 1966). Each wire measures the oxygen pressure in a sphere about 30 μm in diameter. Similar reactions of tissue P_{O_2} have been also described by other authors (Bicher 1973; Nair *et al.* 1975).

To understand these reactions and the influence of flow changes, we should remember that tissue P_{O_2} is a balance between the local O_2 demand of the tissue and the oxygen locally delivered by the adjacent capillaries. If the oxygen demand remains constant—as can be assumed to happen under these conditions—the change in tissue P_{O_2} is mainly influenced by the blood P_{O_2} and flow. The increase in blood P_{O_2} from 90 to 180 mmHg should result in an increase in tissue P_{O_2}. However, only three traces distinctly increase. The others change only a little or not at all. Since such reactions have been found when the measuring wires were only 100 μm apart, the behaviour of tissue P_{O_2} reflects that of the adjacent capillaries. Smaller changes at a low

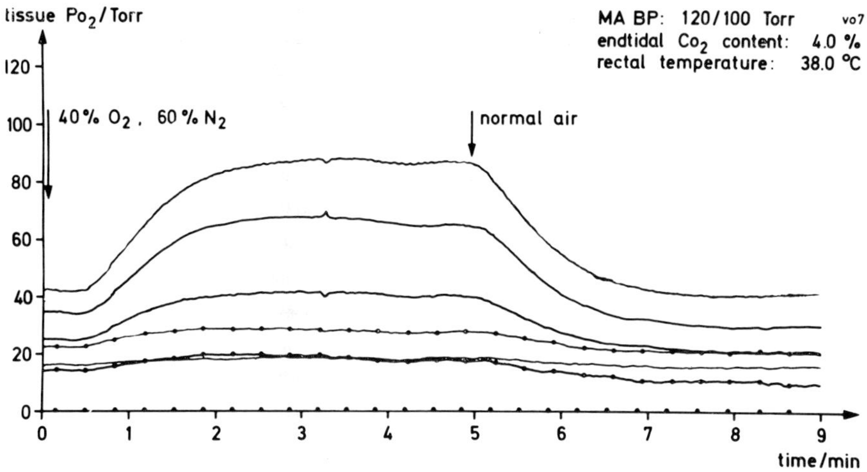

FIG. 2. Original recording of local tissue Po_2 (surface of the grey matter, cat) during exposure to 40% O_2. Tissue Po_2 was recorded at seven sites with a membrane-covered multiwire platinum electrode (diameter of the platinum wire, 15 μm). MABP: mean arterial blood pressure. (Reproduced from Leniger-Follert *et al.* 1975, with permission.)

Po_2 are not in themselves an argument for flow changes since the release of oxygen from haemoglobin makes the reaction of tissue Po_2 non-linear.

To analyse this non-linear behaviour of Po_2, we shall first discuss the changes in the oxygen concentrations in blood, $[O_2]$. Let us assume that a central capillary supplies O_2 to a cylindrical space with homogeneous tissue oxygen consumption. As a consequence of the homogeneous O_2 consumption, the oxygen content of the blood, $[O_2]$, decreases linearly along the length of the capillary, *l*, from the arterial oxygen concentration, $a[O_2]$, to the venous $v[O_2]$ (Fig. 3). Under steady-state conditions, the oxygen delivery to the tissue, $\dot{T}[O_2]$, must match the oxygen consumption, $\dot{A}[O_2]$. Oxygen delivery to the tissue is given by the product 'arterio-venous difference of oxygen content, $\Delta[O_2]$, times flow, $\dot{F}$':

$$\dot{A}[O_2] = \dot{T}[O_2] = \Delta[O_2] \cdot \dot{F} = [a[O_2] - v[O_2]] \cdot \dot{F} \tag{3}$$

and

$$[a[O_2] - v[O_2]] = \frac{\dot{A}[O_2]}{\dot{F}} \tag{4}$$

or

$$v[O_2] = a[O_2] - \frac{\dot{A}[O_2]}{\dot{F}} \tag{5}$$

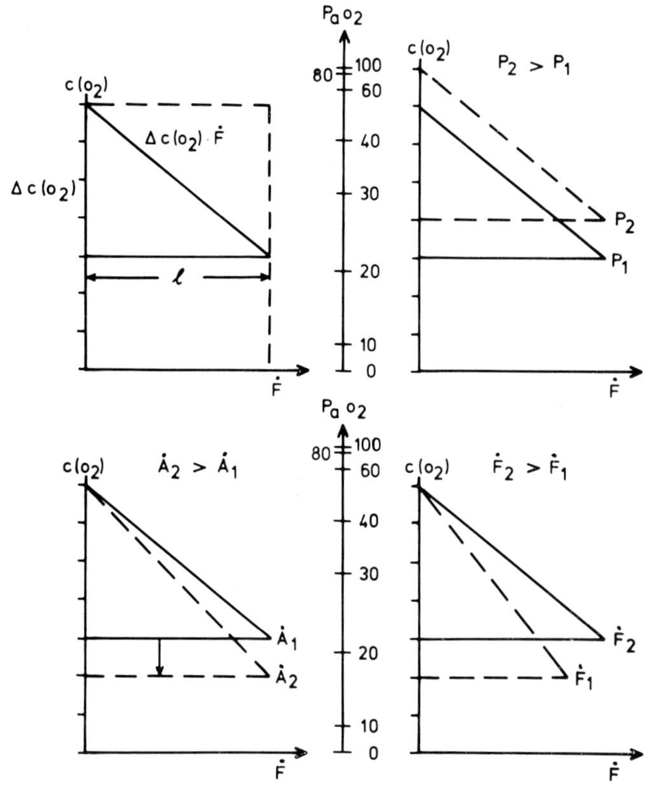

FIG. 3. Influence of changes in arterial oxygen pressure, oxygen consumption and flow on changes in oxygen concentration along the capillary (cat). The oxygen delivered to tissue corresponds to Eq. (3), $\dot{T}(O_2) = \triangle c(O_2)\cdot\dot{F}$. With homogeneous oxygen consumption, $\dot{A}(O_2)$, oxygen concentration decreases linearly along the capillary length, *l*.

The situation is shown before and after changing different parameters: arterial Po_2 ($P_2 > P_1$), oxygen consumption ($\dot{A}_2 > \dot{A}_1$), and flow ($\dot{F}_2 > \dot{F}_1$). y-axis: oxygen concentration $c(O_2)$ (linear) or oxygen pressure Pao_2 (non-linear). x-axis: flow, $\dot{F}$ (and capillary length, *l*).

If the O_2 concentration, $[O_2]$, at a site other than the venous end of the capillary is being discussed, $v[O_2]$ has to be replaced by $c[O_2]$

$$c[O_2] = a[O_2] - \frac{\dot{A}_c[O_2]}{\dot{F}_c} \tag{6}$$

($\dot{A}_c[O_2]$ and $\dot{F}_c$ refer to the tissue volume involved).

Fig. 3 shows how increases in arterial Po_2, ($P_2 > P_1$), tissue respiration ($A_2 > A_1$) and flow ($F_2 > F_1$) affect the changes in blood oxygen concentration, $\Delta[O_2]$.

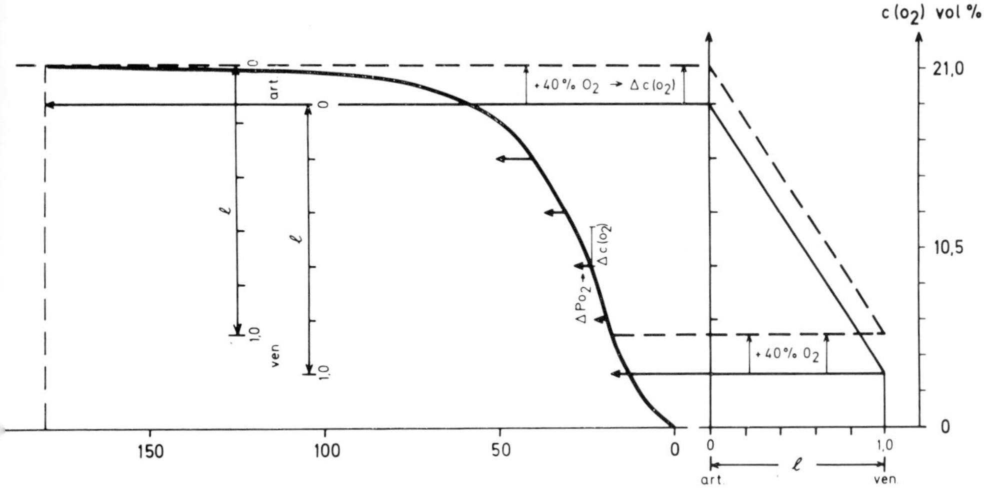

FIG. 4. Influences of changes in arterial P_{O_2} on tissue P_{O_2} (cat). When arterial P_{O_2} increases the arterial oxygen concentration, $c(O_2)$, increases (dashed lines) (see Fig. 3, $P_2 > P_1$); $c(O_2)$ decreases linearly along the capillary length, l. From the oxygen dissociation curve (left), the corresponding blood P_{O_2} values and the increases in these values (arrows) can be seen.

To obtain from the oxygen concentration the corresponding P_{O_2} values the oxygen dissociation curve has to be taken into account:

$$[O_2]_b = k \cdot b(P_{O_2}, P_i) \cdot P_{O_2} \tag{7}$$

(P_i = other factors influencing O_2 dissociation) and, if P_i is constant,

$$[O_2] = k \cdot b(P_{O_2}) \cdot P_{O_2} \tag{7a}$$

If we now experimentally increase the oxygen pressure from 90 to 180 mmHg, the arterial and venous O_2 concentrations increase to the same amount, since the linear slope of the decrease in the oxygen content along the capillary is not changed by this increase. To demonstrate the corresponding P_{O_2} changes, the O_2 dissociation curve has been drawn beside the $[O_2]$ curve (Fig. 4). The linear decrease in $[O_2]$ is accompanied by a non-linear decrease in the blood P_{O_2}. An increase in $a[O_2]$, with concomitant and equal increases along the capillary, brings about different increases in the blood P_{O_2}, as shown in Fig. 4 by arrows of different lengths. With Eq. (7a) we obtain for the arterial P_{O_2}

$$P_{aO_2} = \frac{a[O_2]}{k \cdot b(P_{aO_2})} \tag{8}$$

and using Eqs. (6) and (7a)

$$P_{c}O_2 = \frac{c[O_2]}{k \cdot b(P_{c}O_2)} = \frac{a[O_2] - \dot{A}[O_2]\dot{F}}{k \cdot b(P_{c}O_2)} \tag{9}$$

$$= \frac{k \cdot b(PaO_2) \cdot PaO_2 - \dot{A}(O_2)/\dot{F}}{k \cdot b(P_{c}O_2)} \tag{10}$$

Equations (9) and (10) show that the capillary PO_2 depends on arterial PO_2, oxygen binding curve, tissue O_2 consumption and flow

$$P_{c}O_2 = f\{PaO_2, k \cdot b(PO_2, P_i), \dot{A}[O_2], \dot{F}\} \tag{11}$$

and with $\dot{A}[O_2]$, $\dot{F}$ and P_i constant

$$P_{c}O_2 = f\{PaO_2, k \cdot b(PO_2)\}.$$

Within the tissue, oxygen is transported by diffusion along the oxygen pressure gradient. This gradient is generated by the O_2 consumption of the mitochondria. Since the local PO_2 in the neighbourhood of a mitochondrion can decrease to about 0.05 mmHg without affecting the turnover number of the cytochrome *c* oxidase (EC 1.9.3.1) (Chance *et al.*1966; Starlinger & Lübbers 1973), the cytochrome oxidase reaction with molecular oxygen is a sink that is very effective in generating the PO_2 gradient between tissue and capillary blood. The PO_2 difference, $\Delta PO_2[tis]$, which must be provided for sufficient oxygen transport, can be calculated for a cylindrical space from the Erlang–Krogh equation (Krogh 1919*a*, *b*). When tissue PO_2, P_tO_2 at the border of the cylinder is not smaller than the critical mitochondrial PO_2, $\dot{A}(O_2)$ is independent of the PO_2 and we obtain (Fig. 5)

$$\Delta PO_2[tis] = P_{c}O_2 - PtO_2 = \frac{\dot{A}[O_2]}{2\alpha \cdot D}\, g(r_t, r_c, r_z) \tag{12}$$

with

$$g(r_t, r_c, r_z) = r_z^2 \cdot \ln\left(\frac{r_t}{r_c}\right) - (r_c^2 - r_t^2) \tag{12a}$$

(r_c = radius of capillary; r_t = distance of measuring point from capillary centre; r_z = radius of tissue cylinder; Fig. 5).

$\Delta PO_2[tis]$ depends on oxygen consumption, 'O_2 diffusion times solubility coefficient', and the geometrical distances

$$\Delta PO_2[tis] = f\{\dot{A}[O_2], \alpha \cdot D, g(r_t, r_c, r_z)\} \tag{13}$$

Fig. 5 demonstrates that the tissue PO_2 depends on the arterial PO_2, on the PO_2 decrease along the capillary, $\Delta PO_2[cap]$, and on the PO_2 decrease within

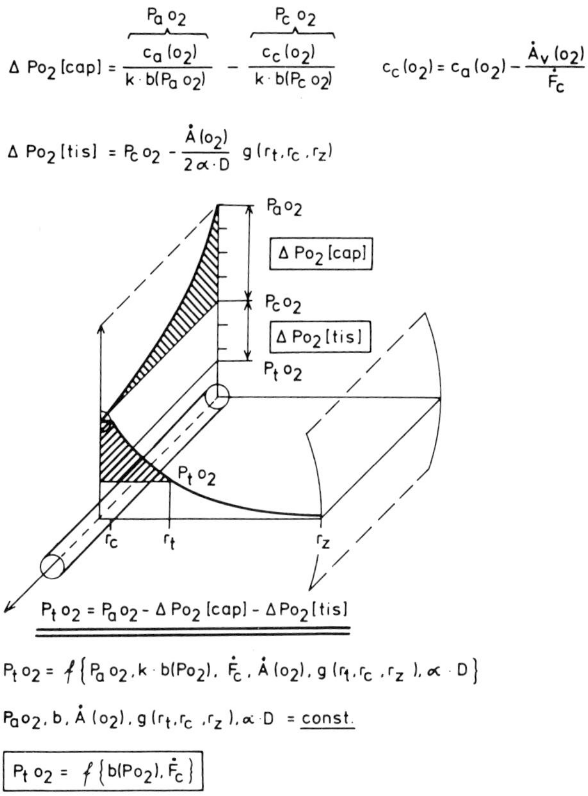

FIG. 5. Dependence of tissue Po_2 on its different parameters (cat). Tissue Po_2 depends on the Po_2 decrease along the capillary, $\triangle Po_2$ [cap], and the Po_2 decrease along the transport path of the oxygen within the tissue, $\triangle Po_2$ [tis]. (For further explanation, see text.)

the tissue, ΔPo_2[tis]. Tissue Po_2 is given by the equation

$$P_tO_2 = PaO_2 - \Delta PO_2[\text{tis}] - \Delta PO_2[\text{cap}] \tag{14}$$

With PaO_2, $\dot{A}[O_2]$, $\alpha \cdot D$, $g(r_t, r_c, r_z)$ constant, the tissue Po_2 is a function of flow, and the actual dissociation curve, $(k \cdot b(Po_2, P_i))$, is

$$P_tO_2 = f\{\dot{F}_c, k \cdot b(Po_2, P_i)\} \tag{15}$$

The flow changes can be calculated by using Eqs. (3), (4) and (7)

$$\frac{\Delta[O_2]_1}{\Delta[O_2]_2} = \frac{\dot{F}_2}{\dot{F}_1} = \frac{k[b(PaO_2) \cdot PaO_2 - b(P_{c1}O_2) \cdot P_{c1}O_2]}{k[b(PaO_2) \cdot PaO_2 - b(P_{c2}O_2) \cdot P_{c2}O_2]} \tag{15a}$$

and

$$P_{t1}O_2 = P_{c1}O_2 - \Delta PO_2[tis]$$
$$P_{t2}O_2 = P_{c2}O_2 - \Delta PO_2[tis]$$

When $\Delta PO_2[tis]$ is not known, only a rough estimation is possible. $\Delta PO_2[tis]$ can be estimated in vasodilated vessels if there is no compensatory flow regulation. In this case, after the increase of arterial $[O_2]$, the increase in tissue PO_2 equals the increase in blood PO_2. In a suitable PO_2 range, this increase depends characteristically on the initial P_cO_2 (see lengths of the arrows in Fig. 4).

In our example, tissue PO_2 should change at least to an amount which would be attained if the electrode were situated in the capillary blood (see Fig. 4). Being in the tissue, P_tO_2 must increase more because of the $\Delta PO_2[tis]$. In any case, when tissue PO_2 does not increase (Fig. 2), one must conclude that flow has decreased to match the increased O_2 concentration of the blood. As a result of our tissue measurements, we find that in at least

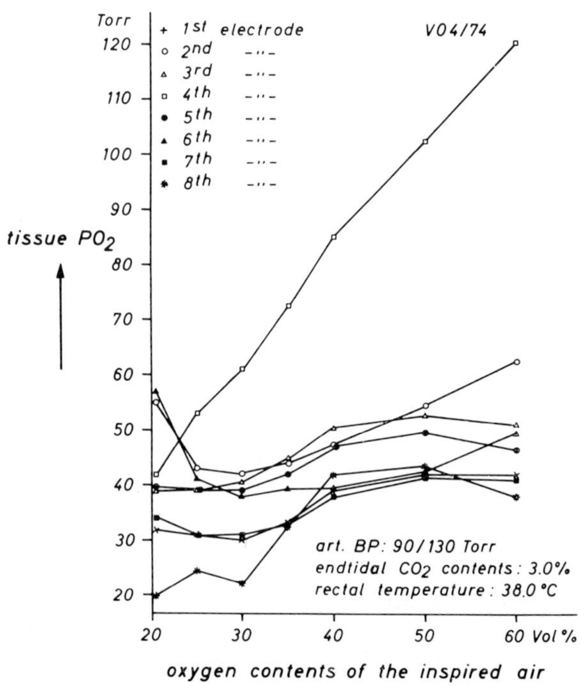

FIG. 6. Response of local tissue PO_2 to gradually increased arterial PO_2 in the cat. Reaction of local P_tO_2 to a stepwise increase in arterial PO_2 recorded at eight sites.

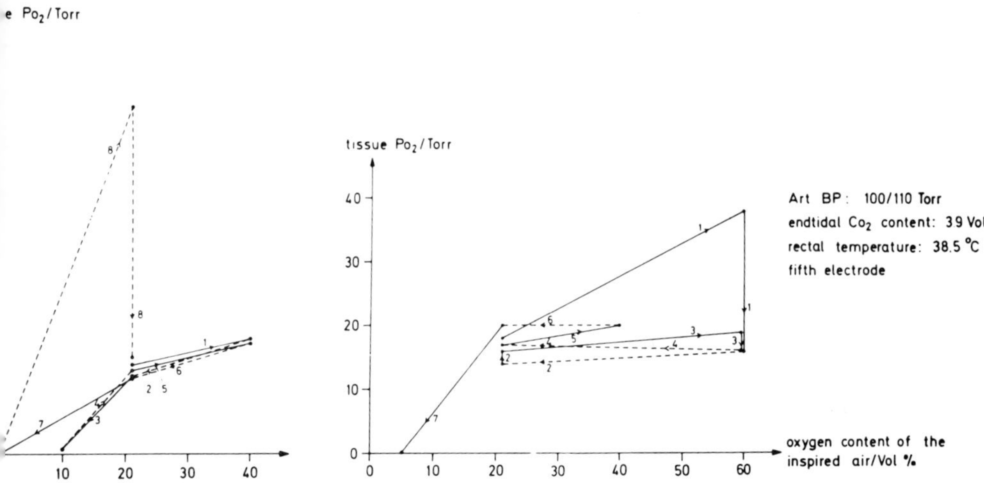

FIG. 7. Response of local tissue P_{O_2} to varying oxygen supply measured at one site (cat). The numerals show the chronological order of the reactions. *Left:* Exposure to 40% O_2 caused only a slight increase (1), while exposure to 10% O_2 caused local tissue P_{O_2} to fall (3). Subsequent respiration with 40% O_2 evoked the same response as was found before 10% O_2 (5). After exposure to N_2 (7), a strong overshoot of tissue P_{O_2} was noticed (8), followed by a gradual re-establishment of the initial values. *Right:* P_{O_2} at first increases but, under the same experimental conditions, later remains constant with changing oxygen content of the inspired air. (Reproduced from Leniger-Follert *et al.* 1975, with permission.)

two-thirds of all sites, a compensatory flow regulation developed (Leniger-Follert *et al.* 1975).

Fig. 6 shows eight tissue P_{O_2} values measured simultaneously during respiration of gas mixtures of different oxygen concentrations. It demonstrates how the compensatory flow regulation can vary at different sites in the tissue. The advantage of the tissue P_{O_2} measurement is that it demonstrates the reactions quicker and even more locally than does H_2 clearance.

The development of the compensatory flow regulation can be directly observed in Fig. 7 (left side). After a short period of anoxia, tissue P_{O_2} rises considerably to a value which corresponds to about the P_{tO_2} without a compensatory flow regulation and then returns to the value before anoxia. The concomitant flow changes can be estimated from Eq. (15a).

There are five types of flow reactions with increasing Pa_{O_2} which can be deduced from the different reactions of tissue P_{O_2}. Fig. 8 schematically summarizes the course of tissue P_{O_2} before and after a short period of N_2 respiration (W. Wrabetz *et al.*, unpublished results). During period A

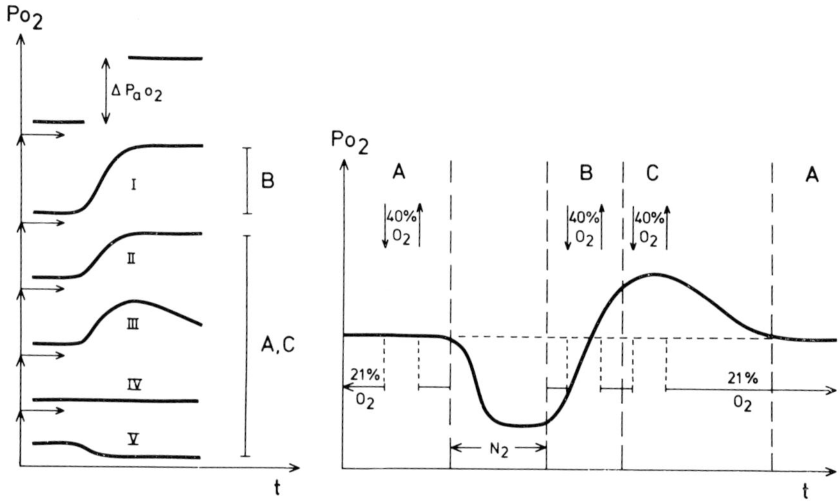

FIG. 8. Course of tissue P_{O_2} before and after a short period of anoxia (cat.). Period A: respiration of 21% O_2 in N_2; Period B: postanoxic hyperaemia first phase; Period C: postanoxic hyperaemia second phase; N_2 = nitrogen respiration. *Left:* reaction patterns (I–V) of tissue P_{O_2} to increases in arterial P_{O_2} ($\triangle P_{aO_2}$). (For further explanation see text.)

(respiration of 21% O_2 in N_2), an oxygen test with 40% O_2 in N_2 can produce four different reactions. In two-thirds of cases, there is either a very small or no reaction (type IV). In one-third, tissue P_{O_2} increases (type II). In a few cases, at first either an increase and then a decrease (type III) or a decrease (type V) is observed. In the postanoxic period, B, the same test leads in all cases to a distinct increase in P_{tO_2}, as shown with the reaction of type I (see also Fig. 6). If the postanoxic maximum has been reached (period C), then the same reaction type as observed in type A is again found. If there was a decrease in A, a decrease has been observed in C as well. There is a characteristic local reaction pattern which remains rather stable.

The response time of the compensatory flow regulation can be in the range of 0.1 to 0.5 s. This points to a mechanism which is situated in the wall of the inflow vessels. Since in period C the same reaction occurs but at a higher local tissue P_{O_2}, this set-point of the inflow regulation must be influenced by the situation within the tissue itself.

Since the reaction pattern may vary from 100 to 100 μm, it is difficult to understand how the arterioles can adjust the regulation of capillary flow so precisely. Therefore, we must discuss whether regulatory mechanisms exist at the capillary level. The reactions of local flow in hypoxia speak in favour of such mechanisms. Fig. 1 also showed that, when there was a marked increase in regional flow, microflow decreased in one capillary region. In 150 anoxic reactions, microflow decreased in a quarter of the sites, in half the sites it followed the blood pressure, and in the remaining quarter it increased without dependence on blood pressure changes.

At first sight, the decrease in flow seems contradictory to the supply situation during tissue hypoxia, since the tissue needs a higher flow when arterial oxygen content and oxygen pressure decrease. Here, other experimental data help us to understand this type of flow reaction. We think it is a physiologically meaningful and useful reaction. From a large number of tissue Po_2 values measured at random, a Po_2 histogram can be drawn which mirrors the tissue oxygen supply (see Lübbers 1969, 1977). As we now know, this histogram has a characteristic bell-shaped form with a steep left side in which the influence of the oxygen binding curve and the normal behaviour of the regulation of microflow is expressed. Comparing the venous Po_2 in sagittal sinus with the tissue Po_2 values recorded in the histogram, it is obvious that the venous Po_2 is higher than predicted from the tissue values. Kessler (1974) pointed out for the liver that without any further assumptions having to be made, different lengths of sinusoids would produce different flows in the sinusoids. Different flows resulting from the different lengths produce differences in the oxygen content and oxygen pressure of the venous capillary blood. Suwa & Takahashi (1971) reported that, indeed, the lengths of the sinusoids vary between 200 μm and 500 μm. So the Po_2 of the venous blood is a mixed venous Po_2. Similar situations have been found in the heart muscle, skeletal muscle, and carotid body.

To assume that the short capillaries are truly responsible for the mixed high venous Po_2 is reasonable but not proved. We may therefore call these capillaries 'functionally superperfused' capillaries. Aside from these superperfused capillaries, capillaries exist in which the flow is well adapted to the demands of the tissue, so that low oxygen tensions in the tissue are produced. As capillaries with metabolically adapted flow, they may be called 'adapted-flow' capillaries. In liver, Kessler (Krumme *et al.* 1975) was able to show that increased metabolism can be accompanied by a flow redistribution, i.e. a flow decrease in the high-flow vessels and an increase where the flow was low. No change was observed in the middle range. It is clear that regional flow can remain constant in spite of considerable changes of microflow.

With the concept of 'functionally superperfused' capillaries, and 'adapted-flow' capillaries, we can easily understand the reactions shown in Fig. 1. The decreased O_2 supply increases the flow in the adapted-flow capillaries and leads to a decreased flow in the functionally superperfused capillaries. In other

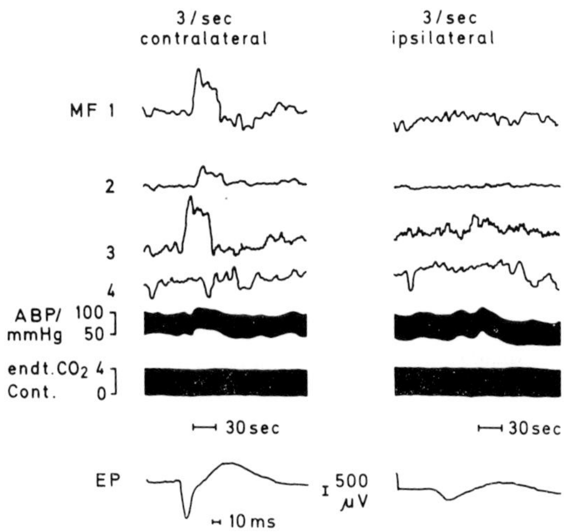

FIG. 9. Simultaneous recording of evoked potentials and microflow in the right somatomotor cortex of the cat during electrical stimulation of both the contralateral and ipsilateral forepaw. Stimulation frequency, 3/s. MF = microflow measured simultaneously at four sites (1–4); EP = evoked potentials; ABP = arterial blood pressure; endt. CO_2 cont = end-tidal CO_2 content. During contralateral stimulation microflow distinctly increases at three sites and remains constant at the fourth site. With ipsilateral stimulation microflow remains constant at all sites. (From Hossmann *et al.* 1977.)

capillaries, functional adaptation on the whole is lost and flow follows the blood pressure changes directly.

This balanced flow regulation in the capillary region leads us to a working hypothesis: we assume that the O_2 supply to the tissue can be subdivided into functional units (probably micro-units in the brain) which are provided with a certain number of functionally superperfused and adapted-flow capillaries. Such a micro-unit could regulate the oxygen supply autonomically by redistribution without affecting regional and main circulation.

The number of capillaries involved in a local flow reaction probably depends on the number of activated cells. Preliminary experiments (Hossmann *et al.* 1977) have demonstrated that the increase in flow which accompanied an evoked potential in the somatocortex of the cat produced, when the forepaw was stimulated by two wires inserted below the skin, a rather sharp edge distinguishing between the activated and non-activated area. This is shown in Fig. 9.

At the moment, it is not known where the regulation of local flow takes place and how it is brought about. It has been suggested that capillaries in the brain might be innervated and could regulate the flow, since innervation has been found in the nucleus caudatus (Rennels & Nelson 1975). Here, myosin could also be detected by immunofluorescence (Owman *et al.* 1977). Observations on the rabbit mesentery led us to another hypothesis: electrical stimulation of capillaries was followed in 80% of all reactions by a flow stop after 2 to 5 s, without visible local changes in the capillary wall. In two cases, we found a funnel-like structure at the branching of the capillary more than 300 μm upstream from the site of stimulation which was responsible for the flow stop (Lübbers *et al.* 1976*b*). However, until now we have had no direct histological evidence for our observation. We only know from histological evidence that the flow stop occurred in capillaries without precapillary sphincters. We should mention that Wolff (Güldner & Wolff 1973) found, at capillary branchings, special seamless cells which are directly perfused. These cells would be well suited for the regulation described. Since the existence of nerves in the capillary walls is still controversial, we have tried to find out by electrical stimulation whether the capillary wall, especially the endothelium, is capable of transducing and conducting the stimulus produced within the tissue to the site of inflow regulation.

If our observations can be further substantiated then the stimulus must have travelled about 300 μm along the capillary wall to its branching, where it produces the regulatory effect. The capillary wall could be considered as a very safe way to reach the right regulatory site and it is well suited for flow regulation in a complicated capillary network. (We must apologize for discussing only working hypotheses but, unfortunately, our knowledge of these basic reactions is very limited.)

To clarify which substances may be involved in the regulation of local flow, we compared the reactions of microflow recorded during and after electrical stimulation with the concomitant changes in tissue P_{O_2}, the redox state of NADH and the activities of hydrogen and potassium ions within the activated area of the brain cortex. Since a change in ion activity and its influence on blood flow will be discussed by Dr Astrup and by Dr Heuser later in this symposium, we shall report on our results very briefly.

We activated an area 5 to 10 mm in diameter in the cat cortex with two silver wires, 300 μm in diameter, fixed to the border of the H_2-P_{H_2} multiwire surface electrode. The cats were anaesthetized with pentobarbital (30–35 mg/kg) and the surface of the gyrus suprasylvius was stimulated. The microflow reaction depended on the parameters of stimulation. With increasing frequency, duration and voltage, the microflow increased from a threshold (4.5 V; 13 Hz/1 ms) to a maximum. A further increase in intensity prolongs the reaction. Microflow increases within 1–2 s and always reaches its maximum after stimulation ends. The initial value was reached again after a period of time of between 30 s and several minutes, according to the intensity of stimulation. Under these experimental conditions, the reaction pattern of microflow was uniform (Leniger-Follert & Lübbers 1976). Leniger (Leniger-Follert 1977; Leniger-Follert & Lübbers 1977*b*) was able to show that in the stimulated area oxygen consumption increased by about 30%–50%. The local O_2 consumption was calculated from the Po_2 decrease attained when brain circulation was suddenly stopped. Measurements of tissue Po_2 under the same conditions, as well as with the combined H_2-PH_2-Po_2 element (Leniger-Follert & Lübbers 1976) showed that P_tO_2 always increased after onset of stimulation with the same time course as microflow. There was no sign of an initial transient hypoxia which might have triggered the flow increase (see Caspers & Speckmann 1972). When we measured the change in haemoglobin content within the stimulated area by reflected light at an isosbestic wavelength of Hb ($\lambda = 445$ nm) and took the change in Hb content as a sign of flow change, then the first flow reaction could be seen after less than 0.5 s (Leniger-Follert *et al.* 1977).

Under the same conditions, extracellular hydrogen activity was measured with a pH microelectrode (Saito *et al.* 1976). The diameter of the tip was between 1 and 4 μm, and the length of the sensitive part was 20–100 μm. The response time of the electrode was 1–3 s for the 90% value. The electrode was inserted into the brain cortex to a depth of 500–1500 μm. The influence of the position of the reference electrode was carefully checked. In some experiments, a reference electrode which was sputtered onto the shaft of the electrode (Baumgärtl & Lübbers 1975; Lübbers *et al.* 1976*a*) was used. The electrodes were mounted on a counterbalanced electrode holder which could follow the movements of the brain. The brain was covered with warm paraffin oil. A similar arrangement was used for potassium measurements. After the beginning of the electrical stimulation, an alkalotic shift occurred which was followed by an acidotic change. Similar changes have been reported by other authors (see Astrup *et al.*, this symposium; Heuser, this symposium). An increase in $[H^+]$ activity could not be seen earlier than 7 s after stimulation (Urbanics *et al.* 1977; Leniger-Follert *et al.* 1977). Fig. 10 shows the changes in microflow, tissue Po_2, and pH on the same time scale during electrical stimulation for varying lengths of time.

The change in extracellular potassium activity was measured by a double-barrelled microelectrode with a tip of 1–3 μm in diameter, prepared as described by Lux & Neher (1973) and others (Kessler *et al.* 1976; Lehmenkühler *et al.* 1976). The sensitivity of the electrode was 45–58 mV/10-fold change in potassium concentration. The second barrel, filled with 150 mM-NaCl, served as the reference and as the d.c. electrode against another surface reference element.

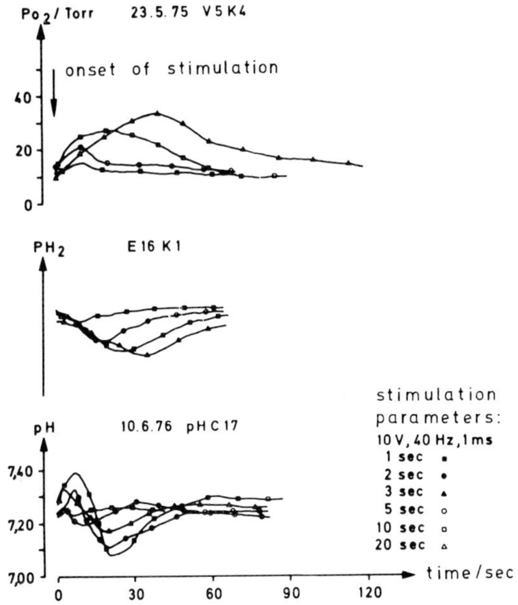

FIG. 10. Behaviour of Po_2, microflow and extracellular [H^+] activity in the brain cortex of the cat during and after electrical stimulation. Time of stimulation was varied, whereas amplitude and frequency remained constant. With the onset of stimulation, local tissue Po_2 (upper trace) and microflow (middle trace, PH_2) increase. pH (lower trace) at first shows an alkalotic, and then an acidotic change. Hydrogen clearance: increase in flow = decrease in PH_2.

Fig. 11 shows that pH, $[K^+]_0$ and d.c. change during stimulation. Extracellular potassium activity increases immediately. This confirms the results of other authors (Astrup *et al.* 1976, and this symposium; Betz & Heuser 1977; Heuser *et al.* 1977; Heinemann *et al.* 1976; Heuser, this symposium). The amplitude depends on the parameters of stimulation. It increases with voltage, frequency and duration. At the end of stimulation, $[K^+]_0$ decreases, often with an undershoot, before it reaches its initial value. pH change shows the course described above.

NADH fluorescence (Rosenthal & Jöbsis 1971) was monitored using the technique developed by K. Harbig *et al.* (1976, unpublished work). To exclude oxygenation changes in haemoglobin, fluorescence and reflected light were determined at an isosbestic point of haemoglobin at $\lambda = 445$ nm. To avoid disturbances to the fluorescence signal from changes in the blood volume, the difference between the fluorescence signal and the reflected light at the same wavelength was recorded after equalizing the change in the reflectance and

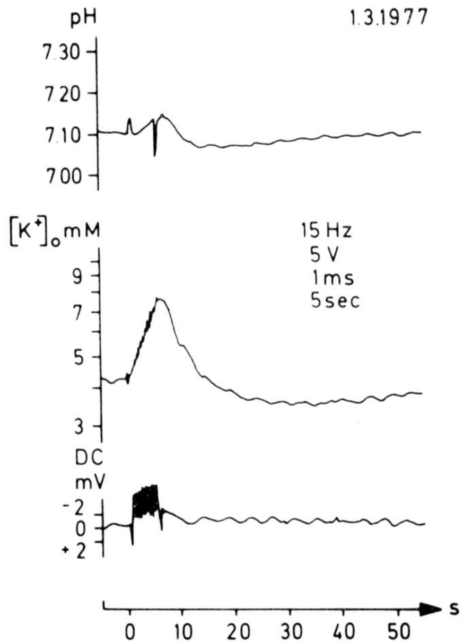

FIG. 11. Simultaneous record of the time course of local extracellular [H^+] and [K^+] activities and d.c. changes during and after direct electrical stimulation of the brain cortex (cat). Similar to Fig. 9, pH shows at first an alkalotic and then an acidotic change (upper trace). $[K^+]_0$ increases very rapidly when stimulation begins and reaches its maximum when stimulation ends. The return to the initial value proceeds with an undershoot (middle trace). The d.c. potential (lower trace) shows a negative shift and the distinct stimulation artifact. (Urbanics *et al.* 1977.)

fluorescence signals during local haemodilution by a saline flush. Disturbances due to brain movements were avoided by inserting a glass window into the bone as described by Harbig *et al.* (1976). Fig. 12 shows that the corrected fluorescence decreased immediately, i.e. within 0.1 s of the beginning of stimulation. The decrease means an oxidation of NADH. Maximum oxidation was reached either when stimulation ended or a few seconds later. NADH fluorescence then returned to its initial level within some minutes, sometimes with an undershoot. The extent of the change depended on the stimulation parameters (Leniger-Follert *et al.* 1977). Under their experimental conditions, Kovách *et al.* (1977) found a reduction in NADH which changed to an oxidation only later during stimulation.

The following conclusions can be drawn from our experiments. Electrical stimulation produces, in the stimulated area of about 5–10 mm, a state of activation of the brain cortex in which O_2 consumption is increased. With

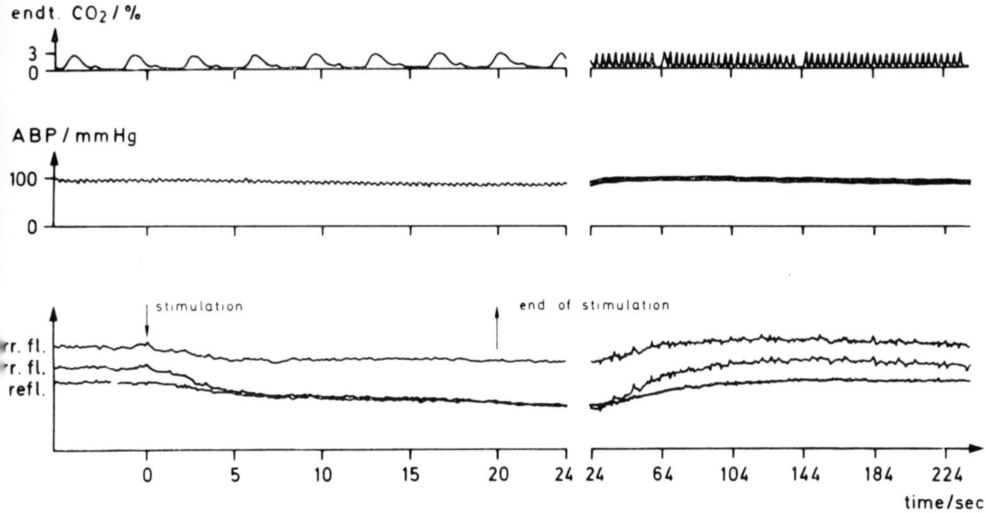

FIG. 12. NADH fluorescence of the brain cortex during electrical stimulation. endt. CO_2= end-tidal CO_2 content; ABP = arterial blood pressure; corr. fl. = corrected fluorescence measured at 445 nm (a decrease means oxidation of NADH); uncorr. fl. = uncorrected fluorescence; refl. = reflectance at 445 nm. Oxidation of NADH starts with the onset of stimulation and reaches its maximum some seconds after stimulation ends. (From Leniger-Follert *et al.* 1977.)

the beginning of stimulation NADH becomes oxidized, which can be taken as a sign of enhanced turnover in the respiratory chain. At the same time, during stimulation extracellular potassium leaves the cells and $[K^+]_0$ increases at first rather steeply; later, probably because of the increased flow, it increases more gradually in most cases. After 0.5 to 1 s, flow starts increasing homogeneously to such an extent that tissue oxygen tension increases concomitantly. We may remember that tissue with an increased O_2 consumption needs a higher tissue Po_2 for the increased rate of oxygen transport (Eq. 12).

The increased flow clears away the extracellular $[H^+]$ ions in the first few seconds, so that pH shifts in the alkaline direction. Later, the release of $[H^+]$ from the cells increases so much that the extracellular $[H^+]$ activity rises, in spite of a high flow. When stimulation ends, $[K^+]_0$ decreases immediately, whereas flow and Po_2 reach their maximum later, and then slowly return to their initial values. The time course of pH changes is very similar to that of the microflow, whereas NADH reduction begins earlier.

Since transient hypoxia was never observed, we think that mitochondrial anoxia can be excluded as a trigger for the flow increase. Potassium ions could trigger, and hydrogen ions maintain, the increase in flow. However, no causal connection should be deduced from the parallel nature of the events. Many other substances may equally well be candidates for regulating flow, the time course of which was not investigated, mainly because of the lack of suitable methods.

In summary, local flow measurements at the capillary level have shown that we must distinguish between local and regional flow reactions. Without changes in regional flow, local flow at the capillary level, as measured directly by the H_2–PH_2 clearance (microflow) or indirectly as tissue PO_2 changes, can react differently at different sites in the same region. Systematic studies of microflow have led to the concept of functional units of microcirculation with 'functionally superperfused' capillaries and 'adapted-flow' capillaries. The functionally superperfused and adapted-flow capillaries may regulate the flow demand by flow redistribution.

The mechanisms which can regulate flow at the capillary level are still unknown. If our findings on the electrical stimulation of the capillaries can be substantiated, then the capillary endothelium must be capable of transmitting the stimulus to the next capillary branching where flow regulation occurs.

At changing values of arterial PO_2 there is a compensatory flow regulation with a time constant of the order of 0.1 to 0.5 s. This short reaction time points to a direct effect on the smooth muscle of the arterioles or metarterioles at the inflow. The set-point of this regulatory mechanism is surprisingly stable and a locally characteristic reaction pattern can be found. Since this pattern can be influenced by the metabolic state of the tissue, we think that the local metabolic demand has a decisive effect on this pattern. During electrical stimulation we observed oxidation of NADH and increases in potassium activity, flow and tissue PO_2. There is no direct evidence that a single ion is responsible for the flow reaction. We have to consider that potassium ions influence not only the smooth muscle but, probably, also the nerves of the vessels. It is possible that potassium ions trigger, and hydrogen ions maintain, the local flow reaction. However, we must state that the signal which evokes the flow response is not known.

References

Acker, H., Lübbers, D. W. & Durst, H. (1977) The relationship between local flow and total flow of the cat carotid body at changes of blood pressure, arterial PO_2 and PCO_2, in *Recent Advances in Basic Microcirculatory Research* (Lewis, D. H., ed.) *(Bibl. Anat. No. 15)*, pp. 395–398 Karger, Basel

Astrup, J., Heuser, D., Lassen, N. A., Nilsson, B., Norberg, K. & Siesjö, B. K. (1976)

Evidence against H^+ and K^+ as the main factors in the regulation of cerebral blood flow during epileptic discharges, acute hyperemia, amphetamine intoxication and hypoglycemia: A micro-electrode study, in *Ionic Actions on Vascular Smooth Muscle* (Betz, E., ed.) p. 110, Springer, Berlin

Astrup, J., Heuser, D., Lassen, N. A., Nilsson, B., Norberg, K. & Siesjö, B. K. (1978) Evidence against H^+ and K^+ as main factors for the control of cerebral blood flow: a microelectrode study, in this volume, pp. 313–332

Baumgärtl, H. & Lübbers, D. W. (1975) Herstellung von Mikro-Po_2- und PH_2-Elektroden mit der Hochfrequenzzerstäubungstechnik. *Naturwissenschaften 62*, 572

Betz, E. (1972) Cerebral blood flow: its measurement and regulation. *Physiol. Rev. 52*, 595–630

Betz, E. & Heuser, D. (1977) Effects of electrical stimulation on vascular walls and perivascular tissue of the arterial brain vessels. *Arzneim.-Forsch./Drug Res. 27*, 1516

Bicher, H. I. (1973) Autoregulation of oxygen supply to brain tissue, in *Oxygen Transport to Tissue* (Bicher, H. I. & Bruley, D. F., eds.) *(Adv. Exp. Med. Biol.*, vol. 37A), pp. 215–222, Plenum, New York

Caspers, H. & Speckmann, E. J. (1972) Cerebral Po_2, Pco_2 and pH: changes during convulsive activity and their significance for spontaneous arrest of seizures. *Epilepsia 13*, 699–725

Chance, B., Schoener, B. & Schindler, F. (1966) The intracellular oxidation reduction state, in *Oxygen in the Animal Organism* (Dickens, F. & Neil, E., eds.), pp. 367–388, Pergamon Press, London

Güldner, F. H. & Wolff, J. R. (1973) Seamless endothelia as indicators of capillaries developed from sprouts, in *Clinical Aspects of Microcirculation (Bibl. Anat. No. 12)*, pp. 120–123, Karger, Basel

Harbig, K., Chance, B., Kovách, A. G. B. & Reivich, M. (1976) In vivo measurement of pyridine nucleotide fluorescence from cat brain cortex. *J. Appl. Physiol. 41*, 480–488

Heinemann, U., Deckstein, W. D. & Lux, H. D. (1976) Biphasic rises in extracellular potassium activity in relation to stimulus-induced psychoactivity in the somatosensory cortex of cats. *Pflügers Arch. Eur. J. Physiol. 365*, R 42

Heuser, D. (1978) The significance of cortical extracellular H^+, K^+ and Ca^{2+} activities for regulation of local cerebral blood under conditions of enhanced neuronal activity, in this volume, pp. 339–348

Heuser, D., Astrup, J., Lassen, N. A., Nilsson, B., Norberg, K. & Siesjö, B. K. (1977) Are H^+ and K^+ factors the adjustment of cerebral blood flow to changes in functional state: a microelectrode study, in *Cerebral Function, Metabolism and Circulation* (Ingvar, D. H. & Lassen, N. A., eds.), pp. 216–217, Munksgaard, Copenhagen

Hossman, K.-A., Leniger-Follert, E. & Lübbers, D. W. (1977) Behaviour of microflow of the somatomotor cortex during specific activation. *Arzneim.-Forsch./Drug Res. 27*, 1518 (Abstr.)

Kessler, M. (1974) Lebenserhaltende Mechanismen bei Sauerstoffmangel und bei Störungen der Organdurchblutung, in *Mitteilungen der Max-Planck-Gesellschaft, München*, pp. 444–463

Kessler, M. & Lübbers, D. W. (1966) Aufbau und Anwendungsmöglichkeiten verschiedener Po_2-Elektroden, *Pflügers Arch. Gesamte Physiol. Menschen Tiere 291*, R 82

Kessler, M., Clark, L. C. Jr., Lübbers, D. W., Silver, I. A. & Simon, W. (eds.) (1976) *Ion and Enzyme Electrodes in Biology and Medicine*, Urban & Schwarzenberg, München

Kovách, A. G. B., Dora, E., Gyulai, L. & Eke, A. (1977) Cerebrovascular and metabolic reactions at the CBF autoregulatory level evoked by electrical stimulation of the cat brain cortex, in *Recent Advances in Basic Microcirculatory Research* (Lewis, D. H., ed.) *(Bibl. Anat. No. 16)*, pp. 270–276, Karger, Basel

Krogh, A. (1919*a*) The rate of diffusion of gases through animal tissues with some remarks on the coefficient of invasion. *J. Physiol. (Lond.) 52*, 391–408

KROGH, A. (1919*b*) The number and distribution of capillaries in muscles with calculations of the oxygen pressure head necessary for supplying the tissue. *J. Physiol. (Lond.) 52*, 409–415

KRUMME, B. A., STREHLAU, R., SCHÖNLEBEN, K. & KESSLER, M. (1975) Redistribution of microcirculation – a new principle of regulation. *Pflügers Arch. Eur. J. Physiol. 359*, R 35

LEHMENKÜHLER, A., SPECKMANN, E.-J. & CASPERS, H. (1976) Cortical spreading depression in relation to potassium activity, oxygen tension, local flow and carbon dioxide tension, in *Ion and Enzyme Electrodes in Biology and Medicine* (Kessler, M. *et al.*, eds.), pp. 311–315, Urban & Schwarzenberg, München

LENIGER-FOLLERT, E. (1977) Direct determination of local oxygen consumption of the brain cortex in vivo, in *Oxygen Transport to Tissue III* (Silver, I. A. *et al.*, eds.). Plenum, New York

LENIGER-FOLLERT, E. & LÜBBERS, D. W. (1975) Interdependence of capillary flow and regional blood flow in the brain, in *Cerebral Circulation and Metabolism* (Langfitt, T. W. *et al.*, eds.), pp. 46–48, Springer, New York

LENIGER-FOLLERT, E. & LÜBBERS, D. W. (1976) Behavior of microflow and local P_{O_2} of the brain cortex during and after direct electrical stimulation, *Pflügers Arch. Eur. J. Physiol. 366*, 38–44

LENIGER-FOLLERT, E. & LÜBBERS, D. W. (1977*a*) Regulation of microflow and behavior of local tissue P_{O_2} during activation and anoxia of the brain cortex, in *Recent Advances in Basic Microcirculatory Research* (Lewis, D. H., ed.) *(Bibl. Anat. No. 16)*, pp. 345–349, Karger, Basle

LENIGER-FOLLERT, E. & LÜBBERS, D. W. (1977*b*) Microflow, local tissue P_{O_2} and metabolism of the brain cortex during and after direct electrical stimulation. *Arzneim.-Forsch./Drug Res. 27*, 1517–1518 (Abstr.)

LENIGER-FOLLERT, E., LÜBBERS, D. W. & WRABETZ, W. (1975) Regulation of local tissue P_{O_2} of the brain cortex at different arterial O_2 pressures, *Pflügers Arch. Eur. J. Physiol. 359*, 81–95

LENIGER-FOLLERT, E., WRABETZ, W. & LÜBBERS, D. W. (1976) Local tissue P_{O_2} and microflow of the brain cortex under varying arterial oxygen pressure, in *Oxygen Transport to Tissue – II* (Grote, J. *et al.*, eds.), pp. 361–367, Plenum, New York

LENIGER-FOLLERT, E., URBANICS, R., HARBIG, K. & LÜBBERS, D. W. (1977) The behavior of local pH and NADH-fluorescence during and after direct activation of the brain cortex, in *Cerebral Function, Metabolism and Circulation* (Ingvar, D. H. & Lassen, N. A., eds.), pp. 214–215, Munksgaard, Copenhagen

LÜBBERS, D. W. (1969) The meaning of the tissue oxygen distribution curve and its measurement by means of Pt electrodes, in *Oxygen Pressure Recording in Gases, Fluids and Tissues* (Kreuzer, F., ed.), pp. 112–123, Karger, Basel

LÜBBERS, D. W. (1972) Physiologie der Gehirndurchblutung, in *Der Hirnkreislauf* (Gänshirt H., ed.), pp. 212–260, Thieme, Stuttgart

LÜBBERS, D. W. (1977) Quantitative measurement and description of oxygen supply to the tissue, in *Oxygen and Physiological Function* (Jöbsis, F. F., ed.), pp. 254–276, Professional Information Library, Dallas, Texas

LÜBBERS, D. W. & STOSSECK, K. (1970) Quantitative Bestimmung der lokalen Durchblutung durch elektrochemisch im Gewebe erzeugten Wasserstoff, *Naturwissenschaften 57*, 311–312

LÜBBERS, D. W., BAUMGÄRTL, H. & SAITO, Y. (1976*a*) Insulation properties and ion-sensitivity of thin layers of dielectrics deposited by RF sputtering on glass surfaces, in *Ion and Enzyme Electrodes in Biology and Medicine* (Kessler, M. *et al.*, eds.), pp. 110–115, Urban & Schwarzenberg, München

LÜBBERS, D. W., HAUCK, G. & WEIGELT, H. (1976*b*) Reaction of capillary flow to electrical stimulation of the capillary wall and to application of different ions, in *Ionic Actions on Vascular Smooth Muscle* (Betz, E., ed.), pp. 44–47, Springer, Berlin

LUX, H. D. & NEHER, E. (1973) The equilibration time course of K^+ in cat cortex. *Brain Res. 17*, 190

NAIR, P., WHALEN, W. J. & BUERK, D. (1975) Po_2 of cat cerebral cortex: response to breathing N_2 and 100% O_2. *Microvasc. Res. 9*, 158–165

OWMAN, CH., EDVINSSON, L., HARDEBO, J. E., GRÖSCHEL-STEWART, U., UNSICKER, K., WALLES, B. (1977) Immunohistochemical demonstration of actin and myosin in brain capillaries, in *Cerebral Function, Metabolism and Circulation* (Ingvar, D. H. & Lassen, N. A., eds.), p. 384–385, Munksgaard, Copenhagen

PURVES, M. J. (1972) *The Physiology of the Cerebral Circulation*, Cambridge University Press, London

RENNELS, M. L. & NELSON, E. (1975) Capillary innervation in the cat brain, in *Blood Flow and Metabolism in the Brain* (Harper, A. M. *et al.*, eds.) pp. 1.10–1.11, Churchill Livingstone, Edinburgh

ROSENTHAL, M. & JÖBSIS, F. F. (1971) Intracellular redox changes in functioning cerebral cortex. II. Effects of direct cortical stimulation. *J. Neurophysiol. 34*, 750–762

SAITO, Y., BAUMGÄRTL, H. & LÜBBERS, D. W. (1976) The RF sputtering technique as a method for manufacturing needle-shaped pH microelectrodes, in *Ion and Enzyme Electrodes in Biology and Medicine* (Kessler, M. *et al.*, eds.) p. 103–109, Urban & Schwarzenberg, München

SKOLASINSKA, K., HARBIG, K., LÜBBERS, D. W. & WODICK, R. (1977) Microflow pattern of the beating heart in response to changes of arterial Po_2. *Pflügers Arch. Eur. J. Physiol.* (submitted for publication).

STOSSECK, K., LÜBBERS, D. W. & COTTIN, N. (1974) Determination of local blood flow (microflow) by electrochemically generated hydrogen: construction and application of the measuring probe. *Pflügers Arch. Eur. J. Physiol. 348*, 225–238

STARLINGER, H. & LÜBBERS, D. W. (1973) Polarographic measurement of the oxygen pressure performed simultaneously with optical measurements of the redox state of the respiratory chain in suspensions of mitochondria under steady-state conditions at low oxygen tensions. *Pflügers Arch. Eur. J. Physiol. 341*, 15–22

SUWA, N. & TAKAHASHI, T. (1971) in *Morphological and Morphometrical Analysis of Circulation in Hypotension in Ischemic Kidney* (Bücher, F., ed.), Urban & Schwarzenberg, München

URBANICS, R., LENIGER-FOLLERT, E. & LÜBBERS, D. W. (1977) Extracellular H^+ and K^+. activities of the brain cortex during and after direct electrical stimulation. *Arzneim.-Forsch./Drug Res. 27*, 1518 (Abstr.)

WODICK, R. (1976) *Möglichkeiten und Grenzen der Bestimmung der Blutversorgung mit Hilfe der lokalen Wasserstoffclearance.* Akademie der Wissenschaften und der Literatur, Mainz, in Kommission bei Franz Steiner, Wiesbaden

Discussion

Plum: Is your microelectrode recording from surface pools, not depth pools?

Lübbers: In the main experiments those were surface elements but with micro Pt-electrodes (tip size of 1–2 μm) we can also register from deeper layers.

Plum: With electrode recordings on the surface, isn't surface Po_2 always higher than venous Po_2?

Lübbers: In the anaesthetized cat brain there is no detectable difference between the Po_2 histograms from the surface and from the tissue itself. We use the surface electrodes because these do much less harm than if we puncture the tissue.

Plum: I am trying to sort out where are the capillary channels which compensate for the low Po_2. You essentially showed that venous tensions are always higher than cortical surface tensions, which means that there must be a region other than where you are recording where the oxygen tension is disproportionately high.

Lübbers: Unfortunately we do not have enough quantitative information about the dimension of the capillary network in the brain. In liver the histogram of capillary length varies between 200 μm and 500 μm. If the hydrostatic pressure gradient along the capillaries remains the same, the flow in the short capillaries is much higher and they supply much less tissue than the longer ones. As I mentioned, the venous Po_2 must be understood as a mixture of different capillary Po_2 values.

Plum: But you require the assumption that none of the shunts are on the surface? Your histogram is essentially totally skewed, the venous Po_2 being higher than all of your sampling points.

Lübbers: In this model there are short capillaries with a high venous Po_2.

Plum: Why didn't you see any of those short capillaries?

Lübbers: Some high Po_2 values are always found in the Po_2 histogram.

Purves: But it is surely almost impossible to disentangle the various factors which make up the skewness of that histogram?

Lübbers: I agree. The main reason for the 'skewed' form of the Po_2 histogram is the haemoglobin. A cumulative histogram in which the different samples are drawn not side by side but one over the other is closely comparable with the oxygen binding curve. By drawing a histogram in such a way, you can get interesting information about the different factors. Together with W. Grunewald we studied the influence of the different parameters on the Po_2 histogram (Grunewald & Sowa 1977).

Siesjö: It would be interesting to know the proportion of the capillaries in any one area which show no increase in blood flow when the oxygen tension is lowered. Is the resolution of your method much superior to that obtained by ^{14}C-autoradiography? The reason I ask is that, to my knowledge, autoradiography does not show regional differences in CBF response to hypoxia.

Lübbers: The smallest dimension in which flow was measured with our technique by Dr H. Acker was a sphere of 80 μm.

Siesjö: But surely the current must be influenced by diffusion of hydrogen gas from neighbouring areas?

Lübbers: The amount of hydrogen we are supplying is small. The size of the volume in which the clearance process is measured follows from the theory (Wodick 1976). Using a diffusion coefficient of hydrogen $D_{H_2} = 2.9 \times 10^{-4}$ $cm^2 \cdot s^{-1}$ the radius along which the hydrogen diffuses is $r = 54$ μm. After

25 s r amounts to 270 μm. For our usual surface element with a wire distance of 250 μm we obtain a volume of about 0.07 mm^3. With smaller evaluation times we measure smaller tissue volumes. By varying the dimension one can adapt the probe to the particular problem under study.

Siesjö: If you give hydrogen gas by inhalation and measure hydrogen clearance, can you also see inhomogeneities with hypoxia?

Lübbers: We have not investigated that systematically.

Siesjö: So essentially these dissimilarities in response to hypoxia are mainly observed when you put electrodes on the surface?

Lübbers: Yes, but we can also observe it by Po_2 measurement with needle electrodes which have a different basis. Similar results are obtained with these different methods. In the liver Kessler (1974) directly showed redistribution measured at the same spot under different conditions.

Purves: In fact the method of estimating flow using the oxygen electrode with all the assumptions involved there, gives the same kind of distribution as with direct measurements.

Jöbsis: On the initiation of hyperoxia some of your traces showed oscillation. Other people have claimed that with oxygen electrodes they observe oscillations even in steady states. Since you have a method with which relatively large areas of up to 0.2 mm can be compared with smaller areas of about 80 μm, can you tell us anything about oscillations in the flow rather than in the oxygen concentration or tension?

Lübbers: Unfortunately we have not made many measurements of flow and oscillation with these micro methods. The oscillations we found depend on the state of narcosis. If we measure in barbiturate narcosis we seldom see oscillations. But if we measure in other kinds of narcosis we often see them. Interestingly enough the oscillations can remain uninfluenced by and during the respiration of 40% oxygen (Leniger-Follert *et al.* 1976; Fig. 1).

Jöbsis: Do the flow oscillations have the same frequency as the oxygen oscillations?

Lübbers: Yes. At least they do in all cases in which we measure both simultaneously.

Jöbsis: Do you think that the oscillations originate as a function of the capillary or vascular system or from a change in activity and thereby of oxygen utilization?

Lübbers: In our conditions they probably originate from the arterioles. It may be the other way round in other situations.

Purves: But you are both talking about oscillations lasting over a minute.

Lübbers: They may have different frequencies. In our case they have a frequency of 1 cycle/min.

Jöbsis: The oscillations in cytochrome a, a_3 reduction state which we occasionally observe have a frequency of 3 or 4 cycles/min.

Lübbers: The frequency depends very much on the state of narcosis and the investigations are not standardized in this respect.

Heuser: Can one conclude from your measurements that two different mechanisms govern blood supply to a certain area of the brain? The results of our own investigations, which I shall present later in this symposium, provide some evidence for the existence of two different mechanisms: one acts very quickly, being responsible for the initiation of flow increase, while the other acts more slowly, being essential for maintenance of increased cerebral blood flow.

Lübbers: The two mechanisms I was talking about concern the site of the sensor. From the time constant of regulation we assume that one has to be in the vessel wall whereas the other one is within the tissue. Additionally a different mechanism may exist for producing vascular dilatation or contraction, as may be deduced from the ion measurements.

Astrup: When you put the surface electrode on the brain you have to squeeze the brain slightly to establish close contact between the tissue and the electrode. Could that introduce slight relative oligaemia just under the electrode and explain why the average tissue Po_2 was substantially lower than the mixed venous Po_2?

Lübbers: If we puncture the brain cortex with the 1 μm microelectrode, we obtain about the same Po_2 histogram within the brain cortex as with the surface electrode. We use a lucite ring covered with filter paper for supporting the electrode. A droplet of solution keeps the electrode in place by the capillary suction of the filter paper. We also tried a counterbalance to reduce the pressure but we don't see any difference between the techniques, so we use the lucite ring.

Astrup: What is the actual pressure on the electrode? What is the surface area?

Lübbers: The data for two electrodes were, for example:

H_2 electrode: diameter 3.1 mm; weight 100 mg; area 7.54 mm^2; pressure 13 mg/mm^2.

PO_2 electrode: diameter 6 mm; weight 2.0 g; area 28.26 mm^2; pressure 70 mg/mm^2.

McDowall: An additional answer to the last question is that the upper limit of Po_2 recorded on the surface of the brain is the same as the arterial Po_2, so we can get some values that read the same as the arterial oxygen tension. Using your electrode, Professor Lübbers, we get the same fit for the oxygen dissociation curve in the cat as you described. With hypotension induced by haemorrhage we saw a large number of electrode points with very low oxygen readings at a mean blood pressure of 30 mmHg. Using drug-induced hypotension to the same level we do not see such a change in distribution of surface Po_2 measurements. Why is it that a certain group of Po_2 measurement areas seems to fall outside the normal oxyhaemoglobin distribution curve with haemorrhagic hypotension but not with drug-induced hypotension? Is there a change in capillary flow distribution between these two different situations?

Lübbers: The Po_2 histograms show first the absolute distribution of oxygen values, so that one knows how many low and high levels there are. But the form of the Po_2 histogram also tells us something about the normality of the microcirculation. If the microcirculation is disturbed the histogram changes in a characteristic way. For example, when microcirculation is disturbed the values are 'dented': some bars are high and some low. That happens especially with hyperoxia. The uniformity of the curve begins to be disturbed. When we measured microflow in hypoxia some of the capillaries reacted with decreased flow, some with increased flow, and some with paralysis.

References

GRUNEWALD, W. A. & SOWA, W. (1977) Capillary structures and O_2 supply to tissue. An analysis with a digital diffusion model as applied to the skeletal muscle. *Rev. Physiol. Biochem. Pharmacol.* 77, 149–209

KESSLER, M. (1974) Lebenserhaltende Mechanismen bei Sauerstoffmangel und bei Störungen der Organdurchblutung, in *Mitteilungen der Max-Planck-Gesellschaft*, München, pp. 444–463

LENIGER-FOLLERT, E., WRABETZ, W. & LÜBBERS, D. W. (1976) Local tissue Po_2 and microflow of the brain cortex under varying arterial oxygen pressure, in *Oxygen Transport to Tissue-II* (Grote, J. *et al.*, eds.), pp. 361–367, Plenum, New York

WODICK, R. (1976) *Möglichkeiten und Grenzen der Bestimmung der Blutversorgung mit Hilfe der lokalen Wasserstoffclearance.* Akademie der Wissenschaften und der Literatur, Mainz, in Kommission bei Franz Steiner, Wiesbaden

Cellular microenvironment in relation to local blood flow

I. A. SILVER

Department of Pathology, Medical School, University of Bristol

Abstract The investigation was designed to identify microenvironmental factors that might be important in the regulation of local blood flow. Cellular microenvironment in terms of Po_2, pH, [K^+], [Cl^-], [Ca^{2+}] and lactate was measured in rat brain by means of specific microelectrodes. Vascular endothelium was stained *in vivo* with Thioflavine S. Local blood flow was measured with micro hydrogen electrodes.

Some intracellular measurements of pH were made in conjunction with extracellular measurements. The main findings were that local autoregulation responses and blood flow changes in response to imposed hypoxic changes were very rapid (1–1.5 s). Microflow responses to changes in local cell activity were limited to a region not more than 250 μm in diameter. Increased blood flow in acute hypoxia occurred within 1–2 s of the fall in tissue Po_2 and was much more rapid than changes in either pH or potassium. Intracellular pH changed within 10 s of the onset of severe hypoxia but in all cases the blood flow followed the Po_2 much more closely than any other parameter. It is suggested that changes in capillary endothelium and local membrane transmission may play a part in autoregulatory mechanisms.

Many reports on general cerebral blood flow (CBF) under conditions of hypotension and shock have been published (see Kovách & Sandor 1976) but very little hard information has been obtained on the control of microflow in brain at the arteriolar–capillary level. Betz and colleagues (Knabe & Betz 1972; Betz 1976; Heuser & Betz 1976) have shown the effects of changes in cerebrospinal fluid (CSF) composition on the smooth muscle of pial vessels and have measured K^+ and H^+ fluxes from the smooth muscle of such arteries in the cat. They found that decreases of [H^+] in the CSF caused arteriolar constriction and increases led to dilatation; similar responses occurred in relation to [K^+] although very high K^+ concentrations caused constriction. Electrical stimulation of pial vessels (10 kHz at 0.5 mA) usually gave constriction but this depended on the extravascular ionic environment. Blocking Ca^{2+} with

EDTA caused dilatation and abolished the constriction response to electrical stimuli. In high concentrations of extracellular K^+ such as those seen during anoxic depolarization (Van Harrevald 1971) or under severe stress (20 mequiv./l), electrically induced constriction was weak, as compared to responses induced in normal (3 mequiv./l), low or very high (100 mequiv./l) K^+ concentrations, and Betz and colleagues also showed an interaction between $[Ca^{2+}]$ and $[K^+]$ on pial arteriolar sensitivity. They concluded that the interference by K^+ with activity of other ions in smooth muscle might be important in autoregulation of flow.

However, the most persistently baffling aspects of local blood flow control are (*a*) the identification of the signal that initiates increase or decrease of local capillary perfusion, (*b*) the site at which this control is exercised, (*c*) the method of transmission of the signal to the effector, and (*d*) the nature of the 'set point' about which the local conditions fluctuate and to which they are returned. In addition, it is not clear what is the exact mechanism whereby the local blood flow is controlled, although it appears to stem from changes in arteriolar diameter with a possible involvement of endothelial participation at the capillary level.

Many publications exist on the control of microflow in muscle because of the historical interest generated by the work of Krogh (1918) and his predictive model on oxygen diffusion and also because of the relative ease of technical approach and analysis of results. This relative ease is due, in part at least, to the parallel arrangement of capillaries in many voluntary muscles, and to the existence of simple methods of imposing large and rapid changes of flow in relation to muscular mechanical activity. In muscle, many factors have been invoked, such as P_{O_2}, pH, potassium, P_i, CO_2, ATP and osmolarity (Haddy & Scott 1975), but there is no clear consensus of opinion on the primary cause of microflow changes. Furthermore, models involving either mesenteric capillary beds, skeletal muscle or even pial vessels are not necessarily appropriate to the study of local control of CBF, although it seems likely that similar mechanisms prevail throughout the body microvasculature.

Bicher *et al.* (1973) have demonstrated the possible existence of an oxygen-sensor-controlled process of autoregulation of blood flow in micro areas of brain associated with a shutdown of cell activity in an apparently protective mechanism, and these findings have been incorporated in predictive models by Reneau *et al.* (1970) and Bruley *et al.* (1971). Opitz & Schneider (1950) predicted the existence of an oxygen sensor and suggested that it was located in the venous end of the capillary bed, but it is not at all clear how such a sensor would pass its information (*a*) to the upstream regulator of flow, or (*b*) to the neurons.

My observations (Silver 1973, 1976*a*, 1977) and similar studies by Moskalenko (1975) have indicated that a sudden increase of cell activity in the brain which leads to a fall in local oxygen tension is compensated within 1.5 to 3 s by an increase in *local* blood flow which does not extend beyond 250 μm from the site of increased activity. These measurements were made with micro platinum electrodes used alternately as hydrogen clearance detectors and oxygen cathodes. While this degree of local control is clearly a useful physiological adaptation, it is difficult to reconcile with the idea that a readily diffusible substance (or substances) is released from an area of activity which affects '*upstream*' effectors and leads to an increase in blood flow in a purposeful manner which is closely confined to the site of demand. Rather, diffusion of vasoactive material would lead to a widespread change of flow and because of washout by capillaries it might tend especially to increase flow *downstream* of the active area; this, of course, would be of little metabolic value and is not what is seen experimentally.

There is no doubt that bursts of cell activity reduce local Po_2 (Silver 1965; Bicher & Knisely 1970; Erdmann *et al.* 1973) and also increase the local potassium levels (Bito & Myers 1972; Prince *et al.* 1973). Cell activity also leads to a release of P_i and H^+, as does hypoxia (Heuser & Betz 1976), but such effects are not directional and neither is the production and diffusion of CO_2. All of these substances diffuse rapidly and widely from the production site yet do not increase flow in a non-excited adjacent area in the concentrations available (Silver 1976*a*, 1977). It is also necessary to consider the time relationships of changes in flow to the appearance of possible mediators of circulatory control. For instance, in local hypoxia in the brain, compensatory flow changes occur within 1–3 s, yet H^+ ion concentration does not change in the extracellular space for about 10 s (Silver 1977), although it changes earlier than this intracellularly. Whatever is postulated as the initial feedback stimulus must obviously be something that changes within the experimentally observed time scale and that, when supplied artificially at the appropriate concentration, will also produce local change (in the right direction) of microflow.

Of course, large changes of CO_2, O_2, K^+, H^+, etc. produce alterations in regional blood flow, but even under extreme conditions of artificially high CO_2, an increase in local nervous activity by evoked or direct stimulation leads to a further rise in strictly local flow although the total cerebral flow is maximal (see Kovách & Sandor 1976). One must, therefore, postulate a factor in control of local flow that is additional to, and independent of, the factors regulating gross cerebral regional blood flow.

The autonomic innervation of large cerebral blood vessels has been convincingly demonstrated by immunofluorescence studies (Harper *et al.*, 1972) as being a noradrenergic system in the larger extraparenchymal vessels. A similar but distinct system has been demonstrated by Hartman *et al.* (1972) and Rennels & Nelson (1975) to innervate or at least to be closely associated with the small intraparenchymal vessels, including capillaries. Because of the innervation of capillaries as well as larger vessels, it has been postulated that these nerves may be associated with transcapillary exchange as well as with control of microflow (Raichle *et al.* 1975). These microanatomical findings lend support to earlier physiological evidence for a brain-stem centre which may influence local blood flow (see Molnas & Szanto 1964; Langfitt & Kassel 1968; Meyer *et al.* 1969). However, the time scale we have observed in the compensation of increased metabolic or electrical activity by change in flow is relatively long (around 1–3 s over a distance of 100–150 μm); this must either involve a long multi-synaptic pathway with extremely local detector and effector coupling, which seems inherently unlikely in view of the diffuse nature of the autonomic system, or the rate of conduction of the transmitted impulse is very slow (much slower than by any other nerve pathway), or there is a long latency in stimulating the detector or in transmission from the excited sensor to the effector. If the very local system is neither controlled by autonomic nerves nor by general diffusion of unknown vasoactive substance(s), we must ask what possible system might be involved that could carry out the necessary closely controlled, moderately fast homeostasis that is observed. The most likely pathways appear to be (*a*) direct membrane conduction from neuron (to glia?) to capillary to effector, or (*b*) a substance diffusing from the neuron to a sensitive site on the adjacent capillary, which then leads to capillary membrane conduction upstream to the effector site, or (*c*) the glial cells detect the metabolic change induced by neuronal activity and stimulate the effector site by direct membrane conduction, or (*d*) there is a mixture of pathways including some autonomic nervous component.

The work reported below was carried out to test the following suggestions: (*a*) that fine control of local CBF is exerted through arteriolar–capillary units and that such units often incorporate a 'preferred route' which may be the only part of the system which remains perfused under some adverse haemodynamic conditions, e.g. local ischaemia or systemic hypovolaemia; (*b*) that initial control of capillary blood flow is dependent upon some local sensor of cellular microenvironment; (*c*) that the sensor detects deviation of environmental conditions from an optimum 'set point' in a 'comparator system'; (*d*) that some effector mechanism controlled by the sensor–comparator adjusts the flow to maintain the tissue conditions as nearly as possible at the optimum; (*e*) that transmission of information is by a highly specific, localized

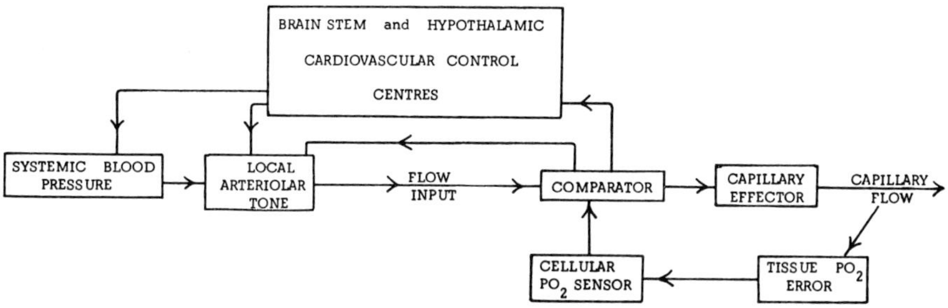

FIG. 1. Block diagram of a possible feedback mechanism for control of local blood flow.

system, probably along membrane pathways; and (*f*) that the sensor mechanism is probably sensitive to a number of factors, among which are Po_2, pH, ionic concentration and intracellular redox state.

A diagrammatic representation of this scheme is set out in Fig. 1.

EXPERIMENTAL FINDINGS

Methods

Local environmental conditions were measured with a variety of microsensing devices which included probes sensitive to pH, based on the designs of Hinke (1959) for extracellular use and of Thomas (1974) and Zeuthen (1976) for intracellular work. Potassium, chloride and calcium were monitored using double or multibarrelled electrodes as described by Zeuthen *et al.* (1974), Kessler *et al.* (1976) and Silver (1976*b*), modified from the design of Walker (1971). Changes in local blood flow were followed either by heat clearance from heated microthermocouples or by hydrogen washout from a hydrogen-generating and detecting system based on that of Lübbers & Baumgärtl (1967) and Stosseck *et al.* (1974). Tissue oxygen tension was followed with platinum–iridium glass-insulated needle electrodes (Silver 1965). Some measurements of local lactate concentration were made with an enzyme microelectrode incorporating pyridine nucleotide and lactic dehydrogenase on the surface of a vitreous carbon fibre (Silver 1977).

The endothelium of capillaries and other vessels was stained *in vivo* by intravenous injection of 0.5% Thioflavine S (Merck, F. G. R.) and examined under incident ultraviolet illumination at $\lambda = 470$ nm.

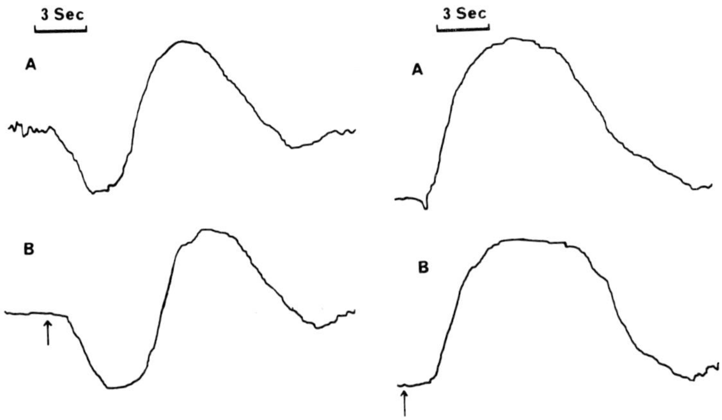

FIG. 2. Local Po_2 changes after multiunit stimulation (at arrows) in rat brain. *Left:* a biphasic response where Po_2 fell significantly before flow compensation occurred. *Right:* monophasic responses with immediate overcompensation (increased Po_2 up).

Results

Response to increased cell activity. Oxygen electrodes in the immediate vicinity of inactive neurons showed either a fall, followed by a rise, of Po_2 when the cell was stimulated, or a rise only. These two types of response are shown in Fig. 2. The biphasic pattern was seen only with very high resolution electrodes placed close to a cell surface. If a group of electrodes was arranged around the stimulation site, the changes in Po_2 could not be detected more than 250 μm from the activated cell(s), which suggested that the increased flow leading to the rise in Po_2 was limited to a very small region around the site of raised metabolism. Records of local blood flow changes from such experiments are shown in Fig. 3.

Hydrogen washout measurements confirmed that the flow changes were very localized. The records also show that the flow did not return to the baseline for many seconds after the end of the stimulus, although the Po_2 was above the resting value.

Stimulation of cell activity also caused a rapid rise in local potassium concentration which could be detected within 100 ms near the cell surface. The change in $[K^+]$ varied between 0.5 and 5 mequiv./l, depending on the anatomical relationship of the cell to the measuring electrode.

pH and calcium changes in the vicinity of *single* cells were very difficult to detect during stimulation. However, falls in pH of the order of 5–20 mV and of $[Ca^{2+}]$ of less than 1 mequiv./l were sometimes obtained when many

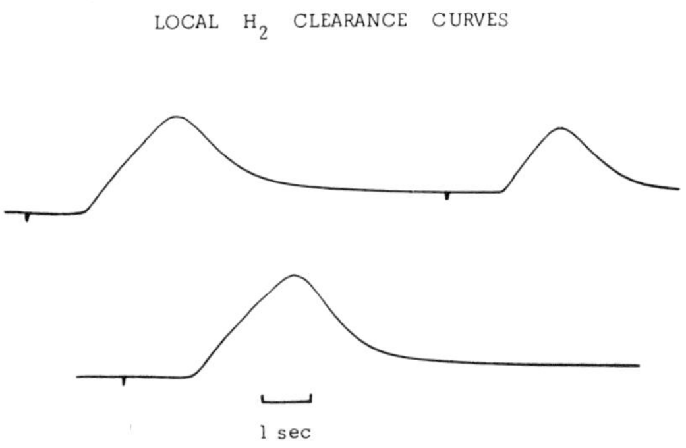

FIG. 3. Hydrogen washout curves (increased blood flow up) after a 1 s stimulation of a single neuron (rat brain) starting at the points marked on the trace.

cells were excited simultaneously over a larger area. The extracellular pH changes were relatively slow compared to the rise in $[K^+]$ or the fall in Po_2 and the increase in blood flow.

Response to hypoxia. Brief periods of arterial hypoxaemia (10–30 s) invariably resulted in a fall in brain Po_2 and a marked increase in local blood flow. During the very early phase of Po_2 fall (1–5 s), there was often a slight increase in cell membrane potential and a *fall* (1–3 mV) in extracellular potassium activity. This was followed by a rapid reversal and a rise in potassium activity to about 2–4 mV above the resting level by 10–15 s (Fig. 4), but little further increase occurred unless the hypoxia was prolonged to 2.5–3.0 min, when the 'anoxic depolarization' (Van Harreveld 1971) phase began with drastic leakage of potassium from, and diffusion of Cl^- into, the cells (Fig. 4).

pH changes in the early stages of hypoxia, whether the animal was maintained in controlled respiration or was allowed to breathe spontaneously with hyperpnoea, always showed an initial rise which appeared to be due to CO_2 washout by the increased blood flow. If hypoxia persisted for more than about 20 s (in the rat), the extracellular pH started to fall (Fig. 5). Thus, blood flow had increased to almost maximal levels early in hypoxia at a time when the extracellular pH was rising, and the potassium concentration first fell and then rose, but only by a slight amount. However, if *intracellular* pH was measured, which is technically difficult even in large cortical cells, an increase in $[H^+]$ could be detected at least 5–10 s earlier than that in the extracellular space. Unfortunately, problems of interpretation of such data may arise not only because the intracellular electrodes have a relatively long response time

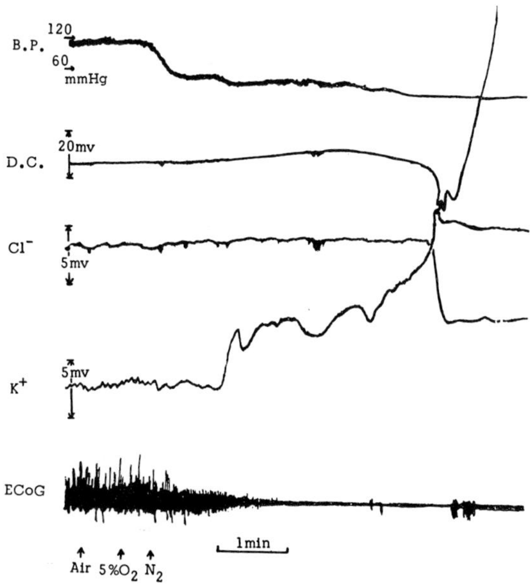

FIG. 4. Simultaneous records from a rat of arterial blood pressure (B.P.), electrocorticogram (ECoG) and extracellular d.c. potential (D.C.), chloride (Cl^-) and potassium (K^+) activity (50 mV log a_{Cl^-} or a_{K^+}) in cortex during normoxia (air breathing) hypoxia (5% O_2) and anoxia (N_2). (Increasing concentration up.)

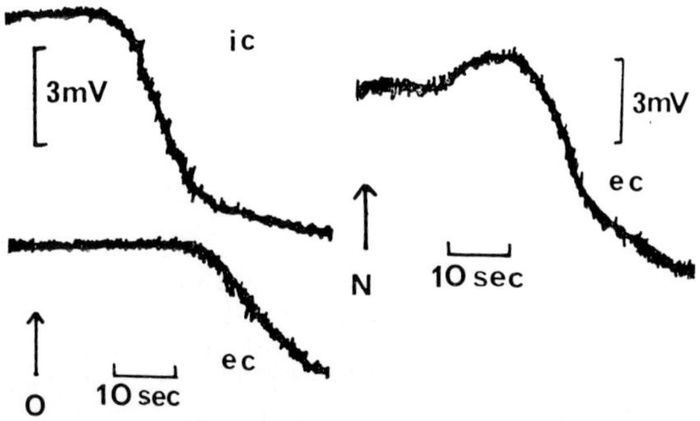

FIG. 5. pH changes (increase up) recorded extracellularly (ec) and intracellularly (ic) during local ischaemia *(left)* in rat. '0' indicates time of occlusion of local artery. *Right:* extracellular pH change during nitrogen breathing (starting at 'N'). Note the initial rise in pH.

but also because the early pH changes may be a reflection of the damage the cell has suffered from the insertion of the electrode.

In *ischaemic* hypoxia after local arterial occlusion, the intracellular pH falls after 5–10 s (see Fig. 5) and, although the extracellular fall may be delayed,

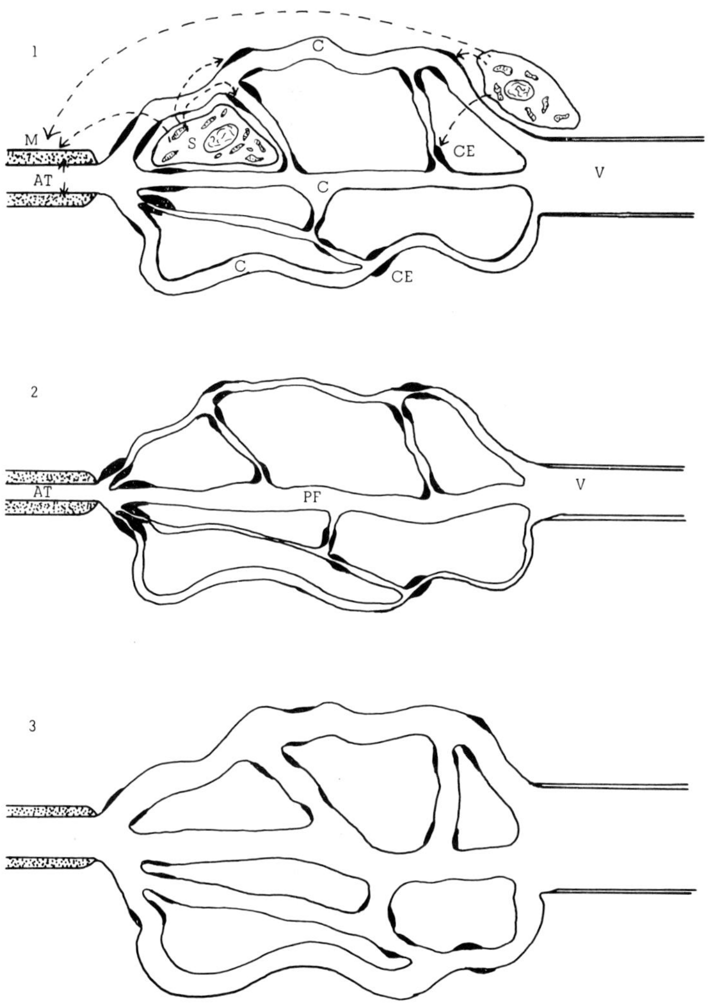

FIG. 6. Diagrammatic reconstruction of an arteriolar–capillary unit. (1) Normal flow; (2) hypovolaemia with preferred route (PF) only, perfused; (3) hyperaemia, all vessels perfused. Key: M, smooth muscle; AT, arteriole; S, sensor cell; C, capillary; CE, possible sites of flow controlling cells; PF, preferred route; V, venule.

there is no preliminary alkalotic response. $[K^+]$ also rises faster in ischaemic hypoxia than in hypoxaemia, which presumably reflects the lack of washout in the former situation as compared to the latter.

In pathological conditions such as hypovolaemic shock, we have observed that in some areas of the brain in some animals, regional blood flow or total brain flow may be maintained at low but not critical levels, yet very low Po_2 values can be found surrounding areas of unusually high Po_2. After injection of Thioflavine S, if such regions are mapped stereotaxically with microelectrodes and reconstructed subsequently from serial sections, it can be demonstrated that the endothelium of only parts of the normal capillary bed is stained and these parts correspond generally to the position of electrodes showing high Po_2 values. Conversely, those areas which had low Po_2 values usually have unstained (and therefore unperfused) capillaries. This suggests that 'preferred' routes may remain open in pathological conditions and allow hyperperfusion of some vessels at the expense of others. A possible explanation for such a situation is that the normal autoregulatory signals in hypoxic tissue fail to elicit the correct local response under conditions of systemic hypovolaemia. In turn, this might imply a systemic over-ride of the local autoregulatory mechanism which is potentially harmful. Fig. 6 shows such changes.

DISCUSSION

While it is clear that a very highly developed mechanism exists for the control of local CBF, it is equally obvious that we have little knowledge of how it operates. On the subject of cellular oxygen tension sensors, there is wide speculation and disagreement (see Reivich *et al.* 1977) but at least there are several credible candidates as possible O_2 detectors. However, it is not at all certain whether microflow is controlled directly by oxygen availability or indirectly by something which is dependent on oxygen, e.g. pH, ionic concentrations or CO_2. It appears from the speed with which arterioles react to hypoxaemia that their smooth muscle is directly sensitive to O_2, but the slower adjustments seen in capillaries suggest a multifactorial mechanism.

Unfortunately, even less information is available on how the 'set point' for tissue Po_2 is determined, what is the nature of the 'comparator' in Fig. 2, or how the signal reaches the effector. As a matter of speculation only, I am inclined to think some form of membrane conduction is involved, possibly along the capillary wall. Kovách (1973) has shown that the α-blocker phenoxybenzamine can prevent 'preferred route' perfusion in hypovolaemic shock, which suggests that, at least under pathological conditions, local sympathetic innervation is important.

Finally, there is little evidence on the nature of the effector mechanism in the redistribution of capillary flow. Three possibilities suggest themselves: (*a*) that the capillary wall is contractile, (*b*) that the endothelial cells at the entrance to capillary branches may be able to swell and occlude the lumen as, for instance, is seen in viral endarteritis, or (*c*) that the elasticity of the endothelium may be altered by the environment or by some nervous mechanism. Most capillaries are slightly smaller than red blood cells and are distorted by their passage. Only a very small biophysical change would be required to 'stiffen' the capillary wall to the point where passage of red cells was prevented. Alternatively, when there was increased flexibility of the wall, resistance to flow would decrease.

A feature of the autoregulation of local blood flow to imposed distortions is that the 'on' mechanism for increasing flow seems more sensitive than the 'off' and overcompensates, at least in terms of oxygen supply, in response to sudden demand. Thus, while O_2 lack may be the 'on' trigger, the 'off' switch may be activated by something other than Po_2 or, alternatively, is rather insensitive. However, where normal metabolic requirements are concerned, the 'set point' is presumably one which has proved functionally successful and about which only slight fluctuations occur. It may be that by imposing sudden drastic changes on the brain under experimental conditions in order to observe obvious environmental alterations, we produce only the more extreme responses of the system rather than those which normally keep the environment constant.

CONCLUSION

Cellular microenvironment in terms of a number of physical factors is important in the control of local blood flow but the precise mechanism by which control operates is still obscure. Such evidence as exists suggests that oxygen may be the most important parameter in regulating arteriolar diameter, but that capillaries are more likely to be controlled by interaction of several factors.

References

BETZ, E. (1976) Pial vascular smooth muscle reactions during perivascular microperfusion with artificial CSF of varying ionic composition, in *Ion and Enzyme Electrodes in Biology and Medicine* (Kessler, M. *et al.*, eds.), pp. 316–319, Urban & Schwarzenberg, Munich

BICHER, H. I. & KNISELY, M. H. (1970) Brain tissue reoxygenation-time demonstrated with a new ultramicro-oxygen electrode. *J. Appl. Physiol. 28*, 387–392

BICHER, H. I., BRULEY, D. F., RENEAU, D. D. & KNISELY, M. (1973) Regulatory mechanisms of brain oxygen supply, in *Oxygen Supply* (Kessler, M. *et al.*, eds.), pp. 180–185, Urban & Schwarzenberg, Munich

BITO, L. S. & MYERS, R. E. (1972) On the physiological response of the cerebral cortex to acute stress (reversible asphyxia). *J. Physiol. (Lond.) 221*, 349–370

BRULEY, D. F., BICHER, H. I., RENEAU, D. D. & KNISELEY, M. (1971) Autoregulatory phenomena related to cerebral tissue oxygenation. *Adv. Bioeng. (CEP Symp. Ser.) 67*, 195–201

ERDMANN, W., KUNKE, S. & KRELL, W. (1973) Tissue P_{O_2} and cell function, in *Oxygen Supply* (Kessler, M. *et al.*, eds.), pp. 169–174, Urban & Schwarzenberg, Munich

HADDY, F. J. & SCOTT, J. B. (1975) Metabolic factors in peripheral circulatory regulation. *Fed. Proc. 34*, 2006–2011

HARPER, A. M., DESCHMUKH, V. D., ROWAN, J. O. & JENNETT, W. B. (1972) The influence of sympathetic nervous activity on cerebral blood flow. *Arch. Neurol. 27*, 1–6

HARTMAN, B. K., ZIDE, D. & UDENFRIEND, S. (1972) The use of dopamine β-hydroxylase as a marker for the central noradrenergic nervous system in rat brain. *Proc. Natl. Acad. Sci. U.S.A. 69*, 2722–2726

HEUSER, D. & BETZ, E. (1976) Measurement of K^+ and H^+ activities by means of microelectrodes in brain vascular smooth muscle, in *Ion and Enzyme Electrodes in Biology and Medicine* (Kessler, M. *et al.*, eds.), pp. 320–330, Urban & Schwarzenberg, Munich

HINKE, J. A. M. (1959) Glass microelectrodes for measuring intracellular activities of sodium and potassium. *Nature (Lond.) 184*, 1257–1258

KESSLER, M., HAJEK, K. & SIMON, W. (1976) Four-barrelled microelectrode for the measurement of potassium-, sodium- and calcium-ion activity, in *Ion and Enzyme Electrodes in Biology and Medicine* (Kessler, M. *et al.*, eds.), Urban & Schwarzenberg, Munich

KNABE, U. & BETZ, E. (1972) The effects of varying extracellular K^+, Mg^{++} and Ca^{++} on the diameter of pial arterioles, in *Vascular Smooth Muscle* (Betz., E., ed.), pp. 83–85, Springer, Berlin

KROGH, A. (1918) The number and distribution of capillaries in muscles with calculation of the oxygen pressure head necessary for supplying the tissue. *J. Physiol. (Lond.) 52*, 409–415

KOVÁCH, A. G. B. (1973) Tissue blood flow and metabolism in control and phenoxy benzamine pretreated animals in experimental shock, in *Traumatic Shock* (Szanto, G. *et al.*, eds.), pp. 163–185, Akademiai Kaido, Budapest

KOVÁCH, A. G. B. & SANDOR, P. (1976) Cerebral blood flow and brain function during hypertension and shock. *Annu. Rev. Physiol. 39*, 571–596

LANGFITT, T. W. & KASSELL, N. F. (1968) Cerebral vasodilatation produced by brain-stem stimulation: neurogenic control vs. autoregulation. *Am. J. Physiol. 215*, 90–97

LÜBBERS, D. W. & BAUMGÄRTL, H. (1967) Herstellungstechnik von palladinierten Pt-Stichelektroden (1–5 μ Aussendruckmesser) zum polarographischen Messung des Wassenstoffdruckes für die Bestimmung der Mikrozirkulation. *Pflügers Arch. Gesamte Physiol. Menschen Tiere 294*, R39

MEYER, J. S., NOMURA, F., SAKAMOTO, K. & KONDO, A. (1969) Effect of stimulation of the brain-stem reticular formation on cerebral blood flow and oxygen consumption. *Electroencephalogr. Clin. Neurophysiol. 26*, 125–132

MOLNAS, L. & SZANTO, J. (1964) The effect of electrical stimulation of the bulbar vasomotor centre on the cerebral blood flow. *Q. J. Exp. Physiol. Cogn. Med. Sci. 49*, 184–192

MOSKALENKO, Y. Y. (1975) Regional cerebral blood flow and its control at rest and during increased functional activity, in *Brain Work* (Ingvar, D. H. & Lassen, N. A., eds.), pp. 133–141, Munksgaard, Copenhagen

OPITZ, E. & SCHNEIDER, M. (1950) The oxygen supply of the brain and the mechanism of deficiency effects. *Ergeb. Physiol. Biol. Chem. Exp. Pharmakol. 46*, 126–260

PRINCE, D. A., LUX, H. D. & NEHER, E. (1973) Measurement of extracellular potassium activity in cat cortex. *Brain Res. 50*, 489–495

RAICHLE, M. E., HARTMAN, B. K., EICHLING, J. O. & SHARPE, L. G. (1975) Central noradrenergic regulation of brain microcirculation, in *Blood Flow and Metabolism in the Brain* (Harper, A. M. *et al.*, eds.), pp. 1.3–1.6, Churchill Livingstone, Edinburgh

REIVICH, M., COBURN, R., LAHIRI, S. & CHANCE, B. (1977) *Tissue Hypoxia and Ischemia*, Plenum Press, New York

RENEAU, D. D., BICHER, H. I., BRULEY, D. F. & KNISELY, M. (1970) A mathematical technique for predicting tissue reoxygenation time as a function of the rate of change of effective blood flow, in *Blood Oxygenation* (Hershey, D., ed.), pp. 175–200, Plenum Press, New York

RENNELS, M. C. & NELSON, E. (1975) Capillary innervation in the cat brain, in *Blood Flow and Metabolism in the Brain* (Harper, A. M. *et al.*, eds.), pp. 1.10–1.11, Churchill Livingstone, Edinburgh

SILVER, I. A. (1965) Some observations on the cerebral cortex with an ultramicro membrane covered, oxygen electrode. *Med. Electron. Biol. Eng. 3*, 377–387

SILVER, I. A. (1973) Local Po_2 in relation to intracellular pH, cell membrane potential and potassium leakage in hypoxia and shock. *Adv. Exp. Med. Biol. 37A*, 233–232

SILVER, I. A. (1976*a*) Tissue response to hypoxia, shock and stroke. *Adv. Exp. Med. Biol. 75*, 325–334

SILVER, I. A. (1976*b*) Multiparameter electrodes, in *Ion and Enzyme Electrodes in Biology and Medicine* (Kessler, M. *et al.*, eds.), pp. 119–122, Urban and Schwarzenberg, Munich

SILVER, I. A. (1977) Ion fluxes in hypoxic tissues. *Microvasc. Res. 13*, 409–420

STOSSECK, K., LÜBBERS, D. W. & COTTIN, N. (1974) Determination of local blood flow (microflow) by electrochemically generated hydrogen. *Pflügers Arch. Eur. J. Physiol. 348*, 225–234

THOMAS, R. C. (1974) Intracellular pH of snail neurones measured with a new pH sensitive glass microelectrode. *J. Physiol. (Lond.) 238*, 159–180

VAN HARREVALD, A. (1971) The extracellular space in the central nervous system, in *Structure and Function of Nervous Tissue*, vol. 4 (Bourne, G. J., ed.), pp. 447–511, Academic Press, London

WALKER, J. L. (1971) Ion specific liquid ion exchanger microelectrodes. *Anal. Chem. 43*, 89A–93A

ZEUTHEN, T. (1976) A double-barrelled Na^+-sensitive electrode. *J. Physiol. (Lond.) 254*, 8P

ZEUTHEN, T., HIAM, R. C. & SILVER, I. A. (1974) Microelectrode recording of ion activity in brain, in *Ion Selective Microelectrodes* (Berman, H. & Hebert, N. C., eds.), pp. 145–156, Plenum Press, New York

Discussion

Owman: Professor Silver mentioned that capillaries may change in size and in configuration. With immunohistochemical techniques we have been able to show directly that there are contractile proteins in the capillary walls (Owman *et al.* 1977). For example, in the rat hypothalamus processed for indirect immunofluorescence the capillaries show myosin immunoreactivity in their walls. We obtain the same picture with actin, showing that actin and myosin are present together, which indicates that the capillary wall is actively contractile. It appears from the fluorescence microscopic analysis that the contractile proteins are present both in the pericytes and in the endothelial cells. We don't know yet how these contractile proteins are oriented in the cells. Theoretically, the cells could either produce changes in capillary lumen size and thereby change the rate of flow through the capillaries, or they could change the 'length' of the cell so that the junctions between the cells open or close, with resulting alterations in permeability.

Rosendorff: Can you see actin or myosin filaments by electron microscopy?

Owman: Microfilaments of a contractile nature have recently been demonstrated with electron microscopic techniques in pericytes (Lebeux & Willemot 1977) and endothelial cells (S. Nag, personal communication) of brain capillaries.

Siesjö: Professor Silver showed a capillary arrangement that made me very happy. At a Princeton conference (Siesjö *et al.* 1973) we reported that with a combination of low blood pressure and hypercapnia we had the paradoxical finding of a higher than normal venous oxygen tension and a disruption of the energy metabolism of the tissue. We postulated that there must be different vessels, some of which are easy to perfuse, being straight and short, whereas others may be long and tortuous and therefore difficult to perfuse. Conceivably, preserved or increased flow through the former type of vessels may explain the high venous P_{O_2}, while cessation of flow in other vessels should lead to regional anoxia, explaining why cerebral energy state was affected.

You said that there may be areas within the tissue that, during hypoxia, have higher than normal P_{O_2}. Did you mean that all vessels were dilated under those circumstances and that the more easily perfused ones were actually stealing blood from the others? Or did you postulate that you get very low P_{O_2} in some spots because vessels do not dilate, or perhaps even show increased resistance, e.g. due to swelling?

Silver: Some vessels were not perfused in those circumstances and others were superfused. I suspect that this local 'superfusion' could have accounted for your findings of high venous P_{O_2} with accompanying tissue hypoxia. Where five or six capillaries arise from an arteriole, some of them may close down completely while one or two show high flow. In the vicinity of the latter, there is a high P_{O_2} but elsewhere it is very low.

Siesjö: That is exactly what we predicted.

Purves: Both of you are really suggesting that redistribution is a very important part of the response and therefore presumably vulnerable.

Lübbers: Some of the vessels showed no reaction any more (Fig. 1 of my paper). They are paralysed, and this too is an important factor. It seems to depend on the state of the metabolic tissue around the capillary. Other vessels react rather strongly.

Silver: In some cases where we induced ischaemia or haemorrhagic shock and subsequently reperfused the area, we saw big changes in pH during the ischaemic period. In some areas, these changes persisted long after the general blood flow of the brain had apparently returned to control values. One may establish normal regional flow and still get small areas of brain which are acidotic.

Rapoport: Is the time constant of your electrodes so short that you can be sure that changes in flow precede changes in extracellular pH?

Silver: No. The intracellular electrodes cannot detect pH changes in less than 2 s, and even that is rather difficult. However, the extracellular pH electrodes are very fast. I am quite sure that the extracellular pH changes are slower than the Po_2 and flow changes because these latter are almost coincidental.

Rapoport: The new evidence that there is actomyosin in the endothelium is important. In skeletal muscle, actomyosin is activated by Ca but H^+ ions can compete with Ca (Portzehl *et al.* 1969). So at the site of actomyosin there may be a multifactorial effect with steady-state tension established by Ca levels and with transient effects produced by slight changes in H^+.

Silver: There may be a very early increase in intracellular H^+ production which is bound and obscured by local intracellular buffering systems. That might act almost immediately and it wouldn't be seen.

Rapoport: K, Ca and pH all may work, depending on initial conditions, at the site of actomyosin or at the cell membrane. Flow therefore might be regulated by several of these factors.

Silver: I am sure there are many factors. The ones we were looking for were the initiating factors. CO_2 obviously is very important in some circumstances, and high K certainly increases flow. However, the autoregulatory changes are very fine and localized. These may be brought about by intracellular pH alterations but the evidence is not good yet.

Jöbsis: I am puzzled by the delay in the extracellular response compared with the intracellular response. One would almost have to postulate a buffering system of quite considerable magnitude in the extracellular space. This may not necessarily be a biochemical buffering system but a 'cellular' buffering system for cells that take up hydrogen ions or CO_2. The responses should be faster, like those in muscle contraction experiments with extracellular electrodes. What do you think causes the long delay of 5 to 8 s?

Silver: I am surprised at the delay too, because our extracellular electrodes are really very fast. A possible explanation is that whenever an electrode is put into a cell, the cell produces a vesicle around the electrode tip and provides a microcosm which the electrode senses. We are probably measuring the conditions in the vesicle which may not necessarily reflect exactly what is happening in the general cytosol of the cell. On the other hand, the delay may merely reflect the efficiency of intracellular buffering. Certainly we have always found this rather long delay of 5 s to 10 s between the beginning of intracellular and extracellular pH change.

Jöbsis: Professor Siesjö, what kind of time relations do you see for lactate production?

Siesjö: We can increase lactate production in the cerebral cortex of the rat by more than fivefold. Normal glucose consumption is about 0.8 μmol g^{-1} min^{-1}, which gives a production of pyruvate of 1.6 μmol g^{-1} min^{-1}. Thus, maximal lactate production is about 8 μmol g^{-1} min^{-1}, or less than 0.15 μmol g^{-1} s^{-1}.

Let me emphasize that one can *increase* pH in the tissue and still see, as Professor Silver says, a circulatory response to hypoxia. The easiest way to increase pH transiently is to lower P_{CO_2} when hypoxia is induced. For a while, the alkalinizing effect of the fall in P_{CO_2} is larger than the acidifying effect of increased lactic acid production. As will be discussed later by Drs Astrup and Heuser (this volume), hypoxia leads to a prompt CBF response even though it may take at least one minute to obtain net acidosis in the tissue. These results correspond well with those reported by Professor Silver.

Plum: Neuropathologically the selective vulnerability of brain cells is not randomly distributed. It tends to occur again and again at the same anatomical site. Do the physiological experiments predict an anatomical distribution where shunts occur and the side channels are closed off?

Lübbers: If a vascular system could be reconstructed on this microcapillary basis I am sure one could predict those events.

Plum: In zones H_1 and H_2 of the hippocampal formation is the capillarity different?

Lübbers: That is the impression I get from the stable reaction patterns we find in certain areas. If the patterns were not so stable I would say that there were stochastic changes of blood flow between one capillary and the next.

Rubio: Professor Silver, what criteria did you use to decide that you actually had an intracellular recording?

Silver: The membrane potential is the criterion. For intracellular recording we always use double-barrelled electrodes so that we don't have a problem with interpretation. The biggest technical problem with the pH electrode is that we have to use a double-barrelled one because otherwise changes in membrane potential may look as if they are pH changes.

Astrup: Dusser de Barenne *et al.* in 1938 had already found transient alkaline shifts, using surface electrodes. It is interesting that with your very elegant and miniaturized pH electrode inserted in the tissue you get similar results. As I shall show later (this volume) we have made observations similar to those of Professor Lübbers and his group. Thus the pH data seem unaltered by the improvements in techniques, so we may conclude that either the observations are correct or we are still making the same error (tissue damage?).

Purves: This poses a very clear problem for you, Professor Lübbers. If you have alkaline shifts this is yet one more factor that you have to account for in the oxygen binding. Can you do that?

Lübbers: Yes, though it is an estimate. We have to use a corresponding oxygen binding curve.

Purves: People have reported various sizes of alkaline shift but they are all agreed on its presence.

Astrup: Professor Silver, did you measure a potassium increase during the brief period of hypoxia?

Silver: Yes. Normally we see a two-stage increase. First there is a small increase (up to about 5 mV) in extracellular potassium activity which lasts for 1 to 2.5 min, then there is massive rise in $[K^+]$ which rapidly becomes irreversible (Zeuthen *et al.* 1974).

Astrup: But what happens in the brief periods of nitrogen inhalation?

Silver: There we get a very small change in potassium, of somewhere between 3 and 5 mV.

Astrup: This corresponds well with what we see: an immediate slight rise in potassium at the onset of hypoxia or ischaemia indicating arousal and activation, especially in lightly anaesthetized animals.

Heuser: Have you also measured Ca^{2+} activity during hypoxia?

Silver: With Professor Simon's calcium-sensitive ligand (Ammann *et al.* 1976) we have seen changes, but I am not satisfied that they were real. We didn't have enough of the material to be sure of the results. But we also tried the calcium-sensitive photoluminescent protein 'obelin' which is much more sensitive, and this showed an extracellular decrease of calcium concentration during the increase of blood flow in early hypoxia.

Heuser: That would fit quite well with our results. We also found a decrease in local extracellular Ca^{2+} activity during cerebral neuronal activation, possibly as a trigger mechanism for the onset of functional hyperaemia.

Rapoport: Insertion of an electrode into brain tissue can damage the capillary bed and thereby disrupt the blood–brain barrier to HCO_3^- ion. Such damage is demonstrated by an alkaline pH change at the cortical surface in response to an intravenous injection of $NaHCO_3$, rather than by an acidic response that occurs with an intact barrier (Rapoport 1964). Do you obtain an alkaline or acidic shift in response to $NaHCO_3$, Professor Silver?

Silver: You mean if we give intravenous sodium bicarbonate? We normally see a fall in pH.

Purves: The bicarbonate flux is a very slow one.

Astrup: We have inserted 100-μm electrodes in the cat cortex. Injection of bicarbonate in the blood gives an acid shift by the pH electrode. The explanation is that the CO_2 driven out in the blood diffuses readily into the brain and gives an initial acid shift for a minute or so (Heuser *et al.* 1975).

Rapoport: So in fact you have not severely disrupted the capillary bed?

Astrup: That is right. We concluded that the inserted electrodes, even those rather large electrodes, do not merely reflect the plasma pH.

Purves: And if you inject lactic acid again, there is similarly a transient change but no long-lasting one?

Astrup: We did not try lactic acid.

Siesjö: Professor Plum asked about the selective vulnerability of the brain. Since a meeting like this is meant to be speculative and provocative, I want to offer a speculative suggestion (see Siesjö 1978). It has been shown that neurons from the locus coeruleus innervate both Purkinje cells in the cerebellum and cells in the hippocampus and the cerebral cortex. Calderini *et al.* (1978*a*, *b*) have shown that after ischaemia and during status epilepticus there is markedly increased noradrenaline synthesis. Perhaps we are dealing with hyperactivity in noradrenergic neurons in the brain, and this hyperactivity may have something to do with selective vulnerability.

References

AMMANN, D., BISSIG, R., CIMERMAN, Z., FIEDLER, U., GUGGI, M., MORF, W. E., OEHME, M., OSSWALD, H., PRETSCH, E. & SIMON, W. (1976) Synthetic neutral carriers for cations, in *Ion and Enzyme Electrodes in Biology and Medicine* (Kessler, M. *et al.*, eds.), pp. 22–37, Urban & Schwarzenberg, Munich

CALDERINI, C., CARLSSON, A. & NORDSTRÖM, C.-H. (1978*a*) Monoamine metabolism during bicuculline-induced epileptic seizures in the rat. *Brain Res.* Submitted for publication

CALDERINI, C., CARLSSON, A. & NORDSTRÖM, C.-H. (1978*b*) Influence of transient ischemia on monoamine metabolism in the rat brain during nitrous oxide and phenobarbitone anaesthesia. *Brain Res.* Submitted for publication

DUSSER DE BARENNE, J. G., MARSHALL, C. S., MCCULLOCH, W. S. & NIMS, L. F. (1938) Observations on the pH of the arterial blood, the pH and the electrical activity of the cerebral cortex. *Am. J. Physiol. 124*, 631–636

HEUSER, D., ASTRUP, J., LASSEN, N. A. & BETZ, E. (1975) Brain carbonic acid acidosis after acetazolamide. *Acta Physiol. Scand. 93*, 385–390

LEBEUX, Y. J. & WILLEMOT, J. (1977) Actin-like filaments in brain pericytes as demonstrated by HMM labeling. *Anat. Rec. 187*, 635

OWMAN, CH., EDVINSSON, L., HARDEBO, J. E., GRÖSCHEL-STEWART, U., UNSICKER, K. & WALLES, B. (1977) Immunohistochemical demonstration of actin and myosin in brain capillaries. *Acta Neurol. Scand. 56, Suppl. 64*, 384–385

PORTZEHL, H., ZAORALEK, P. & GAUDIN, J. (1969) The activation by Ca^{2+} of the ATPase of extracted muscle fibrils with variation of ionic strength, pH and concentration of MgATP. *Biochem. Biophys. Acta 189*, 440–448

RAPOPORT, S. I. (1964) Cortical pH and the blood-brain barrier. *J. Physiol. (Lond.) 170*, 238–249

SIESJÖ, B. K. (1978) *Brain Energy Metabolism*, ch. 15, Wiley, Chichester, in press

SIESJÖ, B. K., EKLÖF, B. & MACMILLAN, V. (1973) Energy metabolism in the brain in ischemia, in *Cerebral Vascular Diseases, 8th Conference* (McDowall, F. H. & Brennan, R. W., eds.), pp. 99–111, Grune & Stratton, New York

ZEUTHEN, T., HIAM, R. C. & SILVER, I. A. (1974) The recording of ion activities in brain with ion-selective microelectrodes, in *Ion Selective Microelectrodes* (Berman, H. J. & Hebert, N. C., eds.), pp. 98–109, Plenum Press, London

Influence of the cerebrovascular sympathetic innervation on regional flow, autoregulation, and blood–brain barrier function

LARS EDVINSSON, JAN ERIK HARDEBO and CHRISTER OWMAN

Departments of Histology and Neurology, University of Lund

Abstract Experiments have been done on rats, rabbits and baboons to elucidate the role of the cranial sympathetic nerves originating in the superior cervical ganglia in the regulation of local cerebral blood flow, including its autoregulation, and in blood–brain barrier functions. Flow was measured by the [^{14}C]ethanol technique, thermoclearance, and xenon-133 clearance. Blood–brain barrier functions were studied by the extravasation of an Evans' blue–albumin complex and by calculation of brain uptake index for two compounds (noradrenaline and inulin). Electrical stimulation of the sympathetic nerves reduces regional flow to a degree that is related to the amount of local perivascular innervation. The breakthrough of autoregulation during induced systemic hypertension is prevented by bilateral stimulation of the superior cervical ganglia. Acute sympathectomy markedly enhances the vascular penetration both at normotension (tested by brain uptake index for noradrenaline and inulin) and rapidly induced hypertension (evidenced by extravasation of Evans' blue). This extravasation of Evans' blue during acute hypertension can be counteracted by sympathetic nerve stimulation. The results give further support for the view that the cranial sympathetic nerves afford an efficient control of the cerebrovascular bed.

The cerebrovascular bed and the regulation of the cerebral circulation display several unique and functionally important features. The cerebral vessels are innervated not only by sympathetic adrenergic and parasympathetic cholinergic nerves but also receive peptidergic nerve fibres. The sympathetic system has so far received the greatest attention and has prompted many investigators to use the classical physiological approaches of denervation and stimulation. Various aspects of amine mechanisms in the cerebral circulation have recently been reviewed extensively by Edvinsson & MacKenzie (1976). Arterioles on the brain surface, observed by the pial window technique (Edvinsson & MacKenzie 1976), were seen to constrict in response to sympathetic nerve stimulation, the effect being inhibited by the α-receptor antagonist, phentolamine. Many workers have reported a reduction in cerebral blood flow (only a few observed no effect), in conjunction with stimulation of the cervical sympathetic trunk. However, the amount of reduction is low in normotension and normocapnia, being only between 10 and 20% in most mammals. A slight increment in cerebral perfusion has been noted after acute superior cervical sympathetic ganglionectomy. It should be noted that these studies have usually measured total flow or a mixture of so-called regional flows. This only gives a net result from a complex flow pattern that may mask pronounced changes in small areas.

The cerebrovascular bed is autoregulated, a phenomenon which may be defined as the intrinsic ability of the brain to maintain a relatively constant blood flow despite moderate changes in perfusion pressure (Häggendal & Johansson 1965; Harper 1966). The autoregulation therefore ensures that the supply of oxygen and glucose to the brain remains constant within fairly wide limits of systemic blood pressure. The constancy of cerebral blood flow is achieved by the dilatation of cerebral arterioles in response to a reduction in perfusion pressure; the converse occurs when perfusion pressure is increased. As perfusion pressure is enhanced there is a point where the increase in cerebrovascular resistance is maximal; further increases in systemic blood pressure result in a breakthrough, that is an increase in the cerebral blood flow. This point is termed the upper limit of autoregulation. A sudden increase in perfusion pressure above the upper limit of autoregulation may result in cerebral oedema and blood–brain barrier damage. Similarly, at the lower limit of autoregulation, a very low systemic blood pressure will result in a reduced cerebral perfusion. Recent studies have indicated that the sympathetic nervous system has important roles in the autoregulation of the cerebral circulation to changing arterial pressure and in the blood–barrier function. The experimental evidence for this assumption will be reviewed below.

MEASUREMENT OF CEREBRAL BLOOD FLOW

The studies have been carried out on rabbits, rats and baboons with the use of three principal techniques for measurement of flow.

Local thermoclearance technique

The experiments were done on giant rabbits (Flanders giant or Belgian giant strains) of either sex, weighing 4 to 7 kg (Sercombe *et al.* 1975).

Chronic recording equipment. In 25 animals under light pentobarbitone–diazepam anaesthesia, supplemented by local anaesthesia with 2% lidocaine, trephine holes were drilled in the skull to allow thermoprobes of 0.7 mm outside diameter (Seylaz *et al.* 1973) to be implanted bilaterally into the caudate nucleus and lateral geniculate body. One thermoprobe was heated by a direct current to a few tenths of a degree above the cerebral tissue temperature. This increment in temperature was maintained at a constant level by negative feedback, and variations in the heating current were recorded that were directly proportional to the variations in blood flow. The contralateral unheated probe measured local brain temperature. The thermal clearance technique for blood flow measurement was fully described by Seylaz (1965). Two weeks after trephination a Teflon catheter (1.5 mm) was placed in the abdominal aorta via the saphenous artery in conjunction with recording of blood pressure, Pa_{CO_2} and Pa_{O_2} (Seylaz *et al.* 1974). After two days' recovery experiments lasting 5 to 8 hours were performed in the non-curarized and usually non-anaesthetized animals; these experiments included continuous registration (Seylaz *et al.* 1973) of relative local blood flow in the caudate nucleus and the lateral geniculate body of one side, brain temperature in corresponding regions on the contralateral side, electrocorticogram, arterial blood pressure, Pa_{CO_2}, and Pa_{O_2}. The blood gases were measured by a mass spectrometer via a probe inserted into the previously implanted Teflon catheter. This probe consisted of a flexible stainless steel tube, 0.4 mm in diameter, perforated and covered with a silastic membrane at the sensitive end (Seylaz *et al.* 1974).

Sympathetic nerve stimulation. Six of the rabbits—equipped with thermal probes, cortical electrodes and aortic catheter—were lightly anaesthetized with pentobarbitone and diazepam. A midline incision was made in the neck and the sympathetic nerve trunks were dissected free of surrounding tissue. Two types of electrodes were used for stimulation of the nerves—either a pair of silver wires, 50 μm in diameter and insulated except for the most distal 0.5 mm, which pierced the trunk below the superior cervical ganglion, or a pair of steel wires, 0.5 mm in diameter, over which the preganglionic nerve trunk was loosely hooked. The silver electrodes were left in place throughout the experiment, with the nerve lying in the extracellular fluid. The steel electrodes, however, were withdrawn between stimuli so that the nerve could be put back into the extracellular fluid. The following square wave stimulation parameters were used: frequency, 10 to 15 Hz; shock duration, 1 ms; stimulus strength, 1 to 10 V. The efficiency of stimulation was checked by observing pupillary dilatation. In some experiments, nerve conduction was blocked by preganglionic sectioning or by a piece of cotton wool, soaked in saturated potassium chloride solution of lidocaine, placed over the nerve trunk.

In two animals, a pair of electrodes were implanted chronically for stimulation under non-anaesthetized conditions. The electrodes consisted of a pair of fine silver wires insulated with silastic tubing. A silicone sheet enclosed the bared ends of these wires together with the sympathetic trunk at the site of stimulation. The leads were passed under the skin and led out under the fibreglass cover (Seylaz *et al.* 1973) on the head.

Arteriovenous oxygen difference method

Anaesthesia was induced in male Wistar rats (300–400 g body weight) with 2–3 % halothane and was maintained on 70 % N_2O and 30 % O_2 (Edvinsson *et al.* 1976*a*). The animals were immobilized and artificially ventilated through a tracheal cannula. The body temperature was kept at 37.4 ± 0.2 °C (mean ± S.E.M.). One femoral artery was cannulated for blood pressure recording and the other for anaerobic sampling of blood for measurement of Pa_{CO_2} and pH. A pair of delicate platinum electrodes were placed around the sympathetic trunk immediately below the superior cervical ganglion (from which the cerebrovascular sympathetic nerves originate) through a neck incision on both sides. A longitudinal skin incision was made over the skull bone, and a burr hole was placed over the superior sagittal sinus for sampling of cerebral venous blood to determine arteriovenous difference in oxygen content (AVD_{O_2}). The cerebral blood flow is inversely proportional to AVD_{O_2} under conditions of constant cerebral metabolic rate of oxygen (CMR_{O_2}) (Hägerdal *et al.* 1975). The mean CMR_{O_2}, determined in separate experiments, was 10.2 ml/(100 g min).

After the operative procedures the animals were allowed to rest for 30 min, after which the physiological variables were measured. Angiotensin II amide was infused intravenously in order to increase systemic mean arterial blood pressure (MABP) to various levels. When a steady level of hypertension had been obtained, AVD_{O_2} was measured again. In six non-stimulated rats the calculated cerebral blood flow increased above a pressure of 180 mmHg. In another group of six animals, the cerebral blood flow was determined in the same manner during angiotensin-induced hypertension. At blood–pressure levels above 180 mmHg, the sympathetic chains in the neck below the superior cervical ganglia were stimulated electrically (frequency 15 Hz, impulse duration 1 ms, 30 V) during the angiotensin injection (a maximum MABP of 205–210 mmHg was induced in both groups).

Intra-arterial ^{133}Xe clearance method

Adult baboons weighing 10–15 kg were anaesthetized with phencyclidine and thiopentone sodium, intubated and ventilated with a mixture of 75% N_2O–25% O_2 in an open circuit. The cerebral blood flow was measured by the intracarotid ^{133}Xe injection method and calculated by the height/area equation (Høedt-Rasmussen *et al.* 1966). The isotope was injected via the linguofacial trunk into the common carotid artery; all other branches of the external carotid artery were ligated. The scalp and the occipital and temporal muscles were removed to avoid contamination from the extracranial vascular bed. Arterial blood pressure and blood gases were frequently measured. Systemic blood pressure levels were increased by intravenous infusion of angiotensin II amide. Some of the baboons were subjected to unilateral sympathetic denervation (Strandgaard *et al.* 1974), and others were studied in conjunction with cervical sympathetic stimulation (MacKenzie *et al.* 1977).

RESULTS ON CEREBRAL BLOOD FLOW

Electrical field stimulation of isolated pial (Bevan & Bevan 1973; Edvinsson *et al.* 1976*b*) as well as intracerebral arterioles (Edvinsson & Owman 1977) produces a frequency-dependent vasoconstriction due to the local release of noradrenaline; the response is blocked by guanethidine or phentolamine. The effect of sympathetic nerve stimulation on pial vessels *in vivo* has also been subject to many studies. It was early found (see Edvinsson & MacKenzie 1976 for references) that pial arteries constricted under these conditions, and the observation has recently been confirmed and extended by Kuschinsky & Wahl (1976), who observed a 15% reduction in vessel diameter during stimulation; the effect was blocked by phentolamine. Many studies have been undertaken to assess the cerebral perfusion in conjunction with sympathetic stimulation in various species, using a variety of techniques. This aspect has also been reviewed recently (Edvinsson & MacKenzie 1976) and there is now little doubt about the cerebral vasoconstrictor ability of the adrenergic sympathetic fibres. However, considerable quantitative variation has been noted, from no effect at all to a reduction in flow varying between 10 and 80%. This variability does not seem to depend only on the precision and reliability of the technique used for measurement of flow, but also on the conditions under which the nerves have been stimulated (Lacombe *et al.* 1977).

Stimulation of the sympathetic nerve trunk during normotension

Unilateral electrical stimulation of the sympathetic nerve trunk between the middle and superior cervical ganglia in normotensive rabbits regularly caused a reduction of the blood flow in the ipsilateral caudate nucleus and

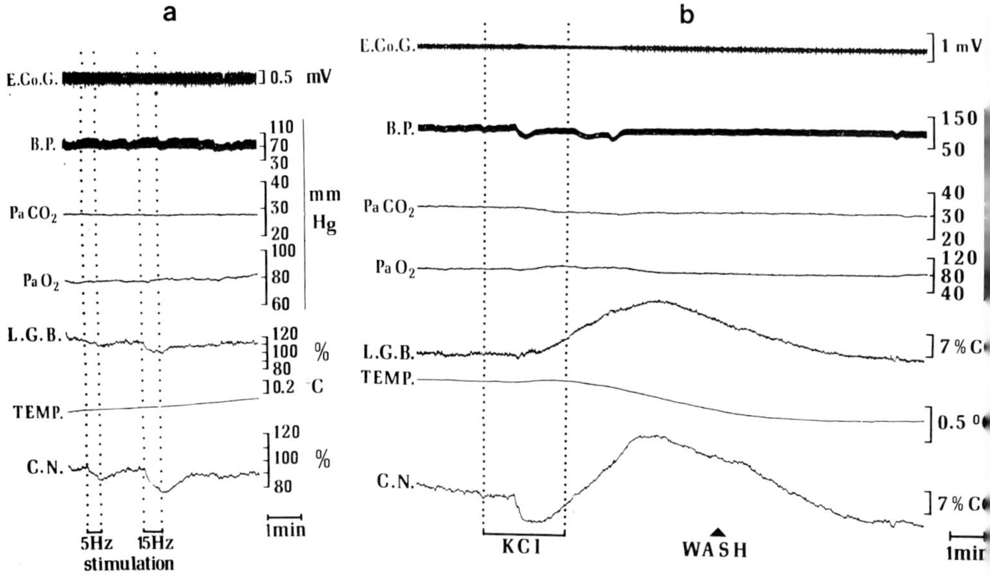

FIG. 1. Measurement of local cerebral blood flow in rabbit by the thermoclearance method. *(a)* Response of blood flow in the lateral geniculate body and the caudate nucleus on one side after preganglionic electrical stimulation of the ipsilateral cervical sympathetic trunk. The flow is expressed in relation to basal flow in the untreated animal, the zero level being obtained after the animal had been killed. The curves show effects of two stimulations of identical intensity but different frequency. Although in both cases there was pronounced pupillary dilatation, the decrease in blood flow in both structures was significantly greater with the higher frequency. *(b)* Effects of blockade of conduction in the preganglionic cervical sympathetic trunk (application of a plug of cotton wool soaked in saturated KCl) on the ipsilateral blood flow and associated variables. The flow levels are related to the effects of inhalation of 7% CO_2 in air. The sharp initial fall in caudate blood flow is probably attributable, in part, to the sudden fall in blood pressure and, chiefly, to stimulation by the KCl (before nerve inactivation). The return to baseline levels was accelerated in the caudate nucleus by washing the nerve with saline solution. E.Co.G., electrocorticogram; B.P., systemic arterial blood pressure; Pa_{CO_2} and Pa_{O_2}, partial pressure of CO_2 and O_2 in the aorta; L.G.B., blood flow in the lateral geniculate body of the right side; TEMP., temperature in the caudate nucleus on the left side; CN, blood flow in the contralateral caudate nucleus.

lateral geniculate body. The amount of reduction varied according to the frequency (Fig. 1*a*) and the intensity of stimulation, but was always relatively greater in the caudate nucleus than in the lateral geniculate body. The size of the relative changes in local flow was estimated by comparison with those induced by inhalations of 5% or 7% CO_2 in air. In some cases, as illustrated in Fig. 1*a*, reference was made to the zero flow level. This was obtained by continuing flow recordings after the animal had been killed. The final level found after cardiac arrest was referred to as zero flow, the resting level before killing being set at 100%. Theoretical and experimental support for the correctness of this means of calibration has been presented by Seylaz (1965). Accordingly, flow was reduced by about 25% in the caudate nucleus and about 15% in the lateral geniculate body during the 15 Hz stimulation of an anaesthetized animal. At frequencies above 15 Hz there seemed to be no further increase in the flow response. Moreover, stimulation for more than about 45 to 60 s sometimes failed to produce a continuing fall in flow, or even a constant reduced level of flow; rather, the flow tended to normalize again before the end of the stimulation.

Effect of sympathetic nerve denervation or blockade

Transection of the sympathetic nerve trunk, or conduction blockade with saturated potassium chloride or lidocaine below the superior cervical ganglion, led to a considerable increase in blood flow in both the lateral geniculate body and the caudate nucleus.

With conduction blockade, the effect was reversible and was sometimes preceded by a fall in flow, notably in the caudate nucleus (Fig. 1*b*). The initial fall in flow was probably caused mainly by stimulation of the fibres by depolarization before full inactivation has been achieved. It was not observed in experiments in which lidocaine was used as the blocking agent. The fall in blood pressure and the slight changes in Pa_{CO_2} and Pa_{O_2} (Fig. 1*b*) could not have accounted for the rise in flow because the alterations were small and, moreover, were in a direction opposite to that which would have been expected to increase the flow.

After nerve division, the mean blood flow remained at a higher level during the rest of the experiment. Moreover, this increase was greater than after chemical blockade of conduction. The proportion of flow changes in the caudate nucleus and the lateral geniculate body was about the same in both types of experiments.

Unilateral sympathetic denervation in the baboon (Strandgaard *et al.* 1974) revealed no difference between perfusion through the two hemispheres at normotension. However, these experiments were on chronically sympathectomized animals and due to an increased sensitivity of the cerebrovascular adrenergic receptors to circulating catecholamines (Edvinsson *et al.* 1971–72) an increased flow may have been masked. The same interpretation seems to apply to a similar study reported by Eklöf *et al.* (1971).

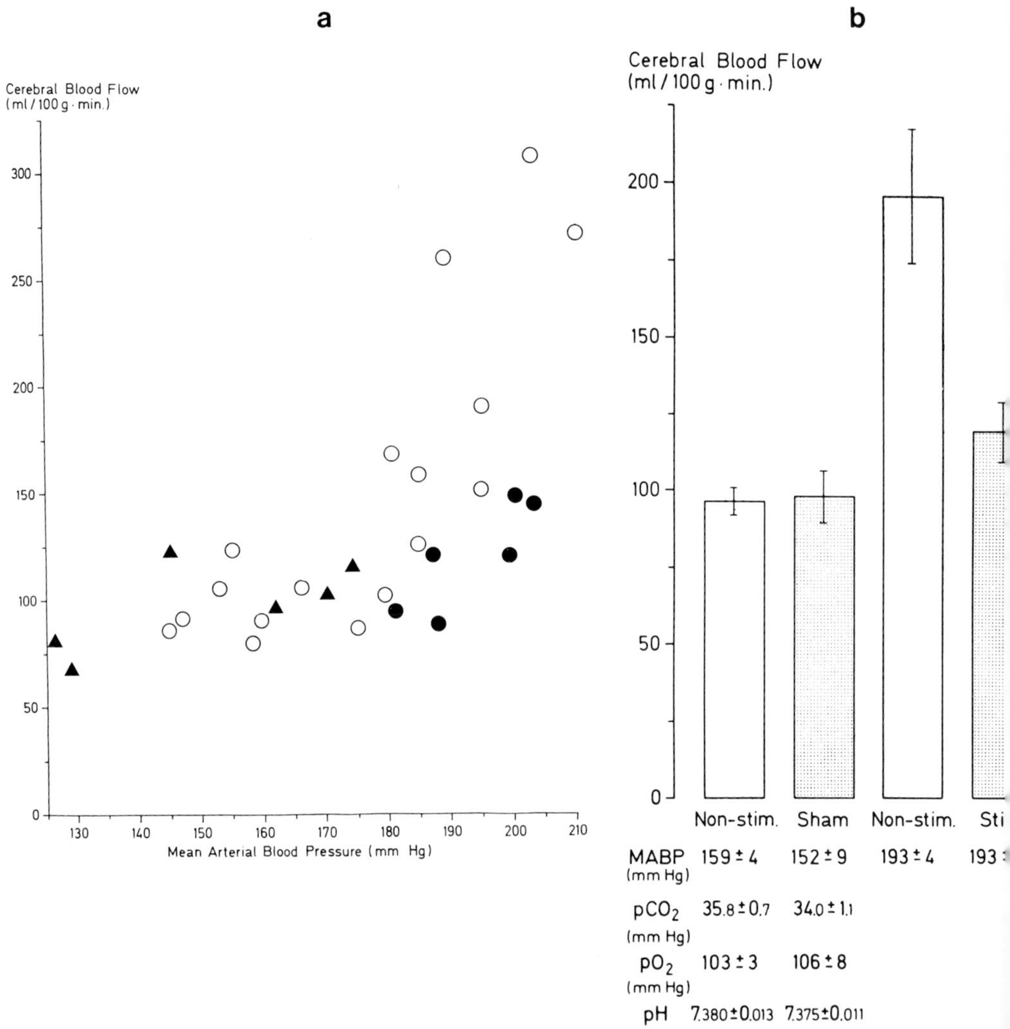

FIG. 2. Measurement of cerebral blood flow in rats with the [^{14}C]ethanol method. *(a)* Individual values for cerebral blood flow at various levels of systemic blood pressure. A desired amount of arterial hypertension was induced by i.v. infusion of angiotensin. Open circles represent determinations in six control animals. Filled symbols represent six animals which had bilateral electrodes on the cervical sympathetic chain for preganglionic stimulation of the superior cervical ganglia; the animals were left non-stimulated at blood pressures below 180 mmHg (filled triangles) but were stimulated electrically (30 V; frequency, 15 Hz; impulse duration, 1 ms) during the various levels of angiotensin-induced hypertension (above 180 mmHg) (filled circles). *(b)* Data on cerebral blood flow and associated physiological variables

(continued on page 77)

Stimulation of the sympathetic nerve trunk in hypertension

In the series of experiments on rats (Edvinsson *et al.* 1976*a*) cerebral blood flow was found to be constant up to a MABP of 180 mmHg, after which the flow increased in proportion to the increment in pressure. The difference in flow measured below and above 180 mmHg was statistically significant. Fig. 2 shows that the manipulation of the sympathetic nerve trunks in the neck that is needed when the stimulation electrodes are inserted had no effect on the cerebral blood flow measured before stimulation. Electrical stimulation of the sympathetic nerves to the cerebrovascular system during arterial hypertension (Fig. 2) almost prevented the cerebral hyperaemia observed in non-stimulated animals as a consequence of the breakthrough in autoregulation that occurs at a MABP of over 180 mmHg.

In another series of experiments the influence of the sympathetic nervous system on the upper limit of autoregulation of cerebral blood flow was studied in anaesthetized baboons by the intracarotid ^{133}Xe technique (MacKenzie *et al.* 1977). Arterial pressure was increased in a stepwise manner by the intravenous infusion of angiotensin II. In the mean arterial pressure range of 130–159 mmHg an average cerebral blood flow increase of $53 \pm 9\%$ was observed. This was significantly higher than the flow increase observed in unilaterally stimulated baboons ($16 \pm 4\%$; $P < 0.01$ according to Student's *t*-test). In these unilaterally stimulated animals there was no significant difference in the cerebral blood flow between the hemispheres from the stimulated and non-stimulated sides. In addition, there was no electroencephalographic change and no blood–brain barrier dysfunction to suggest a side-to-side difference in cerebral blood flow—at any level of mean arterial pressure—in the unilaterally stimulated baboons. Bilateral stimulation of the superior cervical ganglia totally protected ($0 \pm 3\%$; $P < 0.001$) the brain against the breakthrough of the autoregulation.

←

compiled from the data presented in *(a)*. The six non-stimulated controls (open bars) and the six animals bearing electrodes (stippled bars) are grouped on either side of 180 mmHg in mean arterial blood pressure (MABP). The control animals ('Non-stim.') attained a markedly increased flow during hypertension (above 180 mmHg) as compared with the same animals during normotension (Student's *t*-test: $P < 0.001$). The animals bearing electrodes had during normotension the same cerebral blood flow before stimulation ('Sham') as the controls. When electrical stimulation ('Stim') was performed during hypertension there was no significant increase in flow ($P > 0.05$). The marked difference in cerebral blood flow seen during hypertension between the non-stimulated and stimulated groups of animals is significant ($P < 0.01$). There was no significant difference in mean values ($\pm$ S.E.M.) of MABP, arterial CO_2 and O_2 tensions, or pH between controls and animals bearing electrodes on the cervical sympathetic chains.

Comments

It has been discussed for many years whether the sympathetic nervous system can affect cerebral perfusion, and whether any such effects are involved in a physiological control of the cerebral blood flow. It is now quite clear that such a nervous influence exists. The magnitude of this influence appears to be directly related to the degree of sympathetic innervation of the intracerebral arterioles. Since some brain regions are less well innervated (Edvinsson & Owman 1977), heterogeneity in the sympathomimetic flow response can be expected (Sercombe *et al.* 1975). This may well explain the low figures obtained in some experiments on sympathetic stimulation in which net flow is obtained from a mixture of flow levels in various small regions. The brain vessels appear to be under a sympathetic tone that can be revealed by acute denervation. It should be emphasized that *any* type of cerebrovascular effects may be seen after sympathectomy, depending on the time after operation at which the animal is studied, owing to degeneration release of transmitter and subsequent denervation supersensitivity of the vascular receptors (Edvinsson *et al.* 1971–72).

The recent finding of an involvement of the local sympathetic nerves in the autoregulation of cerebral blood flow (Strandgaard *et al.* 1974; Bill & Linder 1976; Edvinsson *et al.* 1976*a*; MacKenzie *et al.* 1977) provides one illustration of the importance of the sympathetic system in a more physiological control function. It means that, provided the intracranial sympathetic nerves are activated, cerebral blood flow can also be kept closer to normal during pronounced arterial hypertension. It is therefore not surprising that it is difficult to detect the upper limit of autoregulation in non-anaesthetized animals in which the induced increase in systemic blood pressure is accompanied by an augmented sympathetic tone. In a corresponding way, our inability to reveal an influence of sympathectomy on the upper limit of autoregulation may be explained by the fact that the anaesthetic agent used will already have reduced sympathetic activity in the non-operated control animals.

METHODS FOR STUDIES OF THE BLOOD–BRAIN BARRIER

A marked acute systemic hypertension is associated not only with impairment of cerebral autoregulation but also with damage to blood–brain barrier functions leading to, for example, cerebral oedema (Johansson 1974). It is assumed that the disruption of the barrier is caused by a pressure-forced overdistension of cerebral microvessels (Johansson *et al.* 1974). In line with the influence of perivascular sympathetic nerves on the cerebrovascular bed, it could be assumed that sympathetic stimulation would help to protect the vessels from overdistension. This was tested in rats by the Evans' blue and brain uptake index techniques to estimate the barrier capacity.

Evans' blue technique

Evans' blue was mixed with blood from the animals and slowly injected intravenously 20 min before the tests (1 ml of a 1.5% solution in Krebs–Ringer buffer). This dye binds with serum proteins *in vivo* and does not, therefore, penetrate the blood–brain barrier under normal conditions. The dye–protein complex can be seen by fluorescence microscopy as a red fluorescence (Steinwall & Klatzo 1966). The animals were killed for macroscopic and fluorescence microscopic examination. The brain was removed and selected regions (frontal, parietal, temporal and occipital cortex with underlying white matter, caudate nucleus, thalamus, mesencephalon, and cerebellum) were frozen rapidly in a propane–propylene mixture cooled to the temperature of liquid nitrogen. After subsequent freeze-drying, the specimens were processed for fluorescence microscopy according to the method of Falck and Hillarp, involving exposure of the tissue to gaseous formaldehyde in dry conditions (Björklund *et al.* 1972).

Brain uptake index method

The brain uptake index (BUI) was studied for noradrenaline and inulin, with ethanol as the highly diffusible standard for comparison. We gave a 1 s injection of 0.04 ml Krebs-Ringer buffer solution (37 °C), containing a mixture of either [7-^{3}H]L-noradrenaline (New England Nuclear; specific activity 3.0 Ci/mmol; concentration 7.5 nmol/ml) or [^{3}H]inulin (Radiochemical Centre, Amersham; specific activity 440 mCi/mmol; concentration 25 nmol/ml) together with [^{14}C]ethanol (Radiochemical Centre, Amersham; specific activity 58 mCi/mmol; concentration 50 nmol/ml). The bolus mixture was infused through a cannula inserted centripetally in the right external carotid artery, thus reaching directly into the brain. The heart of the animal was stopped with saturated potassium chloride 15 s after administration of the bolus, the animal was instantly decapitated, and the head was frozen in liquid nitrogen. Various regions (frontal, parietal and occipital cortex with underlying white matter, caudate nucleus and thalamus) from the injected side were chiselled out in a cryostat at —15 °C, weighed and placed in liquid scintillation vials containing 0.5 ml Soluene (Packard). When the tissue had been dissolved 10 ml of Instagel was added. The tissue samples were counted for β-emissions

TABLE 1

Brain uptake index (BUI) for noradrenaline and inulin in various cerebral regions of anaesthetized rats.

Experimental	*n*	*Frontal cortex*	*Parietal cortex*	*Occipital cortex*	*Caudate nucleus*	*Thalamus*
Noradrenaline						
Unoperated animals	6	3.40 ± 0.29	4.26 ± 0.44	4.46 ± 0.45	2.83 ± 0.38	2.69 ± 0.40
Sham-operated, 3 days	5	3.46 ± 0.18	4.14 ± 0.21	4.12 ± 0.25	3.37 ± 0.19	2.95 ± 0.10
Sympathectomized, 3 days	7	8.07 ± 1.32**	9.85 ± 1.53**	10.27 ± 2.05*	8.53 ± 0.90***	7.11 ± 0.69***
Sympathectomized, 1 month	4	5.09 ± 0.52*	5.48 ± 0.48$^{n.s.}$	5.10 ± 0.24$^{n.s.}$	4.63 ± 0.59*	4.37 ± 0.47*
Inulin						
Unoperated animals	5	1.66 ± 0.06	1.57 ± 0.17	1.70 ± 0.08	1.67 ± 0.13	1.70 ± 0.18
Sympathectomized, 3 days	5	2.67 ± 0.16***	2.91 ± 0.27**	2.73 ± 0.24**	2.70 ± 0.20**	2.75 ± 0.18**

Values are mean ± S.E.M., *n*, number of animals. Student's *t*-test: comparison between unoperated and operated animals * $P < 0.05$; ** $0.05 < P < 0.01$; *** $0.01 < P < 0.001$; n.s. = non-significant.

in a Nuclear Chicago liquid scintillation counter. Quench correction was performed according to conventional principles.

The BUI for noradrenaline and inulin was calculated according to the method developed by Oldendorf (1971):

$$\text{BUI} = \frac{\text{tissue} - {}^{3}\text{H}/\text{tissue} - {}^{14}\text{C}}{\text{mix} - {}^{3}\text{H}/\text{mix} - {}^{14}\text{C}} \times 100$$

RESULTS ON BLOOD–BRAIN BARRIER FUNCTION

Regional variation in blood–brain barrier capacity and the effect of sympathectomy during normotension

The BUI for noradrenaline and inulin in animals with an intact blood–brain barrier varied according to the region studied, as shown in Table 1. The uptake for noradrenaline was slightly higher in the cortical tissue than in the deeper regions of the hemisphere. Three days after excision of the superior cervical ganglia the BUI was enhanced about twofold as compared with unoperated or sham-operated controls. The uptake index for an inert substance, inulin, was similarly enhanced in all the regions studied after sympathectomy (Fig. 3), indicating that the increased uptake was not merely due to a change in local demand for neurotransmitter but more probably reflected a true impairment of blood–brain barrier function.

No brain regions taken from (non-sympathectomized) control animals injected with Evans' blue revealed any macroscopically visible staining of the parenchyma. Fluorescence microscopy revealed a greenish background fluorescence in the brain tissue. The well-known appearance and distribution of the formaldehyde-induced fluorescence in the monoamine neuron systems were recognized. The lumen of vessels everywhere in the brain contained Evans' blue, which could easily be seen by its bright red fluorescence. No Evans' blue could be found in the vascular walls except for a red fluorescence restricted to the intima of the pial vessels. In five out of ten sympathectomized animals injected with Evans' blue, a discrete patchy extravasation of the Evans' blue–albumin complex was noticed in cortical structures on the denervated side. One explanation of these findings is that the barrier properties of the capillary endothelium, which appears to have contractile proteins (Owman *et al.* 1977), are directly influenced by the nerve endings, demonstrated by electron microscopy to be in close association with the capillary wall (Rennels & Nelson 1975). One month after sympathectomy the BUI for noradrenaline was less markedly increased and now amounted to levels only

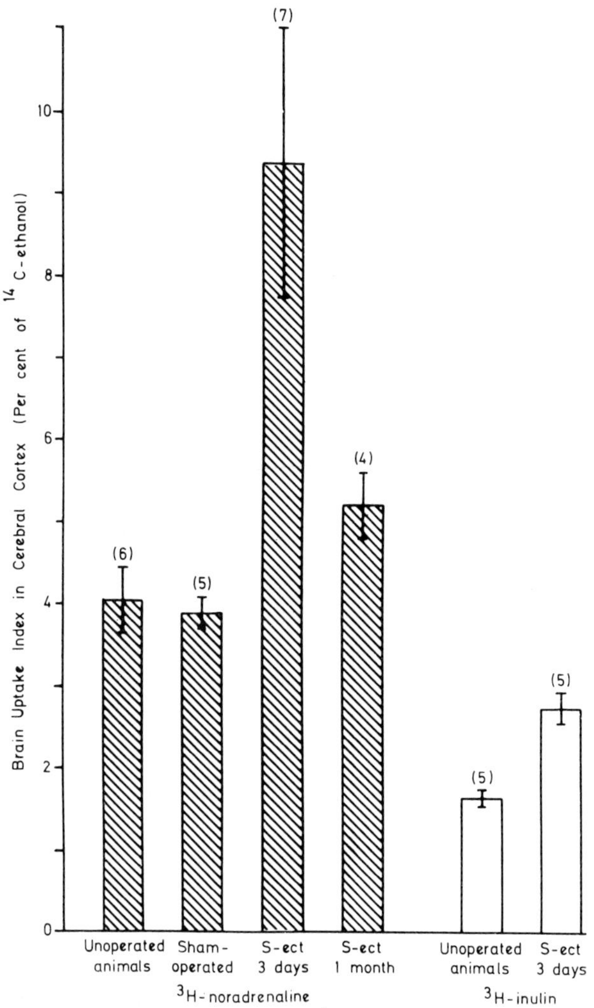

FIG. 3. Brain uptake index (BUI) for [^{3}H]noradrenaline and [^{3}H]inulin in cerebral cortex from rats. [^{14}C]ethanol was used as the highly diffusible standard, and the index is expressed in relation to the uptake of labelled ethanol. Values are means ± S.E.M.; number of animals given within parentheses. Unoperated controls vs. sympathectomy (S-ect) 3 days according to Student's t-test: $P < 0.001$ for both tracers.

slightly different from those of control animals (Table 1). This would favour the direct involvement of the sympathetic nervous system on the blood–brain barrier since it can be anticipated that after chronic sympathectomy there would be a tendency to normalization of the barrier function due to the progressive development of denervation supersensitivity (Fig. 3).

Effect of sympathectomy on blood–brain barrier function during hypertension

Acute arterial hypertension was produced by the model described by Johansson (1974). The anaesthetized rat (with a resting MABP of 140–150 mmHg) was first injected with dihydralazine, a potent dilator, which reduced the blood pressure to 90 mmHg, and hypertension was subsequently induced by intravenous injection of angiotensin II amide, which increased the blood pressure by about 90–110 mmHg. A patchy and dot-like extravasation of Evans' blue was noted macroscopically and to a similar extent in all surface structures; the degree of extravasation of Evans' blue has been estimated semi-quantitatively (Table 2). This barrier damage is believed to be caused by a pressure-forced overdistension of the vessel wall (Johansson *et al.* 1974).

One to three days after unilateral sympathectomy, an acute rise in systemic blood pressure resulted in more marked barrier damage on the sympathectomized side than on the contralateral side of the brain (Table 2). On the other hand, when this acute hypertension was induced during electrical stimulation (30 V, 15 Hz, 1 ms pulse duration) of the right cervical sympathetic chain below the superior cervical ganglion, only minor barrier damage occurred on the stimulated side (Table 2).

Comments

The fact that increased brain uptake of noradrenaline and inulin is seen after sympathectomy even in normotensive animals indicates that the sympathetic nervous system exerts some kind of physiological influence on blood–brain barrier functions. It can be assumed that such an influence is mediated both through the nerve supply to the small arteries and arterioles in the brain (Owman *et al.* 1974) and through the possible innervation of the capillary wall (Rennels & Nelson 1975). This could either be a myogenic mechanism in the endothelium of the larger intracerebral vessels (Majno *et al.* 1969; Robertson & Khairallah 1972; Bevan & Duckles 1975) or in the capillary pericytes and endothelial cells, which have recently been shown to contain contractile proteins demonstrable by immunohistochemistry (Owman *et al.* 1977), or an effect of amines on the vesicular transport in the endothelium (Westergaard 1975). These mechanisms may also be involved in the pathophysiology of blood–brain barrier disruption during acute hypertension, though it is conceivable that the pressure–forced overdistension of the cerebral vessels is primarily counteracted by an increased tone of these vessels mediated by their sympathetic innervation of the muscular media.

TABLE 2

Effect of acute systemic hypertension on blood–brain barrier function as shown by the degree of Evans' blue–albumin extravasation, which is expressed arbitrarily from 0 (no extravasation) to +++ (marked patchy and dot-like extravasation). The hypertension was induced by angiotensin II amide preceded by dihydralazine methane sulphate.

Treatment	*n*	*Initial MABP (mmHg)*	*MABP after dihydralazine (mmHg)*	*MABP increase after angiotensin (mmHg)*	*Blood–brain barrier lesions*							
					Right side				*Left side*			
					+++	++	+	0	+++	++	+	0
Moderate acute hypertension												
Control	20	147 ± 2	88 ± 2	91 ± 2		8	6	6		8	6	6
Right sympathectomy	12	144 ± 5	89 ± 1	94 ± 2	1	11				4	5	3
Marked acute hypertension												
Control	11	145 ± 2	88 ± 1	111 ± 2	8	3			8	3		
Right sympathetic stimulation	11	145 ± 4	89 ± 2	112 ± 2			3	8	1	5	3	2

Values on mean arterial blood pressure (MABP) are means ± S.E.M., *n*, number of animals.

ACKNOWLEDGEMENT

Supported by the Swedish Medical Research Council (Grant No. 04X-732).

References

BEVAN, J. A. & BEVAN, R. D. (1973) Localized neurogenic vasoconstriction of the basilar artery. *Stroke 4*, 760–764

BEVAN, J. A. & DUCKLES, S. P. (1975) Evidence for α-adrenergic receptors on intimal endothelium. *Blood Vessels 12*, 307–310

BILL, A. & LINDER, J. (1976) Sympathetic control of cerebral blood flow in acute arterial hypertension. *Acta Physiol. Scand. 96*, 114–121

BJÖRKLUND, A., FALCK, B. & OWMAN, CH. (1972) Fluorescence microscopic and microspectrofluorometric techniques for the cellular localization and characterization of biogenic amines, in *The Thyroid and Biogenic Amines* (Rall, J. E. & Kopin, I. J., eds.), pp. 318–368, North-Holland, Amsterdam

EDVINSSON, L. & MACKENZIE, E. T. (1976) Amine mechanisms in the cerebral circulation. *Pharmacol. Rev. 28*, 275–353

EDVINSSON, L. & OWMAN, CH. (1977) Sympathetic innervation and adrenergic receptors in intraparenchymal cerebral arterioles of baboon, in *Cerebral Function, Metabolism and Circulation* (Ingvar, D. H. & Lassen, N. A., eds.), Munksgaard, Copenhagen

EDVINSSON, L., NIELSEN, K. C., OWMAN, CH. & WEST, K. A. (1971–72) Sympathetic adrenergic influence on brain vessels as studied by changes in cerebral blood volume of mice. *Eur. Neurol. 6*, 193–202

EDVINSSON, L., OWMAN, CH. & SIESJÖ, B. (1976*a*) Physiological role of cerebrovascular sympathetic nerves in the autoregulation of cerebral blood flow. *Brain Res. 117*, 519–523

EDVINSSON, L., OWMAN, CH. & SJÖBERG, N.-O. (1976*b*) Autonomic nerves, mast cells, and amine receptors in human brain vessels. A histochemical and pharmacological study. *Brain Res. 115*, 377–393

EKLÖF, B, INGVAR, D. H., KÅGSTRÖM, E. & OLIN, T. (1971) Persistence of cerebral blood flow autoregulation following chronic bilateral cervical sympathectomy in the monkey. *Acta Physiol. Scand. 82*, 172–176

HÄGERDAL, M., HARP, J. R. & SIESJÖ, B. (1975) Influence of changes in arterial P_{CO_2} on cerebral blood flow and cerebral energy state during hypothermia in the rat. *Acta Anaesthesiol. Scand. Suppl. 57*, 25–33

HÄGGENDAL, E. & JOHANSSON, B. (1965) Effect of arterial carbon dioxide tension and oxygen saturation on cerebral blood flow autoregulation in dogs. *Acta Physiol. Scand. Suppl. 258*, 27–53

HARPER, A. M. (1966) Autoregulation of cerebral blood flow: influence of arterial pressure on blood flow through the cerebral cortex. *J. Neurol. Neurosurg. Psychiatry 29*, 398–403

HØEDT-RASMUSSEN, K., SVEINSDOTTIR, E. & LASSEN, N. A. (1966) Regional cerebral blood flow in man determined by intra-arterial injection of radioactive inert gas. *Circ. Res. 18*, 237–247

JOHANSSON, B. (1974) *Blood–Brain Barrier Dysfunction in Acute Arterial Hypertension.* Thesis, Department of Neurology, University of Göteborg, Sweden

JOHANSSON, B., STRANDGAARD, S. & LASSEN, N. A. (1974) On the pathogenesis of hypertensive encephalopathy. *Circ. Res. Suppl. 34–35*, 1162–1171

KUSCHINSKY, W. & WAHL, M. (1976) The ability to influence the pial arterial tone by the sympathetic nervous system, in *The Cerebral Vessel Wall* (Cervós-Navarro, J. *et al.*, eds.), Raven Press, New York

LACOMBE, P., SERCOMBE, R., REYNIER-REBUFFEL, A. M., LUSAMVUKU, N. A. T., AUBINEAU, P., PINARD, E. & SEYLAZ, J. (1977) Time course of the effects of cervical sympathetic stimulation on local CBF, in *Cerebral Function, Metabolism and Circulation* (Ingvar, D. H. & Lassen, N. A., eds.), Munksgaard, Copenhagen

MACKENZIE, E. T., MCGEORGE, A. P., GRAHAM, D. I., FITCH, W., EDVINSSON, L. & HARPER, A. M. (1977) Breakthrough of cerebral autoregulation and the sympathetic nervous system, in *Cerebral Function, Metabolism and Circulation* (Ingvar, D. H. & Lassen, N. A., eds.), Munksgaard, Copenhagen

MAJNO, G., SHEA, S. M. & LEVENTHAL, M. (1969) Endothelial contraction induced by histamine-type mediators. An electron microscopic study. *J. Cell Biol. 42*, 647–672

OLDENDORF, W. H. (1971) Brain uptake of radiolabeled amino acids, amines and hexoses after arterial injection. *Am. J. Physiol. 221*, 1629–1638

OWMAN, CH., EDVINSSON, L., FALCK, B. & NIELSEN, K. C. (1974) Amine mechanism in brain vessels, with particular regard to autonomic innervation and blood–brain barrier, in *Pathology of Cerebral Microcirculation* (Cervós-Navarro, J., ed.), Walter de Gruyter, Berlin

OWMAN, CH., EDVINSSON, L., HARDEBO, J. E., GRÖSCHEL-STEWART, U., UNSICKER, K. & WALLES, B. (1977) Immunohistochemical demonstration of actin and myosin in brain capillaries, in *Cerebral Function, Metabolism and Circulation* (Ingvar, D. H. & Lassen, N.A., eds.), Munksgaard, Copenhagen

RENNELS, M. L. & NELSON, E. (1975) Capillary innervation in the mammalian central nervous system: an electron microscopic demonstration *Am. J. Anat. 144*, 233–241

ROBERTSON, A. L. & KHAIRALLAH, P. A. (1972) Effects of angiotensin II and some analogues on vascular permeability in the rabbit. *Circ. Res. 31*, 923–931

SERCOMBE, R., AUBINEAU, P., EDVINSSON, L., MAMO, H., OWMAN, CH., PINARD, E. & SEYLAZ, J. (1975) Neurogenic influence on local cerebral blood flow. *Neurology 25*, 954–963

SEYLAZ, J. (1965) Développement d'une méthode de mesure instantanée localisée et semi-quantitative du débit sanguin *in vivo*. *Biophysik 2*, 330–339

SEYLAZ, J., AUBINEAU, P., CORRÈZE, J. L. & MAMO, H. (1973) Techniques for continuous measurement of local cerebral blood flow, Pa_{O_2}, Pa_{CO_2} and blood pressure in the non-anesthetized animal. *Pflügers Arch. Eur. J. Physiol. 340*, 175–180

SEYLAZ, J., PINARD, E., CORRÈZE, J. L., AUBINEAU, P. F. & MAMO, H. (1974) Quantitative continuous measurement of blood gas tensions by mass spectrometry. *J. Appl. Physiol. 37*, 937–941

STEINWALL, O. & KLATZO, I. (1966) Selective vulnerability of the blood–brain barrier in chemically induced lesions. *J. Neuropathol. Exp. Neurol. 25*, 542–559

STRANDGAARD, S., MACKENZIE, E. T., SENGUPTA, D., ROWAN, J. A., LASSEN, N. A. & HARPER, A. M. (1974) Upper limit of autoregulation of cerebral blood flow in the baboon. *Circ. Res. 34*, 435–440

WESTERGAARD, E. (1975) Enhanced vesicular transport of exogenous peroxidase across cerebral blood vessels induced by serotonin. *Acta Neuropathol. 32*, 27–42

Discussion

Purves: You used the angiotensin to cause hypertension. What is your evidence that it is inert with respect to cerebrovascular smooth muscle?

Edvinsson: I have recently examined the effects of angiotensin II (Hypertensin, CIBA) on intracranial arteries and arterioles. The contractile effect is surprisingly weak, amounting to only about 30–40% of that obtained with, for example, 5-hydroxytryptamine (serotonin). The contraction induced by angiotensin II is not affected by the presence of phentolamine (an α-adrenergic blocking agent) in the organ bath. Furthermore, sympathectomy does not change this *in vitro* response. These results rather tend to support our use of angiotensin II in producing hypertension. In these studies on the upper limit of the autoregulation of the cerebral blood flow, Bill & Linder (1976) found that sympathetic stimulation reduced the risk for regional overperfusion to the same extent whether the hypertension was produced by ligation of the thoracic aorta, or by injection of metaraminol or angiotensin II.

Purves: Most people have found marked tachyphylaxis with the use of angiotensin. So, to achieve relatively high levels of hypertension, you have to use doses perhaps 500 or 1000 times greater than the amount used to test smooth muscle initially. In other words, are the responses which you show simply due to the sympathomimetic or angiotensin-like drugs, or can one generalize and say that the response is a function of hypertension, however caused?

Edvinsson: I think that we have enough evidence now to state in general terms that sympathetic nerve stimulation tends to protect the brain against overperfusion and breakdown of the blood–brain barrier. This evidence has been collected from three separate studies using different techniques in baboons, cats and rats. Furthermore, the hypertension has been produced by different means, avoiding a systematic error.

Pickering: The staining you get may not be due to what you call a breakdown. In 1963 Frank Byrom induced severe hypertension in rats and attributed the leakage of dye into the cortex to vascular spasm and the resultant ischaemia in the cortex. Giese (1964) showed that when angiotensin is injected intravenously a beaded appearance of the arteries in the rat mesentery is produced. If India ink is injected intravenously it appears not in the constricted bits but in the dilated bits. Then Goldby & Beilin (1974) reported that these dilated bits showed the earliest stage of arteriolar necrosis, which of course is the cause of the malignant phase of hypertension. Wilson and I showed in 1938 that this didn't appear in the kidney beyond the clamp. This is part of the evidence for a very high arterial pressure causing the lesion. So what you are studying may be arteriolar damage represented by arteriolar necrosis, which is caused by a greatly raised arterial pressure (Pickering 1968). Did you examine the brain arteries histologically?

Edvinsson: We have never observed any necrosis in the arteriolar wall by light microscopy since the studies were performed in a rather acute way. However, if you are right, leakage of water might occur and we would expect oedema of the brain, which nobody has been able to demonstrate. We did not obtain any oedema of the brain, only extravasation of the tracer.

Pickering: It is very difficult to demonstrate oedema of the brain.

Moskowitz: Are the effects that you observe unilateral?

Pickering: Weren't they bilateral? I thought they were only unilateral if you cut the sympathetic on one side.

Edvinsson: The blood pressure increase is bilateral. Our ability to affect the risk of damage is unilateral. We can minimize the extravasation of the Evans' blue tracer by stimulating the sympathetic system on one side, keeping the other side as a control.

Pickering: If the arteries and arterioles are constricted when the sympathetic is stimulated, one would expect the vessels to be protected distally from the rise in pressure. It is the rise in pressure that produces arteriolar necrosis. If the sympathetic has any action, one would expect the pressure in the arterioles to rise more when the sympathetic is cut and less when the sympathetic is stimulated. Wouldn't that explain what you see?

Edvinsson: That is a possibility.

Sandler: George Cotzias (Cotzias *et al.* 1974) claimed that when he gave an MAO inhibitor to an experimental animal, methylene blue would get across the blood–brain barrier, whereas its passage had previously been impeded. Other amines too, including dopamine in particular, which didn't get across before the inhibitor was given, did so afterwards.

When we consider noradrenaline uptake, perhaps we have all accepted too readily Weil-Malherbe's early data (Weil-Malherbe *et al.* 1959) that parenterally administered catecholamines have extremely restricted access to the brain. It seems to me that these findings need reassessment, not only because bolus injection was employed but also because of other methodological considerations. Did you inject labelled or unlabelled noradrenaline, Dr Edvinsson?

Edvinsson: We injected a bolus containing [^{14}C]ethanol and [^{3}H]noradrenaline into the internal carotid artery ipsilaterally.

Sandler: There is a high affinity, low capacity binding system (Danon & Sapira 1972) which would immediately take up small amounts of carrier-free noradrenaline, if that is what you happened to be injecting. This would complicate one's interpretation of plasma decay curves more than somewhat, and might well prevent tracer amounts, in the absolute sense, gaining access to the brain.

There is a further point. You mentioned propranolol as though it possessed one single action, as a beta-blocker and nothing more. It has well-known membrane effects and other interesting properties are now coming to light (Koch-Weser 1975), unmasked particularly by using the D-isomer (R. Cundall

& P. Bond, personal communication) which seems to be relatively free from beta-blocking activity.

Purves: An odd thing about angiotensin as opposed to a mechanically produced rise in blood pressure is that angiotensin brings about its effect by a fairly heavy activation of sympathetic fibres. Thus we might expect that in the baboon with all the nerves intact, there would already have been a fairly high degree of sympathetic activity, whereas with a mechanical rise in blood pressure you would expect negligible sympathetic activity. So in the baboon made hypertensive with angiotensin, are you electrically stimulating sympathetic nerves which are already activated?

Edvinsson: We were aware of this problem when we did the flow studies but, as I said, these results agree well with those obtained with other modes of producing hypertension. Furthermore, I was intrigued by the poor effect that angiotensin II had on isolated brain vessels.

Rosendorff: We have all used angiotensin and we all think that it is inert in cerebral vessels. But evidence is now accumulating that angiotensin will increase the blood pressure not only by a direct action on peripheral resistance vessels or by releasing aldosterone but also by activating brain-stem centres. If angiotensin is infused into the vertebral arteries, for example, the rise in blood pressure is greater than that produced by the same dose of angiotensin given intravenously (Rosendorff *et al.* 1970). This suggests that there is some area within the distribution of the vertebral artery which responds to angiotensin by affecting vascular dynamics. Joy (1971) reported that this is around the area postrema in the brain stem, which is not far from the nucleus (locus coeruleus) of the intracerebral noradrenergic pathway. Marcus Raichle and his colleagues (1975) have shown that stimulation of the locus coeruleus produces an increase in brain water permeability. Also, we have recently observed changes in cerebral blood flow after stimulation of the locus coeruleus (Rosendorff *et al.* 1976). Therefore, the changes in permeability and blood flow described by Dr Edvinsson may be at least partly due to the activation of some of the brain-stem nuclei by angiotensin, and may be quite independent of the systemic blood pressure effects of angiotensin. At least, it is a possibility that should be looked at.

I think that we all accept that noradrenaline does not get into brain but is stopped by the blood–brain barrier. This begs the question of what the blood–brain barrier for noradrenaline is. This barrier can be disrupted by hyperosmolar urea, which shrinks capillary endothelial cells. However, the blood–brain barrier to noradrenaline can also be disrupted at the arteriolar level by suppression of noradrenaline uptake, or by MAO or catechol *O*-methyltransferase inhibition, or by a combination of these. There is, therefore, not one but a whole family of barriers to noradrenaline passage into the brain.

Owman: Monoamine oxidase is present in the capillary endothelium. One of the ways circulating noradrenaline is broken down and trapped is through this kind of enzymic barrier (Hardebo *et al.* 1976). If monoamine oxidase is inhibited an increased cerebral blood flow can be demonstrated (MacKenzie *et al.* 1975), probably because noradrenaline then goes into the brain, and stimulates metabolism, which invokes an increased flow. I don't quite see the point about whether angiotensin is having other effects on the brain. How would you then explain the fact that electrical sympathetic stimulation in the neck nevertheless moves the breakthrough point of the autoregulation towards higher blood pressure values?

Rosendorff: I am not suggesting that such effects would invalidate these results. But the absolute values for the breakthrough point might be considerably altered if you used some other hypertensive agent which lacked these effects.

Owman: The main object here is to compare two sides of the same animal, to get around this problem.

Purves: Yes, but you are also making a general statement to the effect that sympathetic stimulation will alter the inflection of the pressure/flow curve representing the upper limit of autoregulation. At some stage someone must ask whether this effect is unique, quantitatively and qualitatively, to the infusion of angiotensin or whether it would appear with all other methods used.

Rapoport: Drs Sokoloff, Pappius, Fieschi, Savaki and I (unpublished work) measured regional brain uptake of [^{14}C]2-deoxy-D-glucose after unilateral perfusion of the rat brain by hypertonic mannitol solution. This procedure, which osmotically opens the blood–brain barrier, results in local increases in cerebral metabolism and augmented uptake of the ^{14}C tracer. As osmotic barrier opening alone can influence metabolism, is it not difficult to interpret changes of cerebral blood flow and metabolism, in response to noradrenaline, after the blood–brain barrier has been osmotically opened?

Edvinsson: Dr Pickard and colleagues (1977) have studied the effect of osmotic opening of the blood–brain barrier by urea on the cerebral circulation. They were unable to demonstrate any change in cerebral blood flow, or cerebral metabolic rate of oxygen or glucose. However, after hypertonic urea injections the blood–brain barrier is osmotically opened and agents that are normally barrier-limited, such as noradrenaline, may now have pronounced effects on the cerebral circulation (Pickard *et al.* 1977; Edvinsson *et al.* 1978).

Rapoport: When you show that sympathectomy increases the brain uptake index of both inulin and noradrenaline, are you sure that the effect is due to increased cerebrovascular permeability rather than to a decrease in brain uptake of [^{14}C]ethanol, the reference tracer you use in the BUI method? This method gives the ratio of brain uptake of test to reference tracer and does not provide absolute permeability.

Edvinsson: We have also examined the barrier after administration of Evans' blue after sympathectomy. There was a transient or occasional increase in the penetration of Evans' blue at the normotensive level after denervation. This was never observed in the non-denervated control animals.

Heistad: It seems important to consider reasons why the thermal clearance technique indicates responses to sympathetic stimulation and denervation and some other techniques do not. One possibility is that the thermal clearance technique may be reflecting something in addition to flow, such as capillary surface area. A second possibility is that the blood–brain barrier is injured, and it is clear from Bill & Linder's study (1976) that injury to the blood–brain barrier augments responses. I realize that evidence for damage to the blood–brain barrier has been looked for, but there may still be some damage from the electrode.

I am also concerned about the magnitude of the responses which were observed. For example, it appears that the increase in flow after sympathetic denervation was three times larger than the response to 7% CO_2. Nobody else has found such an enormous increase in flow.

Edvinsson: You are quite right. We are not at all happy with that calibration, but it was done in order to study increases in flow. However, we also calibrated to the zero level of flow after the experiments by stopping the heart with saturated potassium chloride. We set 100% as the control level. A reduction of about 20% was obtained in the caudate nucleus in conjunction with sympathetic nerve stimulation (Sercombe *et al.* 1975). This agrees well with other results obtained during stimulation.

Siesjö: We recently published work that has a bearing on effects of circulating catecholamines on the brain. We measured cerebral blood flow in the rat, using a modified Kety & Schmidt (1948) technique, which is based on the Fick principle, and calculated the oxygen consumption ($CMRo_2$) in the brain (Carlsson *et al.* 1975, 1977). The animals were initially anaesthetized with 70% nitrous oxide. The animals were then padded up in cotton wool, and injected with a local anaesthetic before the nitrous oxide supply was withdrawn. After 5 min CBF and $CMRo_2$ increased to about 140% and in 30 min to 200% of the control levels. The increases in CBF and in $CMRo_2$ could be blocked by prior adrenalectomy or by administration of propranolol. We presumed that we were dealing with a stress response ('immobilization'), possibly mediated by release of catecholamines. But the question is, of course: how can catecholamines penetrate into the brain? I was very interested in what was said about the area postrema and other areas, which have a less efficient blood–brain barrier to amines.

Plum: Dr Edvinsson, you stimulated the sympathetic nerves preganglionically in the neck and measured the blood pressure systemically, showing asymmetry in the hemispheric blood flows in association with a given blood pressure. How were you sure that the differences between the two hemispheres weren't due to intense vasoconstriction of the carotid artery being produced on the same side, thereby reducing the blood pressure in the downflow stream on the side of the sympathetic stimulation?

Edvinsson: Harper has found a pronounced constriction of the internal carotid artery by infusion of 5-hydroxytryptamine. This artery belongs to the inflow tract. This, however, did not change the cerebral blood flow.

Plum: Didn't Meyer *et al.* (1967) show in monkeys prominent vasoconstriction in the extracranial carotid system when the sympathetic nerves were stimulated?

Edvinsson: Even ligation of one of the carotid arteries does not change the cerebral blood flow.

Plum: Ligation means a total redistribution.

McDowall: I don't think ligation affects the blood flow but it may affect the intravascular pressure.

Purves: Earlier you suggested, Professor Plum, that stimulation could affect ipsilateral sympathetic nerves right down to very small vessels; so, effectively the changes in pressure are being pushed downstream.

Plum: I am not sure that the experiment tells us anything more than that the external common carotid system has reduced its flow.

Edvinsson: We observe extravasation of the tracer, which offers further information about the function and protection of the blood–brain barrier.

McDowall: If you used supramaximal electrical stimulation on a denervated carotid, might you not still get a constriction of the carotid wall? There is still a plexus running with the carotid after the cervical sympathetic nerve has been divided. If that plexus is stimulated you may well get constriction which has nothing to do with the physiological control of the carotid.

Heistad: We have evaluated the responses of large cerebral arteries with a preparation which I shall be describing later (this volume). We found that electrical sympathetic stimulation does not constrict the large arteries between the carotid and vertebral arteries (Heistad *et al.* 1977). I think therefore that the mechanism proposed by Dr McDowall is unlikely.

Reis: Dr Edvinsson, you showed that stimulation of the cervical sympathetic reduced blood flow in the caudate nucleus. That is a rather tantalizing finding. Does it mean that the blood flow in the hemisphere has been reduced through control of pial vessels, with the reduction being reflected in the caudate? Or are you proposing that the nerves from the superior cervical ganglion are actually penetrating the brain down into the caudate nucleus. If so do they release transmitter onto neurons as well as on blood vessels?

Edvinsson: Pial vessels as well as intraparenchymal vessels are innervated by sympathetic fibres (Edvinsson 1976). We may therefore obtain vasoconstriction of the entire cerebrovascular bed including the caudate nucleus. You are probably confused by the intraparenchymal innervation which Hartman & Udenfriend (1972) have shown. These nerve fibres emanate from brain-stem nuclei and project towards cerebral capillaries and come in close apposition with the vessels in, for example, the caudate nucleus. Stimulation of these fibres may change the flow (Raichle *et al.* 1975).

Reis: Do you think that a vessel in the caudate nucleus is constricting because you are stimulating the superior cervical ganglion? That would mean that peripheral sympathetic nerves are actually reaching down to that depth of the brain. Or does the finding merely reflect a reduction of permeating flow from the cortex which is seen as a reduction of flow but which is not due to constriction of the vessels within the caudate?

Edvinsson: I see it from two points of view. First, there is an extrinsic innervation system which comes from the sympathetic nerves and influences the cerebral circulation. Second, there is an intrinsic system of nerve fibres running only within the brain and when these are activated there may be more localized changes in flow and metabolism.

Reis: I understand that, but you stimulated the extrinsic supply and produced a profound effect in a bed which I would consider was receiving intrinsic innervation.

Owman: We have related the flow responses in the lateral geniculate body, which were compared with responses of the caudate nucleus, to the amount of sympathetic innervation to the arterioles in the regions that we were measuring (Sercombe *et al.* 1975). More than 50% of the total number of arterioles in the caudate nucleus receive sympathetic nerves, whereas about 20% of those in the lateral geniculate body are innervated by sympathetic fibres. We are implying that the sympathetic stimulation produces its effects on local flow by an effect mediated by the perivascular sympathetic nerve fibres.

Reis: You mean that 50% of the innervation of the blood vessels in the caudate nucleus disappears?

Owman: All of the perivascular adrenergic nerves disappear after sympathectomy.

Reis: Is there any reason to believe that this innervation may have some consequences not only in the blood vessels but also on the metabolism of basal ganglia?

Owman: The sympathetic nerves have a close relation to the vessels and it can be assumed that the release of noradrenaline from those fibres would affect only the vessels and not the parenchyma.

Keatinge: I was particularly interested in your evidence that adrenaline or noradrenaline produce different effects when applied to the lumen than when applied outside, Dr Edvinsson. Have you checked that by the more direct experiment of injecting noradrenaline or adrenaline into the brain substance, rather than just trying to get it in indirectly? In experiments of that kind on muscle blood vessels, Grant (1964) found the exact counterpart of what you described but in reverse; he could only get dilatation with internal adrenaline while adrenaline applied to the outside of the muscle arterioles produced vasoconstriction.

Edvinsson: That particular experiment has been done. Intraventricular infusion of noradrenaline produces an increased cerebral blood flow and an enhanced cerebral metabolism (MacKenzie *et al.* 1976).

References

BILL, A. & LINDER, J. (1976) Sympathetic control of cerebral blood flow in acute arterial hypertension. *Acta Physiol. Scand. 96*, 114–121

BYROM, F. B. (1963) The nature of malignancy in hypertensive disease. *Lancet 1*, 516

CARLSSON, C., HÄGERDAL, M. & SIESJÖ, B. K. (1975) Increase in cerebral oxygen uptake and blood flow in immobilization stress. *Acta Physiol. Scand. 95*, 206–208

CARLSSON, C., HÄGERDAL, M., KAASIK, A. E. & SIESJÖ, B. K. (1977) A catecholamine-mediated increase in cerebral oxygen uptake during immobilisation stress in rats. *Brain Res. 119*, 223–231

COTZIAS, G. C., TANG, L. C. & GINOS, J. Z. (1974) Monoamine oxidase and cerebral uptake of dopaminergic drugs. *Proc. Natl. Acad. Sci. U.S.A. 71*, 2715–2729

DANON, A. & SAPIRA, J. D. (1972) Binding of catecholamines to human serum albumin. *J. Pharmacol. Exp. Ther. 182*, 295–302

EDVINSSON, L. (1976) Neurogenic mechanisms in the cerebrovascular bed. Autonomic nerves, amine receptors and their effects on cerebral blood flow. *Acta Physiol. Scand. 96, Suppl. 427*, 1–35

EDVINSSON, L., HARDEBO, J. E., MACKENZIE, E. T. & OWMAN, CH. (1978) Effect of exogenous noradrenaline on local cerebral blood flow after osmotic opening of the blood-brain barrier in the rat. *J. Physiol. (Lond.)*, in press

GIESE, J. (1964) *The Pathogenesis of Hypertensive Vascular Disease*, Munksgaard, Copenhagen

GOLDBY, F. S. & BEILIN, L. J. (1974) The evolution and healing of arteriolar damage in renal-clip hypertension in the rat. An electron microscope study. *J. Pathol. 114*, 139–148

GRANT, R. T. (1964) Direct observation of skeletal muscle blood vessels (rat cremaster). *J. Physiol. (Lond.) 172*, 123–137

HARDEBO, J. E., EDVINSSON, L., FALCK, B., LINDVALL, M., OWMAN, CH., ROSENGREN, E. & SVENGAARD, N.-AA. (1976) Experimental models for histochemical and chemical studies of the enzymatic blood-brain barrier for amine precursors, in *The Cerebral Vessel Wall* (Cervós-Navarro, J. *et al.*, eds.), pp. 233–244, Raven Press, New York

HARTMAN, B. K. & UDENFRIEND, S. (1972) The application of immunological techniques to the study of enzymes regulating catecholamine synthesis and degradation. *Pharmacol. Rev. 24*, 311–330

HEISTAD, D. D., MARCUS, M. L., SANDBERG, S. & ABBOUD, F. M. (1977) Effect of sympathetic nerve stimulation on cerebral blood flow and on large cerebral arteries of dogs. *Circ. Res. 41*, 342–350

JOY, M. D. (1971) The intramedullary connections of the area postrema involved in the central cardiovascular response to angiotensin II. *Clin. Sci. (Oxf.) 41*, 89–100

KETY, S. S. & SCHMIDT, C. F. (1948) The nitrous oxide method for the quantitative determination of cerebral blood flow in man: theory, procedure and normal values. *J. Clin. Invest. 27*, 476–483

KOCH-WESER, J. (1975) Non-beta-blocking actions of propranolol. *N. Engl. J. Med. 293*, 988–990

MACKENZIE, E. T., MCCULLOCH, J., PICKARD, J. D. & HARPER, A. M. (1975) Cerebral circulatory and metabolic effects of endogenous noradrenaline, in *Blood Flow and Metabolism in the Brain* (Harper, M. *et al.*, eds.), Churchill Livingstone, Edinburgh

MACKENZIE, E. T., MCCULLOCH, J., O'KEANE, M., PICKARD, J. D. & HARPER, A. M. (1976) Cerebral circulation and norepinephrine: relevance of the blood-brain barrier. *Am. J. Physiol. 231*, 483–488

MEYER, J. S., YOSHIDA, K. & SAKAMOTO, K. (1967) Autonomic control of cerebral blood flow measured by electromagnetic flow meters. *Neurology 17*, 638–648

PICKARD, J. D., DURITY, F., WELSH, F. A., LANGFITT, T. W., HARPER, A. M. & MACKENZIE, E. T. (1977) Osmotic opening of the blood-brain barrier: value in pharmacological studies on the cerebral circulation. *Brain Res. 122*, 170–176

PICKERING, G. W. (1968) *High Blood Pressure*, Churchill, London

RAICHLE, M. E., HARTMAN, B. K., EICHLING, J. O. & SHARPE, L. G. (1975) Central noradrenergic regulation of cerebral blood flow and vascular permeability. *Proc. Natl. Acad. Sci. U.S.A. 72*, 3726–3730

ROSENDORFF, C., LOWE, R. D., LAVERY, H. & CRANSTON, W. I. (1970) Cardiovascular effects of angiotensin mediated by the central nervous system of the rabbit. *Cardiovasc. Res. 4*, 36–43

ROSENDORFF, C., MITCHELL, G., SCRIVEN, D. R. L. & SHAPIRO, C. (1976) Evidence of a dual innervation affecting local blood flow in the hypothalamus of the conscious rabbit. *Circ. Res. 38*, 140–145

SERCOMBE, R., AUBINEAU, P., EDVINSSON, L., MAMO, H., OWMAN, CH., PINARD, E. & SEYLAZ, J. (1975) Neurogenic influence on local cerebral blood flow. Effect of catecholamines or sympathetic stimulation as correlated with the sympathetic innervation. *Neurology 25*, 954–963

WEIL-MALHERBE, H., AXELROD, J. & TOMCHICK, R. (1959) Blood-brain barrier for adrenaline. *Science (Wash. D.C.) 129*, 1226–1227

WILSON, C. & PICKERING, G. W. (1938) Acute arterial lesions in rabbits with experimental renal hypertension. *Clin. Sci. (Oxf.) 3*, 343

Experimental attempts to unmask effects of neural stimuli on cerebral blood flow

DONALD D. HEISTAD, MELVIN L. MARCUS and FRANCOIS M. ABBOUD

Cardiovascular Division, Department of Internal Medicine and Cardiovascular Center, University of Iowa College of Medicine, and Veterans Administration Hospital, Iowa City, Iowa

Abstract The purpose of this study was to determine whether neural stimuli affect cerebral blood vessels. Microspheres were used to measure total blood flow to the brain and the distribution of flow within the brain (to cerebral grey and white matteı, cerebellum and brain-stem). Reflex stimuli did not affect cerebral vessels. Stimulation or denervation of carotid baroreceptors or chemoreceptors in dogs did not alter flow to the brain. Electrical stimulation of sympathetic pathways did not constrict cerebral vessels, even when cerebral blood flow was increased during hypercapnia. When brain blood flow was increased during severe hypertension, electrical stimulation of sympathetic pathways produced cerebral vasoconstriction which was minimal in dogs but marked in cats. During neurogenic hypertension in cats, physiological stimulation of sympathetic pathways produced modest cerebral vasoconstriction. These studies indicate that (1) several neural stimuli do not alter cerebral blood flow in the normotensive state, (2) electrical stimulation of sympathetic nerves during hypertension produces a small decrease in cerebral blood flow in dogs and a marked decrease in cats, and (3) intense physiological stimulation of sympathetic pathways during neurogenic hypertension produces a small decrease in cerebral blood flow. It is concluded that neural stimuli have a much less important role in regulation of blood flow to the brain than to other organs.

The role of nerves in the regulation of cerebral blood flow continues to be controversial. Although cerebral vessels are richly innervated, it has been difficult to demonstrate that neural factors are important in the control of cerebral vessels. In this paper we shall describe our attempts to uncover the effects of nerves on cerebral vessels. Four topics will be considered.

First, because it is difficult to measure cerebral blood flow accurately, and because questions about methods for measuring flow appear to be central to the controversy concerning neural control, we shall examine the labelled microsphere method that we use to measure cerebral blood flow, and describe the advantages and limitations of the technique.

Secondly, the effects of reflex stimuli on cerebral vessels will be considered. Provocative studies by Ponté & Purves (1974) suggested that carotid chemoreceptors and baroreceptors play a major role in cerebral vascular responses to hypoxia and hypertension. Others have found only a minor role (Eidelman *et al.* 1976) or no effect (Bates & Sundt 1976). Our studies provide the first data on the effects of reflex stimuli on regional, as well as total, cerebral blood flow.

Thirdly, the effects of stimulation of sympathetic pathways on cerebral vessels will be described. We have summarized some of the large number of studies which have dealt with this topic (Heistad & Marcus 1978). Briefly, estimates of the reduction in cerebral blood flow during electrical stimulation of sympathetic pathways range from 80% (D'Alecy & Feigl 1972) to no effect (Alm & Bill 1973). We shall describe our attempts to unmask constrictor responses to sympathetic stimulation by examining responses when cerebral vessels are dilated during hypercapnia or severe hypertension.

Fourthly, we shall examine the role of large arteries in responses to neural and other stimuli. Harper (1975) has suggested that sympathetic nerves may constrict large cerebral arteries but autoregulatory dilatation of distal vessels might maintain a constant flow. We have used the method of Rapela & Martin (1975) to examine responses of large arteries. Our findings suggest that large cerebral arteries do not respond to sympathetic stimulation but, surprisingly, they participate in autoregulatory responses.

MEASUREMENT OF CEREBRAL BLOOD FLOW WITH MICROSPHERES

Rudolph & Heymann (1967) reported that microspheres labelled with isotopes could be used to measure blood flow to many organs as well as distribution of flow within organs. Studies by Utley *et al.* (1974) and Tripp *et al.* (1977) have suggested that the technique provides valid measurements of total and regional myocardial blood flow.

We and others have used radioactively labelled microspheres to measure blood flow to the brain. Labelled carbonized microspheres 15 μm in diameter are injected into the left atrium of experimental animals. The spheres are extracted in one circulation through the brain, because they are too large to pass through capillaries. Microspheres can be labelled with several gamma-emitting isotopes which can be separated with differential spectroscopy so that repeated measurement of flow can be made in the same animal. During and after injection of microspheres, a 'reference' blood sample is withdrawn from an artery at a precisely determined rate. At the end of the experiment the brain is removed, dissected according to tissue or region (e.g. cerebral grey and white matter, cerebellum, brain-stem), and the brain and arterial blood samples are counted in a gamma counter. Blood flow to the brain is determined from the equation: brain blood flow/radioactivity in the brain = rate of withdrawal of reference arterial blood sample/radioactivity in the blood sample.

The microsphere technique has two fundamental advantages over other methods used to measure cerebral blood flow. First, flow to cerebral and extracerebral tissues can be measured separately without ligating any vessels. Secondly, regional as well as total cerebral blood flow can be measured repeatedly in both anaesthetized and unanaesthetized animals.

Several important assumptions are made in the use of microspheres to measure blood flow to an organ: (1) the spheres mix adequately with arterial blood so that streaming does not occur; (2) they are extracted during one circulation through the organ so that shunting of spheres through arteriovenous anastomoses will not cause underestimation of flow; (3) they do not cause significant haemodynamic alterations, i.e. they do not alter the flow which they are being used to measure; and (4) the rheological characteristics of the spheres do not distort the regional distribution of blood flow within the organ. Results of experiments in our laboratory suggest that these assumptions are reasonable if microspheres 15 μm in diameter are used to measure cerebral blood flow (Marcus *et al.* 1976).

EFFECTS OF REFLEX STIMULI ON CEREBRAL BLOOD FLOW

It has been thought that local factors, such as changes in periarteriolar pH, regulate cerebral vascular resistance during changes in blood gases and arterial pressure. This concept was challenged by the report of Ponté & Purves (1974) that carotid chemoreceptors and baroreceptors are essential for cerebral vascular responses to hypoxia and hypertension.

We have re-examined the role of carotid chemoreceptors in the regulation of cerebral blood flow (Heistad *et al.* 1976). Carotid chemoreceptors in dogs were stimulated chemically with nicotine, or physiologically with hypoxic and hypercapnic blood. Chemoreceptor stimulation produced the expected cardiovascular responses (vasoconstriction in muscle, kidney, and bowel), which indicates that the reflex was intact in our preparation, but it did not alter cerebral blood flow. We considered the possibility that the normal responsiveness of cerebral vessels was impaired by the experimental preparation. However, systemic hypercapnia produced marked increases in cerebral flow, which indicates that the cerebral vessels were capable of dilating in the presence of appropriate stimuli.

The question of the role of chemoreceptors was then approached in another

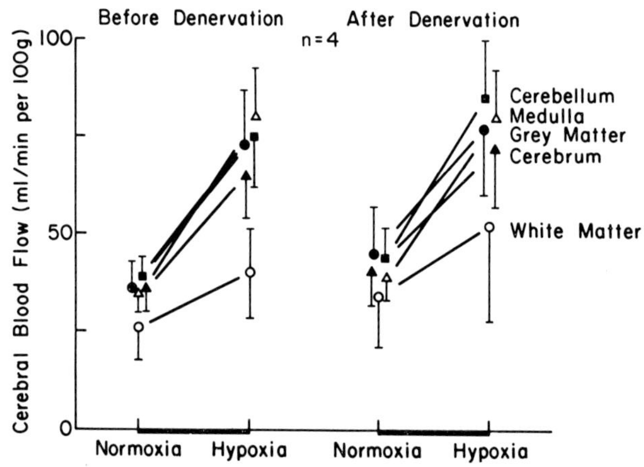

FIG. 1. Cerebral vasodilator responses to systemic hypoxaemia in monkeys were not altered by denervation of arterial chemoreceptors. Values are mean ± S.E.

way. We measured cerebral vasodilator responses to systemic hypoxaemia in dogs and monkeys, before and after denervation of carotid and aortic chemoreceptors. If chemoreceptors were important in the regulation of cerebral resistance, denervation of chemoreceptors would reduce or abolish responses to hypoxia. However, systemic hypoxaemia produced similar increases in flow before and after denervation of arterial chemoreceptors (Fig. 1).

Next we examined the role of baroreceptors in regulation of cerebral blood flow (Heistad & Marcus 1976). Carotid baroreceptors were stimulated by raising pressure in the isolated perfused carotid sinuses of dogs. Stimulation of baroreceptors produced marked bradycardia and vasodilatation in skeletal muscle, but did not alter flow to the brain. Furthermore, cerebral vascular responses to changes in systemic arterial pressure were not altered by denervation of arterial baroreceptors.

Our findings conflict with those of Ponté & Purves (1974) and support the traditional concept that reflex mechanisms are unimportant in the regulation of cerebral blood flow. The possibility of reflex control of cerebral vessels has not yet been excluded, but subsequent studies (Hoff *et al.* 1977) tend to support our view.

EFFECT OF STIMULATION OF SYMPATHETIC PATHWAYS

Despite many years of intensive study, the role of sympathetic nerves in

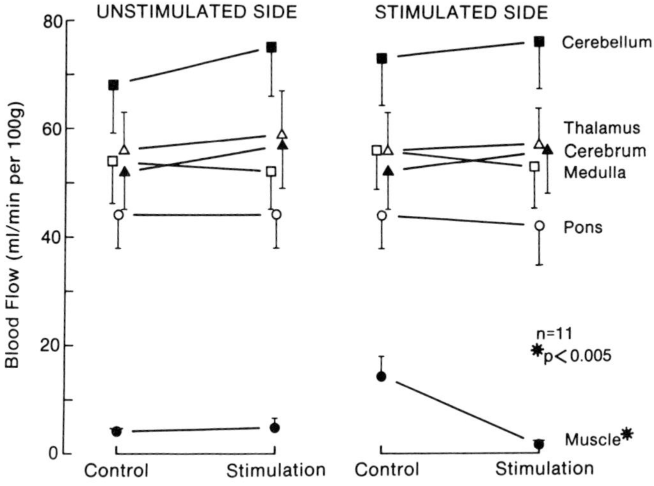

FIG. 2. Stimulation of the left superior cervical sympathetic ganglion in dogs reduced blood flow to cranial muscle on the same side but did not alter flow to the brain.

the regulation of cerebral blood flow remains unclear. Examples of conflicting results abound in the literature. D'Alecy & Feigl (1972) measured cerebral venous outflow and reported that sympathetic stimulation reduces cerebral flow by 80%. However, Traystman & Rapela (1975) found no response, and demonstrated that failure to separate intra- and extracranial veins could account for the findings of D'Alecy & Feigl. Using clearance of inert gas to measure cerebral flow, James *et al.* (1969) found that sympathetic stimulation decreases cerebral flow during normocapnia but Harper *et al.* (1972) found no response.

Results obtained with microspheres, in contrast to those obtained with other techniques, have been entirely consistent. Studies in three laboratories (Alm & Bill 1973; Meyer *et al.* 1977; Heistad *et al.* 1977) have shown that sympathetic stimulation at normal levels of arterial pressure does not decrease cerebral blood flow (Fig. 2). Similar results were obtained in dogs, cats and monkeys.

Our feeling is that there is now sufficient evidence to conclude that sympathetic stimulation, under normal conditions, produces little if any reduction in cerebral blood flow. A reasonable hypothesis is that sympathetic stimulation might have more constrictor effect when cerebral vessels are dilated, for example during hypercapnia. The findings of Harper *et al.* (1972) support this hypothesis, but Alm & Bill (1973) and Traystman & Rapela (1975) found

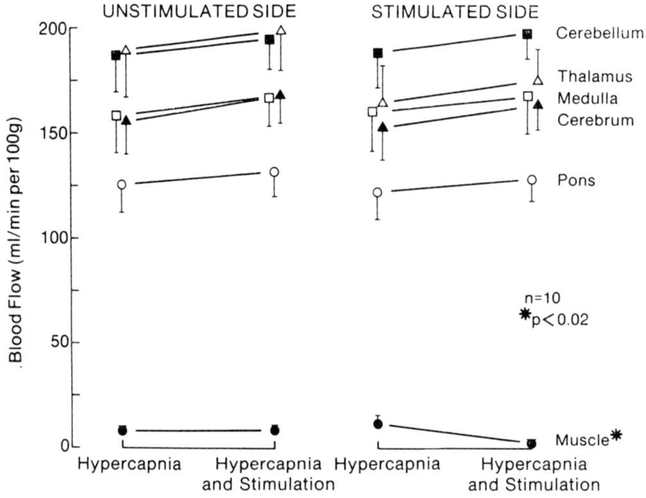

FIG. 3. Systemic hypercapnia increased cerebral blood flow, but even when cerebral vessels were dilated they did not constrict during stimulation of the left superior cervical sympathetic ganglion.

no response to sympathetic stimulation during hypercapnia. During hypercapnia, we have been unable to detect cerebral vasoconstrictor responses to reflex stimuli (Heistad & Marcus 1976) or to sympathetic stimulation (Heistad *et al.* 1977) (Fig. 3).

In the series of studies described above, we found no cerebral vascular response to reflex stimuli or stimulation of sympathetic nerves. However, recently we have at last been able to detect neural effects on cerebral vessels. The critical factor which allowed us to detect neural effects was the examination of responses during severe hypertension. Bill & Linder (1976) suggested that during severe hypertension, when the autoregulatory capacity of cerebral vessels is exceeded and the vessels dilate, sympathetic stimulation then constricts the vessels.

We first measured responses to sympathetic stimulation during hypertension in dogs. When arterial pressure was raised to 230 mmHg with noradrenaline (norepinephrine) or angiotensin, sympathetic stimulation reduced flow in the ipsilateral cerebrum by 9% (Fig. 4). Our conclusions from these studies in dogs were that sympathetic stimulation during severe hypertension produces a small decrease in flow, and that this effect is limited to vessels in cerebral grey matter and in the brain-stem. However, Bill & Linder (1976) had reported much greater responses to sympathetic stimulation during hypertension in

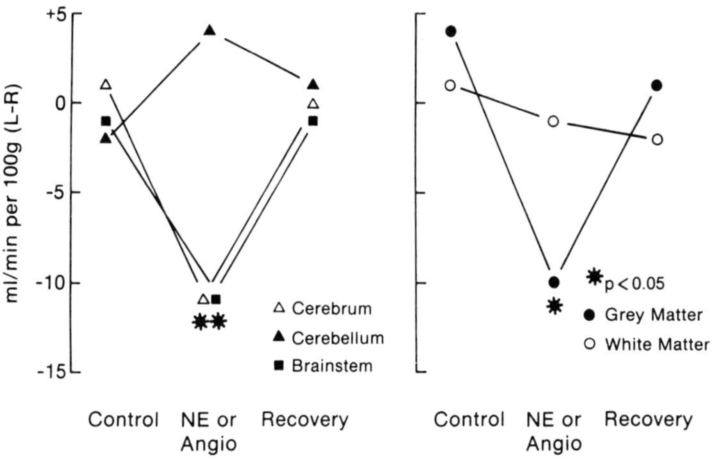

FIG. 4. Difference in blood flow between the two sides of the brain in dogs during control period, hypertension induced by noradrenaline (NE) or angiotensin (Angio), and recovery period. During hypertension the right superior cervical sympathetic ganglion was stimulated electrically, so a decrease indicates constriction in the stimulated hemisphere. Sympathetic stimulation during severe hypertension produced modest constriction in cerebral grey matter and in the brain-stem.

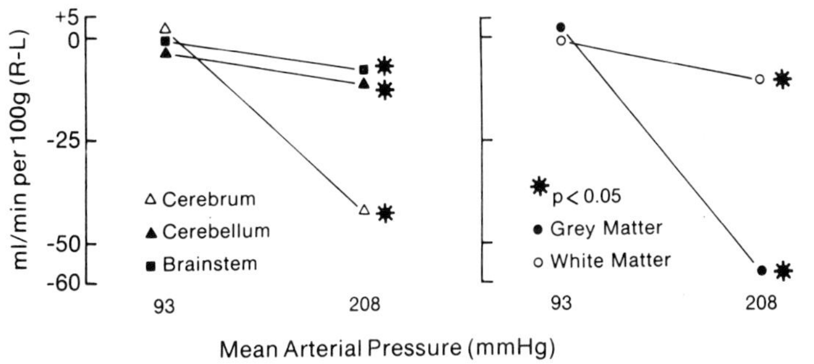

FIG. 5. Difference in flow between the two sides of the brain in cats during control period and during hypertension induced by noradrenaline or angiotensin. Sympathetic stimulation during hypertension produced marked constriction of vessels in cerebral grey and modest constriction in cerebral white matter, cerebellum and brain-stem.

their studies in cats. We therefore performed additional studies in cats to determine whether there is a species difference. When mean arterial pressure was raised to 210 mmHg, sympathetic stimulation reduced flow in the ipsilateral cerebrum by 38% (Fig. 5). There was marked constriction in cerebral grey matter, and slight constriction in white matter, cerebellum and brain-stem. Our conclusions were that sympathetic stimulation constricts cerebral vessels during severe hypertension, that this effect is much greater in the cat than in the dog, and that the effect on distribution of flow in the brain differs somewhat in the two species.

Although these studies indicated that intense *electrical* stimulation of sympathetic nerves constricts cerebral vessels during severe hypertension, the physiological significance of these findings was not clear. We wanted to know whether physiological stimulation of sympathetic pathways could constrict cerebral vessels during hypertension. The experimental model that we used to answer this question was the sinoaortic deafferented cat. These studies were done in collaboration with Paul M. Gross, M. Randall Strait, and Michael J. Brody. Baroreceptors were deafferented by cutting both aortic depressor and carotid sinus nerves. In most cats baroreceptor denervation causes intense activation of sympathetic pathways with severe but transient hypertension (Strait & Brody 1977). We compared cerebral blood flow in one hemisphere, in which the sympathetic nerves were intact, with that in the other hemisphere, in which the superior cervical ganglion had been removed.

At the peak of hypertension, blood flow to the innervated hemibrain was slightly lower than flow to the denervated side. However, blood flow to selected areas of cerebral grey matter (areas that were found at autopsy to be stained with Evans' blue dye) was much less on the innervated than on the denervated side (Fig. 6). As pressure returned towards normal several minutes later, there was a significant difference in flow to the entire cerebrum as flow was significantly less on the innervated side. Later, blood pressure was normal and flow to the two sides was similar. An incidental, unexplained observation was that blood flow to the cerebellum was greater on the innervated side during hypertension. The important finding is that physiological stimulation of sympathetic pathways during hypertension caused modest constriction of cerebral vessels. The modest, transient cerebral vasoconstriction is in sharp contrast with marked, sustained constriction in other vascular beds.

In addition to measuring blood flow in these studies, we evaluated the role of sympathetic stimulation in protection of the blood–brain barrier during hypertension. Evans' blue dye was injected at the start of the experiments. This dye binds to albumin and does not normally pass the blood–brain barrier and stain the brain. Because it extravasates during severe hypertension, it can be used as a rather crude index of the severity of disruption of the blood–brain barrier (Bill & Linder 1976). In dogs, there was only slight staining of the brain by Evans' blue, which indicates that there was minimal disruption of the blood–brain barrier during hypertension. The staining was slightly

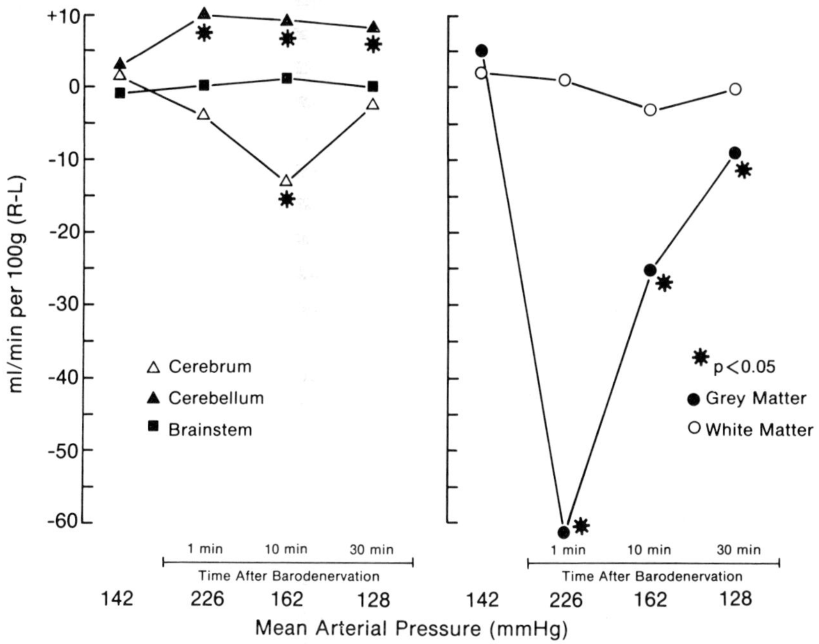

FIG. 6. The right superior cervical sympathetic ganglion was removed in cats and the flow to the two sides of the brain was compared during control period and 1, 10 and 30 min after barodenervation. Arterial pressure during these four measurements is indicated at the bottom of the graph. After baroreceptor denervation, blood flow to selected areas of cerebral grey matter was lower in the hemisphere in which sympathetic nerves were intact. An incidental observation was that blood flow to the cerebellum was higher on the side in which sympathetic nerves were intact.

less in the hemisphere which received sympathetic stimulation. In cats, there was usually deep blue staining of the cerebrum. The staining was consistently less in the hemisphere which received either electrical or physiological stimulation of sympathetic pathways, although the protective effect was much greater during electrical stimulation. Bill & Linder (1976) have also found that electrical stimulation of sympathetic nerves protects the blood–brain barrier during severe hypertension, and our studies indicate that physiological stimulation has a similar (but quantitatively much smaller) effect.

In summary, the effect of sympathetic nerve stimulation on cerebral vessels apparently depends on both the experimental conditions and the species. Under normal conditions, sympathetic stimulation has little or no effect. When vessels are dilated during hypercapnia, sympathetic stimulation still has little or no effect. However when cerebral vessels are dilated during severe hypertension, sympathetic stimulation produces significant vasoconstriction. Electrical stimulation of the nerves produces slight constriction in dogs and marked constriction in cats, with protection of the blood–brain barrier. Physiological stimulation of sympathetic pathways during neurogenic hypertension in cats caused modest constriction of cerebral vessels. Although the physiological activation of sympathetic pathways was intense, the effect on cerebral vessels was small, especially when compared with other vascular beds. The responses to sympathetic stimulation during hypertension convince us, for the first time, that neural stimuli can affect cerebral blood flow, but the physiological importance seems to be rather minor.

ROLE OF LARGE ARTERIES

Arterioles have generally been thought to regulate cerebral vascular resistance, and large arteries have been thought to have little role. This view now seems untenable in light of the significant pressure gradient along large cerebral arteries. Stromberg & Fox (1972) have reported that when systemic pressure is 100 mmHg in cats, pressure in pial arteries 300 μm in diameter is about 70 mmHg. Moreover, the diameter of large cerebral arteries has been reported to vary during changes in arterial pressure (Magun 1973).

We have used a method described by Rapela & Martin (1975) to evaluate responsiveness of large arteries. Catheters are inserted into both vertebral arteries in dogs and advanced until they wedge (Fig. 7). With both vertebral arteries occluded, almost all of the blood flow to the brain is through the carotid arteries. The pressure gradient along the large arteries which supply the brain can then be determined by subtracting vertebral artery wedge pressure from carotid artery pressure. Resistance of large arteries is calculated by dividing this pressure gradient by cerebral blood flow.

Serotonin was used to examine the responsiveness of large arteries. Grimson *et al.* (1969) and Rapela & Martin (1975) had reported that intracarotid infusion of serotonin constricts large arteries. We found that infusion of serotonin into both carotid arteries reduced vertebral artery wedge pressure markedly, and increased the pressure gradient across large arteries. Resistance of large arteries increased almost threefold in five dogs. This confirms the finding that serotonin constricts large arteries which supply the brain, and demonstrates that this technique can detect responses of large arteries.

Does sympathetic stimulation constrict large cerebral arteries? Harper (1975) proposed that sympathetic stimulation could constrict large arteries without reducing blood flow. This could happen if sympathetic stimulation constricted

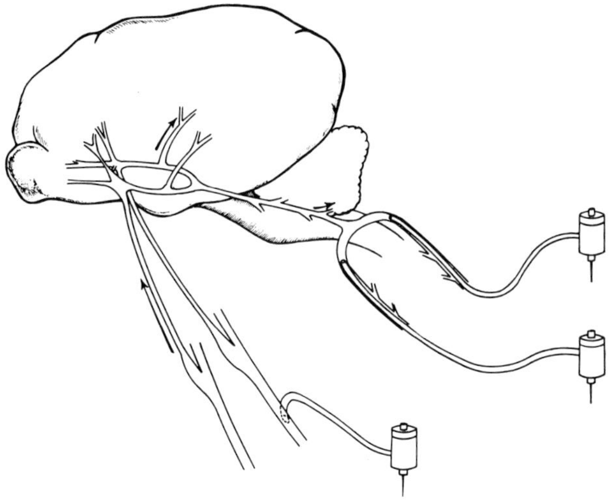

FIG. 7. Method of Rapela & Martin (1975) for evaluation of responsiveness of large cerebral arteries. With both vertebral arteries occluded, the direction of blood flow is indicated by the arrows. The pressure gradient between the carotid artery and the vertebral artery in this preparation is an index of resistance of large arteries.

large arteries and thereby decreased pressure in distal vessels, but autoregulation by small arteries maintained a constant flow. However, bilateral stimulation of both superior cervical ganglia does not increase resistance of large arteries in dogs during normotension (Heistad *et al.* 1977). It is possible that responses of large arteries to sympathetic stimulation would be detectable during hypertension, especially in cats.

Finally, there is the question of the effects of other stimuli, presumably not neural, on large cerebral arteries. The studies of Stromberg & Fox (1972) and Magun (1973) suggest that large cerebral arteries participate in the autoregulatory response to hypotension. However, resistance of large arteries could not be quantitated since blood flow was not measured.

We have tested the hypothesis that large cerebral arteries autoregulate during haemorrhagic hypotension. In 10 dogs, measurements were made during a control period, during two levels of hypotension produced by haemorrhage, and during a recovery period. Cerebral vessels autoregulated perfectly, since flow did not decrease even though mean arterial pressure was reduced to 58 mmHg (Fig. 8). Total cerebral resistance decreased and kept blood flow constant. The pressure gradient across large arteries narrowed during hypotension (Fig. 9). Resistance of large cerebral arteries decreased

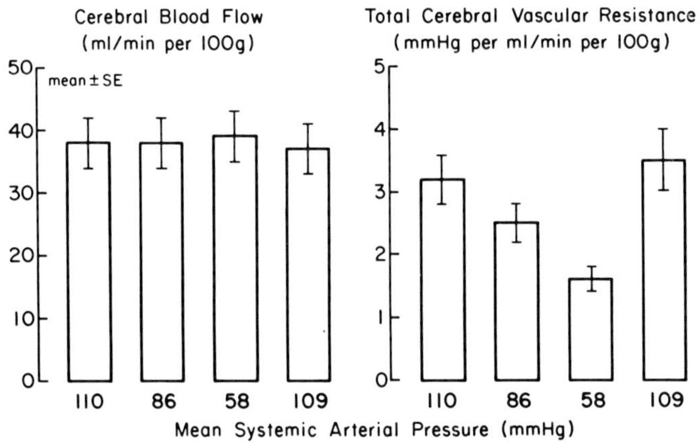

FIG. 8. Haemorrhage decreased arterial pressure from 110 to 58 mmHg, but cerebral vessels dilated, maintaining a constant blood flow.

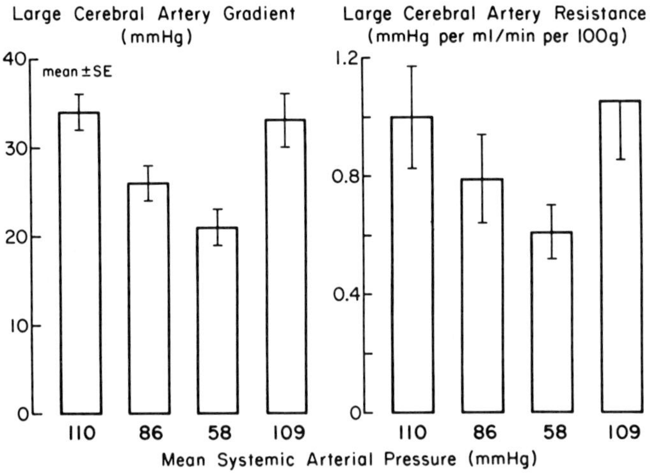

FIG. 9. The pressure gradient along large cerebral arteries (i.e. the difference between carotid and vertebral artery pressure) decreased during hypotension, and the large artery resistance decreased significantly. Therefore large cerebral arteries dilated during hypotension.

significantly during hypotension, which means that large cerebral arteries autoregulate during changes in arterial pressure.

It appears from these studies that large cerebral arteries play an important role in physiological regulation of cerebral resistance. Large arteries constrict during serotonin infusion, dilate during hypotension, but do not respond to sympathetic stimulation.

CONCLUSION

We should like to draw several conclusions from these studies. First, labelled microspheres offer important advantages in measurement of cerebral blood flow. The technique appears to provide valid measurements of flow. Secondly, reflex stimuli have not been shown to affect cerebral blood flow. Thirdly, sympathetic stimulation does not constrict cerebral vessels during normal conditions, but it does produce constriction during severe hypertension. The magnitude of the response during intense physiological stimulation is small. Fourthly, large cerebral arteries play an important role in regulation of cerebral blood flow, but we have not been able to detect any effects of neural stimuli on large cerebral arteries.

As investigators have evaluated the effects of neural stimuli on cerebral vessels, the pendulum has taken several swings. Reflex stimuli or sympathetic nerves have been thought by some investigators to have profound effects on cerebral vessels, and other investigators have suggested that these stimuli have no effect. Our studies now favour the middle region between these two extremes. Under most conditions neural stimuli are unimportant, but under at least one condition (hypertension) sympathetic nerves are potentially important. Our studies provide the first evidence that physiological stimulation of sympathetic pathways produces a protective response in cerebral vessels, but compared with other vascular beds the response of cerebral vessels to neural stimuli is small.

ACKNOWLEDGEMENTS

These studies were supported by Research Career Development Awards HL-00041 and HL-00328, Research Grants HL-16066 and HL-20827, and Program Project Grant HL-14388 from the National Heart and Lung Institute, and by Research Grant MRIS 3546 from the Veterans Administration. We thank Donald Piegors and Judith Donnell for technical assistance, Dr James Ehrhardt for assistance with isotope separation, Patti Young for preparation of the manuscript, Paul M. Gross, M. Randall Strait, and Dr Michael Brody for assistance with studies of neurogenic hypertension, and Dr Allyn Mark for critical review of the manuscript.

References

ALM, A. & BILL, A. (1973) The effect of stimulation of the cervical sympathetic chain on retinal oxygen tension and on uveal, retinal and cerebral blood flow in cats. *Acta Physiol. Scand. 88*, 84–94

BATES, D. & SUNDT, T. M. (1976) The relevance of peripheral baroreceptors and chemoreceptors to regulation of cerebral blood flow in the cat. *Circ. Res. 38*, 488–493

BILL, A. & LINDER, J. (1976) Sympathetic control of cerebral blood flow in acute arterial hypertension. *Acta Physiol. Scand. 96*, 114–212

D'ALECY, L. G. & FEIGL, E. O. (1972) Sympathetic control of cerebral blood flow in dogs. *Circ. Res. 31*, 267–283

EIDELMAN, B. H., MCCALDEN, T. A. & ROSENDORFF, C. (1976) The role of the carotid body in mediating the cerebrovascular response to altered arterial carbon dioxide tension. *Stroke 7*, 72–76

GRIMSON, B. S., ROBINSON, S. E., DANFORD, E. T., TINDALL, G. T. & GREENFIELD, J. C., Jr. (1969) Effect of serotonin on internal and external carotid artery blood flow in the baboon. *Am. J. Physiol. 216*, 50–55

HARPER, A. M., DESHMUKH, V. D., ROWAN, J. O. & JENNETT, W. B. (1972) The influence of sympathetic nervous activity on cerebral blood flow. *Arch. Neurol. 27*, 1–6

HARPER, A. M. (1975) Autonomic control of cerebral blood flow, in *Cerebral Vascular Diseases* (Whisnant, J. P. & Sandok, B. A., eds.), pp. 27–47, Grune & Stratton, New York

HEISTAD, D. D. & MARCUS, M. L. (1976) Total and regional cerebral blood flow during stimulation of carotid baroreceptors. *Stroke 7*, 239

HEISTAD, D. D. & MARCUS, M. L. (1978) Neural mechanisms do not have important effects on cerebral blood flow. *Circ. Res.*, in press

HEISTAD, D. D., MARCUS, M. L., EHRHARDT, J. C. & ABBOUD, F. M. (1976) Effect of stimulation of carotid chemoreceptors on total and regional cerebral blood flow. *Circ. Res. 38*, 20–25

HEISTAD, D. D., MARCUS, M. L., SANDBERG, S. & ABBOUD, F. M. (1977) Effect of sympathetic nerve stimulation on cerebral blood flow and on large cerebral arteries of dogs. *Circ. Res. 41*, 342–350

HOFF, J. T., MACKENZIE, E. T. & HARPER, A. M. (1977) Responses of the cerebral circulation to hypercapnia and hypoxia after 7th cranial nerve transection in baboons. *Circ. Res. 40*, 258–262

JAMES, I. M., MILLAR, R. A. & PURVES, M. J. (1969) Observations on the extrinsic neural control of cerebral blood flow in the baboon. *Circ. Res. 25*, 77–93

MARCUS, M. L., HEISTAD, D. D., EHRHARDT, J. C. & ABBOUD, F. M. (1976) Total and regional cerebral blood flow measurement with 7-10-, 15-, 25-, and 50-μm microspheres. *J. Appl. Physiol. 40*, 501–507

MAGUN, J. G. (1973) The effect of pharmacologically increased blood pressure on brain circulation. *Z. Neurol. 204*, 107–134

MEYER, M. W., SMITH, K. A. & KLASSEN, A. C. (1977) Sympathetic regulation of cephalic blood flow. *Stroke 8*, 197–201

PONTÉ, J. & PURVES, M. J. (1974) The role of the carotid body chemoreceptors and carotid sinus baroreceptors in the control of cerebral blood vessels. *J. Physiol. (Lond.) 237*, 315–340

RAPELA, C. E. & MARTIN, J. B. (1975) Reactivity of cerebral extra and intraparenchymal vasculature to serotonin and vasodilator agents, *Blood Flow and Metabolism in the Brain* (Harper, M. *et al.*, eds.), pp. 4.5–4.9, Churchill Livingstone, Edinburgh

RUDOLPH, A. M. & HEYMANN, M. A. (1967) Circulation of the fetus in utero: methods for studying distribution of blood flow, cardiac output and organ blood flow. *Circ. Res. 21*, 163–184

STRAIT, M. R. & BRODY, M. J. (1977) Contrasting changes in arterial pressure and sympathetic discharge following sinoaortic deafferentation. *Fed. Proc. 36 (abstr.)*, 547

STROMBERG, D. D. & FOX, J. R. (1972) Pressures in the pial arterial microcirculation of the cat during changes in systemic arterial blood pressure. *Circ. Res. 31*, 229–238

TRAYSTMAN, R. J. & RAPELA, C. E. (1975) Effect of sympathetic nerve stimulation on cerebral and cephalic blood flow in dogs. *Circ. Res. 36*, 620–630

TRIPP, M. R., MEYER, M. W., EINZIG, S., LEONARD, J. J., SWAYZE, C. R. & FOX, I. J. (1977) Simultaneous regional myocardial blood flows by tritiated water and microspheres. *Am. J. Physiol. 232*, H173–H190

UTLEY, J., CARLSON, E. L., HOFFMAN, J. I. E., MARTINEZ, H. M. & BUCKBERG, G. D. (1974) Total and regional myocardial blood flow measurements with 25μ, 15μ, 9μ, and filtered 1–10μ diameter microspheres and antipyrine in dogs and sheep. *Circ. Res. 34*, 391–405

Discussion

Owman: It is disturbing that with different techniques and different experimental animals some investigators get an effect of electrical stimulation on flow and others don't. It is hard to believe that such differences would reflect a difference in fundamental biological functions of the various animal species. Of course, the effect of sympathetic stimulation on vasoconstriction is not a very physiological parameter: it could be that in the brain the mechanism for readjustment after vasoconstriction is particularly efficient, so that immediately vasoconstriction occurs metabolic factors will tend to normalize the flow. If the various methods differ in that they do or do not measure changes in flow very discretely and very rapidly, sympathetic stimulation may indeed cause pronounced vasoconstriction, but vasoconstriction which is extremely short-lasting because of the very efficient adjustment mechanisms. Thus, detection of the vasomotor response may be difficult with techniques which either use a steady-state condition or which are not truly regional.

Heistad: I think that is unlikely. The techniques that have shown responses to sympathetic stimulation, such as thermal clearance (Sercombe *et al.* 1975) and venous outflow (D'Alecy & Feigl 1972), have indicated that responses are sustained for at least 1–2 min. We wait 40 s after starting sympathetic stimulation and then inject microspheres. From other studies we would predict that at that point there would be persistent constriction, so I think it is unlikely that we are missing a transient response.

Another possibility that intrigues me is that the microsphere technique may be measuring total blood flow and the thermal clearance technique may be measuring nutritional flow.

Purves: So those people, including myself, who have been able to find fairly consistent but not spectacular changes may really be investigating these effects in animals in which the ability to respond to constriction, which may be intracerebral, is in some way compromised. Are you suggesting that normally there is rapid dilatation and adjustment and that those who have found fairly consistent changes are dealing with preparations that are deteriorating or compromised in some way?

Owman: The problem is when people consistently obtain *negative* results on flow after sympathetic stimulation. There are several reasons for predicting that flow changes *will* occur with sympathetic activation, and what I am saying is that I believe it to be a purely methodological rather than a biological problem.

Siesjö: What form of anaesthesia did you use, Dr Heistad?

Heistad: All animals were anaesthetized with chloralose and urethane. In addition the monkeys were sedated with phencyclidine.

Siesjö: Is there any indication that anaesthesia may affect the response of vessels to sympathetic stimulation?

Heistad: We have also studied unanaesthetized dogs (Marcus *et al.* 1977). A very small effect of sympathetic denervation is detectable during haemorrhage in unanaesthetized dogs which is not detected in anaesthetized dogs.

Keatinge: There is undoubtedly a difference between the dog carotid artery and sheep and other species in the ability to respond to noradrenaline. The dog carotid is much less responsive to noradrenaline and sympathetic nerve stimulation than the sheep carotid.

Heistad: We saw marked differences between dogs and cats. In dogs there was very little disruption of the blood–brain barrier when arterial pressure was raised to 220 mmHg. The same pressure in cats almost always produced marked staining of the brain by Evans' blue. So both in flow responses to sympathetic stimulation and in disruption of the barrier there is a marked species difference.

Edvinsson: At the Stockholm symposium on neurogenic control of the cerebral circulation, Dr J. A. Bevan presented evidence of marked species differences in conjunction with electrical stimulation of isolated pial vessels. Some vessels were unresponsive, others were highly reactive. We were perhaps lucky to be using the baboon and the rat in our stimulation studies. The dog may not be as suitable for studying the sympathetic system. However, the cerebral vessels in all these species are innervated by sympathetic nerves.

Heistad: There are species differences, I think, but the conditions under which responses are studied are also important. The cat in normal conditions does not respond to sympathetic stimulation (Alm & Bill 1973), even though it responds very well to sympathetic stimulation during hypertension (Bill & Linder 1976).

Edvinsson: But there are also differences between the techniques used. Harper *et al.* (1972) studied the effect of nerve stimulation and injection of noradrenaline in the baboon. During hypercapnia they found marked constriction, with a 17% reduction in cerebral blood flow. That is another indication of the species variations.

Heistad: I don't think that is due to species variation. Alm (1975) looked at responses to sympathetic stimulation during normocapnia in monkey, using microspheres to measure flow, and found no response. I think the difference in results in this situation has more to do with differences in techniques.

Purves: Professor Owman suggested that some system, possibly involving intracerebral vessels, may respond to alterations in flow or pressure in the larger vessels and so keep nutrient flow constant. Has anyone who has investigated intracerebral flow or functions of it stimulated the sympathetic? Have you done that, Professor Silver?

Silver: About 15 years ago, B. A. Cross and I (Cross & Silver 1962) did some experiments on changes in intracerebral oxygen tension in the rabbit after sympathetic stimulation. When we stimulated the central end of one cervical nerve, we saw a slight bilateral rise in intracerebral oxygen tension which was almost certainly due to the rise in blood pressure. It was autoregulated but we could just see it. However, when we stimulated the peripheral end of the nerve we saw a very sharp ipsilateral fall in cortical and hypothalamic Po_2. We suggested that there might be some nervous control of intracerebral flow, but this was not well received. I am interested to hear now that it might have been true, but one must be aware of species differences.

Heuser: Regarding sympathetic stimulation in hypercapnia, I would like to emphasize the significance of changes in local ion activities for the effectiveness of transmitter action. From experiments with the perivascular perfusion technique (Csornai 1976; Kuschinsky & Wahl 1976) it is known that the response of pial arteries to noradrenaline is attenuated or even abolished in acid or alkaline media and at high potassium levels. Accordingly one could not expect changes in cerebrovascular resistance under those conditions.

Heistad: I am not surprised either that responses to sympathetic stimulation are not augmented during hypercapnic acidosis. The factor that would perhaps favour a response to sympathetic stimulation would be the fact that the cerebral vessels are dilated. But I agree that in most vascular beds acidosis inhibits constriction. Edvinsson & Sercombe (1976) showed that acidosis *in vitro* inhibits responses to noradrenaline in cerebral vessels.

Reis: E. Mackenzie, M. Mori and I have been interested in trying to alter the cerebral blood flow through excitation of an intrinsic neuronal system of brain. Our studies may throw light on some of the questions about the role of a sympathetic system in regulating cerebral blood flow. We looked at two intrinsic neuronal systems within the brain-stem which when electrically stimulated will profoundly raise the blood pressure. The first of these is a system which is organized in the rostral portion of the fastigial nucleus, a system on which we have worked for many years (Miura & Reis 1970; Doba & Reis 1972, 1974). In the cat, rat, monkey and dog electrical stimulation of the fastigial nucleus produces a profound increase in systolic blood pressure associated with tachycardia. The resultant cardiodynamic pattern is stereotyped. As analysed with electromagnetic flowmeters in the cat the pattern consists of a marked vasoconstriction of the renal, femoral and mesenteric arteries. However, flow in the common carotid artery is passively increased (Doba & Reis 1972), an observation which suggested the possibility that stimulation of the fastigial nucleus in some manner arrested cerebral autoregulation. During this past year we examined this effect on the cerebral circulation of stimulation of the fastigial nucleus in anaesthetized paralysed rabbits. Cerebral blood flow was measured by a hydrogen washout technique, recording from cerebral cortex. The normal autoregulation curve was plotted for 22 rabbits. The blood pressure was varied either by infusing phenylephrine or by controlled haemorrhage. We found there was good autoregulation. The breakpoint was at about 60 mmHg to the lower extreme and about 140 mmHg at the upper extreme. Stimulation of the fastigial nucleus completely abolishes autoregulation, and results in a profound increase in cerebral circulation. This effect is not influenced at all by transection of the sympathetic preganglionic fibres to the superior cervical ganglion. It is also not influenced at all by transection of the spinal cord at the first cervical segment. In fact transection of the spinal cord increases the flow, suggesting some inhibitory influences on the system ascending from the spinal cord. In contrast to the total independence of the cerebral vasodilatation elicited from the nucleus from the sympathetic innervation is the effect of stimulating another blood-pressure-regulating system in dorsal tegmentum of the medulla oblongata. This system, which Dampney, Kumada and I have investigated, appears to mediate the cerebral ischaemic response (Reis *et al.* 1977; Dampney *et al.* 1978). Electrical stimulation elicits a rise in blood pressure and a slowing of the heart rate—associated with a decrease of flow and increased resistance in the femoral and renal arteries. The pressor response elicited from the medulla differs from that elicited by stimulation of the fastigial nucleus by virtue of a very widespread activation of the sympathetic system. For example, fastigial nucleus stimulation does not produce any effect on the pupils whereas medullary stimulation produces wide pupillary dilatation.

When the medullary pressor area is stimulated autoregulation of cerebral blood flow is maintained, the only observation being that the breakpoint is shifted up to the right (i.e. autoregulation is maintained up to 160–170 mmHg). When we remove the cervical sympathetic from these animals, however, we completely abolish autoregulation and convert the cerebrovascular response into a totally unregulated system similar to that elicited from fastigial nucleus.

From these studies we propose that in the brain there may be a very powerful vasodilator system which is counterbalanced by sympathetic neurons in the superior cervical ganglion. In regions of brain, such as the medulla, electrical stimulation coactivates both the vasodilatation system and the sympathetic innervation of the cerebral vessels, thereby nullifying the increase in cerebral blood flow. In contrast, stimulation of the fastigial nucleus, which does not coactivate sympathetic innervation of the cerebral vessels, unmasks the pure vasodilatation.

Plum: The general region of the brain-stem where one sees degenerative changes in advanced human diseases is not in the fastigial nucleus but in the immediately surrounding zone, isn't it? I am talking about the fastigial changes, not the pressure changes. The first series of experiments you did were very close to the zone of the brain-stem where one sees degenerative changes in man. Perhaps this begins to close the link between the experimental and human changes.

Reis: The area of importance that you refer to is the nucleus of the solitary tract (nucleus tractus solitarii, NTS).

Sandler: We are talking in terms of manipulating the noradrenergic supply in isolation. Isn't there, I recall, a cholinergic supply to these blood vessels in addition?

Purves: There is a cholinergic supply which is very difficult to get at. It is exactly the sort of cholinergic supply or dilator supply that might be inferred from what Dr Reis described; that is, in the absence of the sympathetic control it is unopposed.

There are one or two small fragments of information about this interaction. The sympathetic nerves at low blood pressure in hypotension may actually be opposing a predominantly dilator response, because if the sympathetic fibres are cut, blood flow is uniformly higher. More directly, if the cholinergic pathway is stimulated, there is a very clear increase in blood flow which can be abolished by atropine. This implies the existence of muscarinic receptors on smooth muscle. The cholinergic pathway has been much less clearly studied than the adrenergic pathway, which is unfortunate for our discussion. For, as most people have pointed out, the principal response to hypoxia and hypotension is a dilator one.

Siesjö: What absolute pH value is required for noradrenaline to have an effect and at what pH do you see no effect?

Edvinsson: We have studied *in vitro* the effects of changing the pH from 7.0 to 7.8 (Edvinsson & Sercombe 1976). The contractile response to noradrenaline was reduced by about 40% at pH 7.0; on the other hand, the response was enhanced threefold at pH 7.8. Variations in carbon dioxide tension of the buffer solution produced no consistent change, provided the pH remained constant.

Rosendorff: We (Rosendorff *et al.* 1976, 1977) have been looking at the effects of stimulating the intracerebral noradrenergic pathway (INP). This tract originates in the locus coeruleus, and possibly some other nuclei in the brain-stem, and its nerve terminals are found in the hypothalamus and cerebral cortex. It appears to be independent of the 'conventional' sympathetic system, in the sense that the INP remains intact after superior cervical ganglionectomy.

We used the conscious restrained rabbit, with headplates fitted to the top of the skull to allow stereotaxic access to the hypothalamus on either side of the midline. We chose the hypothalamus because it is in the intracerebral pathway, and is a homogeneously perfused and relatively large region of subcortical grey matter. Local hypothalamic blood flow is measured by the clearance of small (5 μl) volumes of xenon-133 in saline injected, via a stereotaxically placed cannula, directly into hypothalamic tissue. Stimulation of the INP in the brain-stem on one side caused a significant ipsilateral increase in mean hypothalamic blood flow of about 8 ml 100 g^{-1} min^{-1}, which is of the order of 11% of the mean resting hypothalamic blood flow. This vasodilatation, not unexpectedly, is quite unaffected by cervical sympathectomy, but is completely abolished by chemical sympathectomy, in the hypothalamus or in the brain-stem, with 6-hydroxydopamine.

There are two possible mechanisms for these effects. Either the INP is a direct vasodilator pathway which has terminals on vascular smooth muscle, or this pathway in some way activates neurons and the vasodilatation is secondary to the increased neuronal metabolic activity. We examined these possibilities using glutamate and barbiturate, neither of which have any direct effect on vascular smooth muscle sensitivity to noradrenaline. Glutamate is well known to produce non-specific neuronal activation; that is, it will increase the firing rate of almost all cells examined in the nervous system. Barbiturate is a non-specific neuronal depressant. We showed that injection of glutamate into the hypothalamus increased hypothalamic blood flow by the same order of magnitude as that induced by INP stimulation. Barbiturate injection into the hypothalamus reduced hypothalamic blood flow and blocked the glutamate-induced vasodilatation.

Siesjö: What is the absolute level of flow?

Rosendorff: About 60–80 ml 100 g^{-1} min^{-1}. Now we come to the really interesting bit. The hypothalamic vasodilator effect of stimulating the INP in the brain-stem is completely abolished by the simultaneous injection of barbiturate into the hypothalamus. It is of course possible that barbiturate as well as switching off neurons also in some way inhibits the vascular response to stimulation, as suggested by Altura & Altura (1975). However, we were unable to show any effect of barbiturate on the noradrenaline sensitivity of an isolated rabbit femoral artery (constant flow, variable pressure) system. We think, therefore, that the INP vasodilatation is due to neuronal activation by the INP, with a secondary increase in local blood flow in response to an increase in the firing rate of perivascular neurons.

There may be three separate ways in which catecholamines can affect cerebrovascular tone. The first is a direct sympathetic vasoconstriction of resistance vessels, an action mediated by alpha-receptors. We have unequivocally demonstrated these receptors; they respond to noradrenaline in high doses, or when the blood–brain barrier to noradrenaline is disrupted, and to tyramine, which releases endogenous noradrenaline, and are blocked by conventional alpha-antagonists. Second, there are undoubtedly beta-adrenoreceptors in cerebral resistance vessels which mediate the dilator response to noradrenaline in low doses, when the noradrenaline blood–brain barrier is intact, or isoprenaline. Third, stimulation of brain-stem nuclei, including the locus coeruleus, will, we think, switch on neurons around the resistance vessels by activating both alpha- and beta-receptors on the neurons. It is the secondary metabolic products of neuronal activation which causes the vasodilatation that we see after stimulation of the INP. We do not know whether any direct vasodilator activation of the vessels occurs from this pathway.

References

ALM, A. (1975) The effect of stimulation of the cervical sympathetic chain on regional cerebral blood flow in monkeys. *Acta Physiol. Scand. 93*, 483–489

ALM, A. & BILL, A. (1973) The effect of stimulation of the cervical sympathetic chain on retinal oxygen tension and on uveal, retinal and cerebral blood flow in cats. *Acta Physiol. Scand. 88*, 84–94

ALTURA, B. T. & ALTURA, B. M. (1975) Pentobarbital and contraction of vascular smooth muscle. *Am. J. Physiol. 229*, 1635–1640

BILL, A. & LINDER, J. (1976) Sympathetic control of cerebral blood flow in acute arterial hypertension. *Acta Physiol. Scand. 96*, 114–121

CROSS, B. A. & SILVER, I. A. (1962) Some factors affecting oxygen tension in brain and other organs. *Proc. R. Soc. Lond. B Biol. Sci. 156*, 483–499

CSORNAI, M. (1976) The effect of serotonin and noradrenaline on the pial arteries, in *Ionic Actions on Vascular Smooth Muscle* (Betz, E., ed.), pp. 83–86, Springer, Berlin

D'ALECY, L. G. & FEIGL, E. O. (1972) Sympathetic control of cerebral blood flow in dogs. *Circ. Res. 31*, 267–283

DAMPNEY, R. A. L., KUMADA, M. & REIS, D. J. (1978) Central neural mechanisms of the cerebral ischemic response: cardiovascular responses to cerebral ischemia in rabbit. *Circ. Res.*, in press

DOBA, N. & REIS, D. J. (1972) Changes in regional blood flow and cardiodynamics evoked by electrical stimulation of the fastigial nucleus in cat: similarity to orthostatic reflexes *J. Physiol. (Lond.) 227*, 729–748

DOBA, N. & REIS, D. J. (1974) Role of the cerebellum and the vestibular apparatus in regulation of orthostatic reflexes in the cat. *Circ. Res. 34*, 9–18

EDVINSSON, L. & SERCOMBE, R. (1976) Influence of pH and pCO_2 on alpha-receptor mediated contraction in brain vessels. *Acta Physiol. Scand. 97*, 325–331

HARPER, A. M., DESHMUKH, V. D., ROWAN, J. O. & JENNETT, W. B. (1972) The influence of sympathetic nervous activity on cerebral blood flow. *Arch. Neurol. 27*, 1–6

KUSCHINSKY, W. & WAHL, M. (1976) Interactions of norepinephrine with H^+ and K^+ at pial arteries of cats, in *Ionic Actions on Vascular Smooth Muscle* (Betz, E., ed.), pp. 87–89, Springer, Berlin

MARCUS, M. L., MUELLER, S. M. & HEISTAD, D. D. (1977) Effects of sympathetic nerves on the regulation of cerebral blood flow during hemorrhagic hypotension in awake and anesthetized dogs, in *Cerebral Function, Metabolism and Circulation* (Ingvar, D. H. & Lassen, N. A., eds.), pp. 42–43, Munksgaard, Copenhagen

MIURA, M. & REIS, D. J. (1970) A blood pressure response from fastigial nucleus and its relay pathway in brainstem. *Am. J. Physiol. 219*, 1330–1336

REIS, D. J., DAMPNEY, R. A. L., DOBA, N. & KUMADA, M. (1977) Central control of blood pressure: a proposed localization of the 'tonic vasomotor center' of the medulla, in *Arterial Hypertension*, pp. 6–8. ICS 410, Excerpta Medica, Amsterdam

ROSENDORFF, C., MITCHELL, G., SCRIVEN, D. R. L. & SHAPIRO, C. (1976) Evidence of a dual innervation affecting local blood flow in the hypothalamus of the conscious rabbit. *Circ. Res. 38*, 140–145

ROSENDORFF, C., MITCHELL, G. & MITCHELL, D. (1977) Adrenergic innervation affecting local cerebral blood flow, in *Neurogenic Control of the Brain Circulation* (Owman, C. & Edvinsson, L., eds.), Pergamon Press, Oxford

SERCOMBE, R., AUBINEAU, P., EDVINSSON, L., MAMA, H., OWMAN, C., PINARD, E. & SYLAZ, J. (1975) Neurogenic influence on local cerebral blood flow. *Neurology 25*, 954–963

General discussion

Purves: I would like to return to the properties of vascular smooth muscle which you introduced earlier, Professor Keatinge. It may be worth emphasizing that your studies have been on comparatively large, extracranial arteries and it is uncertain how far these are involved in the changes of cerebrovascular resistance or indeed whether they have precisely the same properties as vessels inside the brain. However, if we assume that they do, then we presume that they share the property of responding to changes in transmural pressure, apparently without the benefit of nerves but as part of a myogenic response. This is particularly important in the cerebral vascular bed. Would you like to comment on this phenomenon?

Keatinge: Theories of autoregulation have been around for many years. One is that when blood pressure increases, arteriolar smooth muscle is stretched and it develops increased electrical activity which causes it to contract. That process cannot operate without some additional mechanism, since for autoregulation to take place, the arteries and arterioles have to contract, and sustain, a smaller diameter than they possessed before the pressure was increased. At that stage they are no longer being stretched, so direct stretch cannot be maintaining the stimulus. In theory, one possible answer is that a segment of the vessel has little smooth muscle but fires action potentials when stretched. If these were conducted to the resistance section of the arteriole the latter could contract to provide effective autoregulation. No such mechanism has in fact been demonstrated, although stretch can sometimes induce electrical activity in isolated arteries.

The other main theory of autoregulation is the metabolic one, that a fall in P_{O_2} or a rise in P_{CO_2} or adenosine increases blood flow. Again, most of the smooth muscle in resistance vessels is exposed to arterial blood chemicals rather than to tissue metabolites, so that some kind of transmission system is needed. The nerves present in the artery wall do not seem well arranged to provide such a system, but a myogenic system is possible.

Purves: So you are suggesting that there may be a rather odd kind of positive feedback, and from the traditional point of view that would be rather inconvenient. The other question is, what are the intermediate ways in which the mechanical events in smooth muscle actually respond to changes in tension or changes in transmural pressure? Is this electrical or an influx of calcium or what?

Keatinge: Two things may cause an artery to contract more strongly in response to a given stimulus when it is stretched than when it is short. Stretch can induce local electrical activity, resulting in Ca^{2+} influx. Also arterial, like cardiac, actomyosin produces a more powerful contraction in response to a given stimulus when it is elongated than when it is short. But while these processes cause the artery to resist stretch they cannot on their own make it contract to less than resting size and produce autoregulation.

Purves: Has anyone any evidence from other sources that could be extrapolated to smooth muscle?

Rapoport: The excitation–contraction process in muscle is a complex series of events each of which might be influenced so as to alter muscle contraction. In skeletal muscle, for example, depolarization of the surface membrane by electrical excitation or by an increased K^+ concentration induces release of calcium by the sarcoplasmic reticulum, activation of myofibrillar ATPase, and a resultant contraction and consumption of ATP. We demonstrated that tetanized single muscle fibres can become fatigued, despite a high ATP concentration, due to interference with a step in the excitation–contraction process (Nassar-Gentina *et al.* 1976). Interference could possibly be due to H^+ accumulation, to alterations in intracellular Ca kinetics, or to other factors. If one extrapolates these observations to cerebrovascular smooth muscle, it is entirely possible that under certain conditions Ca is critical for regulating blood flow, under other conditions pH is important, and yet in other cases K^+ or energy availability may play a role, as all these factors can influence the excitation–contraction process.

Moskowitz: One additional phenomenon, namely the phosphorylation of specific proteins within muscle cells, may be important for the coupling of excitation events (e.g. membrane depolarization) to contraction of muscle. Phosphorylation of troponin and other calcium-binding proteins has been shown to occur after membrane depolarization, activation of protein kinase, and induction of 3′, 5′-cyclic AMP. Phosphorylation apparently alters the affinity of these protein molecules for the calcium ion and thereby promotes the interaction of actin and myosin (see reviews by Haddy 1976; Kretsinger 1976).

Purves: Do you think this is relevant to the predominant relaxation that seems to be the unusual feature of the cerebral circulation?

Moskowitz: These experiments utilized cardiac muscle, and I am not certain to what extent this information applies to the smooth muscle surrounding cerebral blood vessels. One possibility, of course, is that contraction of smooth muscle in some instances causes dilatation of blood vessels by a mechanism similar to that which has been described for opening and closing the iris diaphragm. In this example, contraction of a specific layer of iris muscle (those cells innervated by sympathetic nerve terminals) causes dilatation of the pupil. At least some of the muscle cells surrounding blood vessels would require such an orientation in order to cause widening of the vessel lumen upon contraction. I am not certain to what extent this has been studied in vascular smooth muscle.

Reis: Several years ago Honig & Frierson (1976) described some intramural ganglion cells in the femoral artery of the dog and postulated that this may mediate some of the cholinergic sympathetic vasodilatation. This brings us back to the problem of whether nerves intrinsic in the brain may have a role of this sort.

Is it conceivable that the nerve plexus which you postulated is itself sensitive to pressure distortions? Could it in fact be depolarized when the pressure is sufficiently increased? Then some local antidromic transmission might be mediated over strips of vessel segments, so that in a sense the axon becomes a system of integration in this neural system.

Keatinge: It would be perfectly possible, in theory, to have a myogenic transmission system of this kind, or a nerve-mediated system or a system using transmission in the endothelium. Any such system could provide the kind of final result one sees, but we have no direct information that any one of them is operating.

Purves: Have you seen anything remotely resembling a plexus, Professor Owman: not just the adventitial plexus which you have described but a plexus such as that described in the smooth muscle of gut which can apparently operate autonomously?

Owman: I don't see why such a nerve plexus is necessary. There is a plexus of at least three or four types of fibres on the vessel surface, together with all the structural requirements for a low resistance coupling between the smooth muscle cells, allowing for myogenic propagation of the stimulus and thus serving as a kind of local reflex mechanism. Judging from electron microscopic studies, that specific type doesn't exist in brain vessels, either at the surface of the brain or in the parenchymal vessels.

Keatinge: From your work, Professor Lübbers, it seems that some of the autoregulation is extremely local, involving segments of often only 10–100 μm. So, if an electrically transmitting system is responsible, we know we are looking for something that conducts over the terminal arterioles for only a short distance.

Lübbers: The distances can be 500–800 μm along the capillary. I prefer the idea that the endothelium itself is involved in the transduction/conduction of this stimulus. We have no evidence on this point.

Keatinge: Another possible mechanism is suggested by the account of contractile protein in the endothelial cells. Is this organized in filaments, allowing contraction of these cells?

Owman: Besides our own immunohistochemical findings of actomyosin in the wall of brain capillaries (Owman *et al.* 1977) there is now recent ultrastructural evidence for the presence of an abundance of contractile microfilaments, both in the pericytes (Lebeux & Willemot 1977) and endothelial cells (S. Nag, personal communication) of brain capillaries.

Lübbers: As I mentioned, we stimulated capillaries in the rabbit mesentery, electrically, using microelectrodes of 1 μm diameter. In 80% of all cases the flow stopped. It took about 1 to 3 s for flow to stop, sometimes 5 s. Flow was later released rather quickly and it resumed in the same channels as before. I don't know if by electrical stimulation or iontophoresis of calcium we are producing artifacts. We are trying to find these changes in structure electron microscopically.

Keatinge: How widely was the contraction conducted?

Lübbers: With iontophoretically applied calcium it was very difficult to find the right dosage. Mostly calcium stopped the flow very quickly and completely, but locally we saw no change in the vascular diameter.

Keatinge: Your evidence would suggest that the capillaries are not contracting.

Lübbers: Not the ordinary capillary wall. There are special structures, especially on the capillary branchings, which change their form after stimulation. In cold-blooded animals the capillaries also contract.

Rapoport: Zweifach (1961) pointed out that endothelial cells in peripheral capillaries are amoeboid and constantly change their relative positions. They have actomyosin filaments which can be demonstrated by electron microscopy and immunocytohistochemistry (Becker & Shustak 1972). On the other hand, contractile protein has not been demonstrated in cerebrovascular endothelial cells except in one instance of malignant hypertension (C. Becker, personal communication).

Lübbers: Did Zweifach show that the endothelial cells were actually contracting?

Rapoport: Zweifach (1961) demonstrated amoeboid activity under *in vivo* conditions, which presumably occurs because of intracellular contractile proteins. Another point: how can cerebrovascular endothelia transmit electrical or chemical information to each other? They are connected by tight rather than by gap junctions.

Lübbers: But nobody has measured the resistance in the capillary walls. We know for example that in other endothelial cells changes in calcium concentration close or open the junctions.

Rapoport: As far as I know, tight junctions do not transmit electrical or chemical information. Gap junctions can form functional connections that are affected by Ca, but do not appear between cerebrovascular endothelial cells.

Raichle: Gap junctions have recently been demonstrated between endothelial cells in brain vessels and the overlying vascular smooth muscle cells (E. Nelson & M. Rennels, unpublished work).

Rapoport: Smooth muscle is not capillary endothelium.

Raichle: But pericytes are seen surrounding brain capillaries (Rennels & Nelson 1975) and some people would like to believe that this cell is a smooth muscle analogue (Forbes *et al.* 1977). It contains contractile proteins and all the intracellular apparatus necessary to regulate dynamics. Thus there is a system there that has been defined and documented. There are gap junctions, and contractile proteins, so the system would appear quite capable of responding. The question is, to what?

Purves: We are now asking what the nature of the effector or the sensor or the comparator is. Could you put some labels on your scheme now, Professor Silver?

Silver: One thing that seems definitely to be sensed is oxygen. The fast response, where the diameter of the terminal arteriole is modified, must be mediated through an oxygen sensor. It seems to be too rapid for anything else. In the capillary bed we get into a much more dubious area. Several things clearly affect the flow through the capillaries, among which oxygen may well be important, but I am sure it is not the only thing. There is a pH effect and ionic effects from Ca^{2+}, K^+ and probably Cl^- and P_i, but what the nature of the sensor is I have no idea, although it must be sensitive either to Po_2 or to something closely dependent on it. As far as the transmission system is concerned, I agree with Professor Lübbers that there is probably transmission along the endothelium, but we have no direct evidence for it. One might perhaps be able to use a charge-sensitive fluorescent dye which localized on endothelium to see if a relatively slow potential wave spreads along the cells.

Lübbers: The trouble is that these dyes, such as merocyanin, for example, are so insensitive.

Purves: If you are effectively measuring gradients in capillaries rather than larger vessels, the responses suggest that the time constants are very small indeed.

Lübbers: I would distinguish between two different types of regulation. One I like to call the 'inflow regulation' and this is a very quick regulation. The sensor may be inside the vascular wall because there are reaction times of only 0.1 s. So the site of inflow regulation may be in small arterioles. After anoxic hypoxia the set point of the reaction is changed without changing the time constant. This means that there must be an influence from processes —probably metabolic—in the tissue which affect the set point of 'inflow regulation'. The time constant for this effect is in the range of 10 s. We may call it 'metabolic regulation'. Since it is difficult to understand how metabolic products or ions can diffuse in this time over a distance of about 500 μm against the stream of the tissue water, we think that a special organization or special structure must be behind it.

Siesjö: If hypoxia is induced in rats by lowering the arterial P_{O_2} to about 25 mmHg, which corresponds to inhalation of about 5% oxygen, cerebral blood flow increases to about four or five times the normal. This is very critical for the survival of the cells. In experiments by Salford *et al.* (1973*a*) one carotid artery was ligated before animals were exposed to this degree of hypoxia. We measured flow using [^{14}C]ethanol as diffusible tracer and showed that flow on the ligated side increased, not five times, but only 2.5 times (Salford & Siesjö 1974). Histological analysis of tissue treated in this way shows that many neurons fail to survive (Salford *et al.* 1973*b*). In the light of these results, isn't it odd that there should be no increase in flow in some capillary areas?

Lübbers: We did not study hypoxia under this special condition which produces a reduction of maximum blood flow in some areas of the brain. We studied only short hypoxic and anoxic periods with normal circulation.

Siesjö: Is the difference in response to hypoxia between different 'microflow areas' a transient phenomenon?

Lübbers: We do not understand why some of the capillaries seem to be paralysed.

Siesjö: But in the long run, if hypoxia is maintained for, say, 60 s to 120 s, would there be an increase in all microflow areas?

Lübbers: No, not necessarily. If the oxygen supply is decreased in the superperfused area and increased in the other area they reach the same level; probably they have the same reduced oxygen supply.

Siesjö: Is total flow increased by four to five times?

Lübbers: The total flow increased, but I have no parallel measurements of local and total flow.

Plum: May I see if I understand? You got a 400% increase in flow, even at very low partial pressure of oxygen, but unless I'm mistaken, the driving force of oxygen outside that capillary zone can't be calculated. How do you calculate oxygen diffusion to the tissue cylinder outside the capillary?

Lübbers: Oxygen transport capacity is reduced dramatically, so we are increasing capillary transport in one area and decreasing it in another. Superfused capillaries take up a lot of blood, relatively, because they are short and fewer capillaries are needed to get an overflow.

Siesjö: But is it really possible to differentiate this in a single capillary? Aren't we discussing microflow areas which may have several or many capillaries?

Lübbers: I am talking about a microcirculation where there may be 100 capillaries or so.

Siesjö: My only point is that if you have a microflow area that may consist of 10 capillaries then changes in flow must affect a relatively large group of cells.

Lübbers: We measured this reaction 150 times. In 25% of all sites we got a strong increase, and in 50% of our experiments we got paralysis of the vessels.

Siesjö: Is it possible to confirm these measurements by using intracerebral microelectrodes?

Lübbers: We didn't do that.

Reis: Is it possible that some of these effects are mediated by nerves? There is no way of knowing but it is conceivable that the hypoxia could be stimulating some of the central areas that are hypoxia-sensitive.

Lübbers: You just need something that affects the circulation as a connecting link. It is completely open.

Silver: I have been looking at very small areas, particularly in relation to single or multineuronal activity or localized hypoxia. My impression is that the flow-regulation mechanisms are very local with respect to nervous activity. I cannot see how a diffuse system like the sympathetic nervous system can be so precise as to adjust a single capillary–arteriolar unit. It may be true but, if it is, the brain must be full of autonomic nerves with very precise distribution and local sensor mechanisms.

Siesjö: Professor Silver, have you seen local changes in the reaction of the microcirculation to hypoxia or do you find by intracerebral measurements a more generalized response?

Silver: In local hypoxia we nearly always see an increase in flow. With the microelectrodes that I used, I very rarely got situations where apparently nothing happened.

Lübbers: We didn't believe our own experiments so we did more until we realized that it was a consistent finding.

Keatinge: A conducted vasodilatation is known in peripheral blood vessels. It was studied particularly by Hilton (1959). We all seem to agree that it is necessary to postulate at least a local conducted vasodilatation in order to explain a whole range of the phenomena which we have discussed so far. The difficulty is that none of the three elements that could be mediating this seems well adapted to do so. The endothelial cells have the wrong kind of junctions. The smooth muscle cells are wrongly aligned for optimal conduction, since they run circularly. Nerves on the whole are also not well distributed to provide an optimal system. Nevertheless, widespread conducted vasodilatation has been detected in some arterial trees. The nature of the arterial conducting systems is one of the major problems holding up advances, and its elucidation merits a high priority.

Lübbers: Have you a good method?

Keatinge: Microelectrode records are quite possible, though difficult, in arteries. We are very short of microelectrode recordings from blood vessels in the brain.

Lübbers: A nice dye is needed to demonstrate these fibres first.

Keatinge: In theory it should be possible to track all nerve fibres present by electron micrographs. It is technically difficult but all of these things are possible with time and patience.

Purves: The 2 μm cells are becoming a little bit easier, aren't they?

Silver: It is very difficult to spike 2 μm cells in a jelly with no firm background, with an 0.5 μm electrode.

Purves: So it seems to be the ability of vessels to dilate which is unusual and which will need the most careful and concerted study.

References

Becker, C. G. & Shustak, C. R. (1972) Contractile protein in endothelial cells; comparison of cerebral capillaries with those in heart and skeletal muscle and liver sinusoids. *Circulation (Suppl. 2)*, 87

Forbes, M. S., Rennels, M. L. & Nelson, E. (1977) Ultrastructure of pericytes in mouse heart. *Am. J. Anat. 149*, 47–69

Haddy, F. J. (1976) Excitation-contraction coupling in cardiac and vascular smooth muscle. *Fed. Proc. 35*, 1272–1306

Hilton, S. M. (1959) A peripheral conducting system underlying vasodilatation. *J. Physiol. (Lond.) 149*, 93–111

Honig, C. R. & Frierson, J. L. (1976) Neurons intrinsic to arterioles initiate postcontraction vasodilatation. *Am. J. Physiol. 230*, 493–507

Kretsinger, R. (1976) Calcium-binding proteins. *Annu. Rev. Biochem. 45*, 239–266

Lebeux, Y. J. & Willemot, J. (1977) Actin-like filaments in brain pericytes as demonstrated by HMM labeling. *Anat. Rec. 187*, 635

Nassar-Gentina, V., Passonneau, J. V., Vergara, J. L. & Rapoport, S. I. (1976) Relation of fatigue state in frog single muscle fibers to concentrations of glycogen, phosphocreatine (PCr) and ATP. *Biophys. J. 16*, 206a

OWMAN, CH., EDVINSSON, L., HARDEBO, J. E., GRÖSCHEL-STEWART, U., UNSICKER, K. & WALLES, B. (1977) Immunohistochemical demonstration of actin and myosin in brain capillaries. *Acta Neurol. Scand. 56, suppl. 64*, 384–385

RENNELS, M. L. & NELSON, E. (1975) Capillary innervation in the mammalian central nervous system: an electron microscopic demonstration. *Am. J. Anat. 144*, 233–241

SALFORD, L. G. & SIESJÖ, B. K. (1974) The influence of arterial hypoxia and unilateral carotid artery occlusion upon regional blood flow and metabolism in the rat brain. *Acta Physiol. Scand. 92*, 130–141

SALFORD, L. G., PLUM, F. & SIESJÖ, B. K. (1973*a*) Graded hypoxia-oligemia in rat brain. I. Biochemical alterations and their implications. *Arch. Neurol. 29*, 227–233

SALFORD, L. G., PLUM, F. & BRIERLEY, J. B. (1973*b*) Graded hypoxia-oligemia in rat brain. II. Neuropathological alterations and their implications. *Arch. Neurol. 29*, 234–238

ZWEIFACH, B. W. (1961) Biological properties of vascular endothelium. *Angiology 12*, 507–510

Cerebral energy consumption and provision: the predominance of neuronal oxidative metabolic processes

FRANS F. JÖBSIS* and MYRON ROSENTHAL+

*Department of Physiology, Duke University, Durham, North Carolina and
+Departments of Neurology and Physiology, University of Miami, Miami, Florida

Abstract Glucose, the preferred substrate in cerebral metabolism, is broken down anaerobically to three carbon moieties with a small net gain in available energy in the form of two ATP molecules for each glucose molecule utilized, or, under anoxic conditions, one ATP molecule for each lactate molecule produced. By the O_2-dependent reactions of the tricarboxylic acid cycle and of the respiratory chain a yield of 34 ATP molecules per glucose molecule is provided. The mitochondrial apparatus for the handling of these oxidative reactions is located almost exclusively in the neurons; the glial components contain less than 10% of these enzymic pathways. Anaerobic glycolysis, the other possible pathway contributing free energy, might well predominate in the glia, but the over-all contribution to cerebral free energy provision under normoxic conditions is less than 1%. Thus neuronal oxidative metabolism is by far the most important mechanism for free energy provision. But the glycolytic capacity of the glial system may serve an important function in pathophysiological situations of hypoxia–anoxia and oligaemia–ischaemia.

Continued cerebral function in stress conditions is dependent on the flux in the oxidative metabolic apparatus rather than on readily available free energy stores (ATP, CrP, glycogen) in the tissue. For this reason, and because of the complete dependence of normal function and metabolism on the integrity of the organ, non-invasive optical techniques are of major importance for the study of functional–metabolic relationships.

Normal functioning of the central nervous system (CNS) depends most sensitively on the adequacy of the energy supply and circulatory perfusion of the system. The energy consumption of the brain is closely related to its electrophysiological activity and the two processes are tightly coupled on a moment-to-moment basis. Problems associated with changes in the relationship of these processes occur throughout the life cycle in vertebrates. Injuries from anoxia and ischaemia are common clinical experiences with readily apparent consequences. More subtle changes in intellectual or motor functioning are less easily recognized, yet alterations in the intimate connections between oxidative metabolism and electrophysiological activity may have their consequences. Likewise, pharmacological alterations in this relationship are clinically apparent and insights into the nature of these alterations must be actively sought. The very rapid disappearance of EEG activity and consciousness and the early onset of deterioration in total anoxia signals the importance of energy in the CNS.

Brain tissue consumes about 20% of the total body oxygen and receives about 15% of the total cardiac output. Thus, brain energy utilization far exceeds its proportional weight, which is only 2–3% of the body total (Schmidt 1964). But this disproportion is large—there are other organs with a similarly high energy consumption. Although an understanding of the reactions of oxidative metabolism is of utmost importance in accounting for the physiological function of any tissue, this is even more applicable to brain because of its complete and sensitive dependency on oxidative metabolism for proper function and viability. Also, the central role of the brain lends great significance to the satisfaction of its energy requirement. In addition, brain has a non-homogeneous vascularity, a capillary supply relatively lower than kidney, liver or adrenals, and low energy reserves (Nair *et al.* 1960). For normal functioning and viability of the brain the relations between energy metabolism, electrophysiological activity and circulatory perfusion are therefore even more critical than for other organs; this supports the concept that proper insight into cerebral function requires simultaneous information on each of these aspects.

ENERGY CONSUMPTION

Little is known of the energy-consuming processes of brain, the proportion of energy utilized by each, and their cellular location, i.e. neurons or glia, soma or dendrites, etc., of each process. It is appropriate, however, that these areas are under increasingly active investigation since they are basic to an understanding of brain activities. Early insights into energy utilization extend from the recognition that there is a gradient of sensitivity to oxygen deprivation which increases from the spinal cord rostrally to the cerebellum and cerebrum. This gradient closely parallels the rate of oxygen consumption. However, no unified concept of energy utilization based on cell types and functioning has yet emerged.

Metabolic energy is believed to be spent in several ways: first, in the transport of ions across the membranes of inactive cells, in maintaining their resting ionic gradient and consequently the resting membrane potential; second, in the transport of ions to restore their distribution to steady-state levels after this distribution has been changed by activity; third, in other transport processes such as those conceived for glucose, amino acids, Ca^{2+} and Cl^-; fourth, in the production and perhaps storage, release, elimination or re-uptake of transmitter substances; fifth, in the maintenance of axoplasmic flow; sixth, in basic metabolic processes such as synthesis of the macromolecular components of membranes and cell inclusions; seventh, in cell growth and regeneration, which is a somewhat controversial topic as far as the CNS is concerned; and eighth, in the function of the smooth muscle cells of the cerebral circulatory system. From this, the dependence of the CNS on oxidative energy is not surprising.

The weight of evidence favours cation transport against electrochemical gradients as accounting for much or most of the energy expenditure of brain. A direct relationship between these was demonstrated by the restoration, by ATP injection, of Na^+ transport in cyanide-poisoned giant axons of the squid, *Loligo* (Caldwell *et al.* 1960). In non-myelinated mammalian nerve fibres, a decrease in transport activity produced by ouabain or substitution of Li^+ for extracellular Na^+ abolished the increase in oxygen consumption produced by stimulation (Ritchie 1967). In addition, increased extracellular K^+ or the addition of other monovalent cations increased the rate of transport and oxygen consumption of resting fibres to approximately the same extent as did stimulation (Rang & Ritchie 1968).

The very large surface-to-volume ratio of brain cells makes these studies particularly relevant in the CNS. In early investigations, Whittam (1961) showed that ouabain or replacement of Na^+ by choline reduced oxygen consumption in brain and kidney slices by about 50%. Since *in vivo* oxygen consumption and transport activity are likely to be above those of the slice, it seems that the 50% figure would be a minimal estimate of the total energy expenditure for Na^+ and K^+ transport. Recently, the development of optical techniques for recording oxidative metabolic activities in intact CNS tissues and of potassium-selective microelectrodes for recording changes in the activity of extracellular potassium has allowed simultaneous comparisons of changes in these parameters under a variety of conditions. Morris (1974) reported that extracellular potassium increased linearly with levels of hypoxia, and other studies showed a close correlation between the response of oxidative metabolism (NADH and cytochrome a,a_3 oxidation) and the increase in potassium activity provoked by stimulation of the cerebral cortex, hippocampus and spinal cord (Lewis & Schuette 1975; Lothman *et al.* 1975; Yamada *et al.* 1977). These data suggest that energy utilization and the extracellular potassium load are tightly linked and that increases in extracellular potassium (presumably with high intracellular Na^+) constitute the major demand for increased energy supply.

In contrast, only a small proportion of brain energy expenditure is likely to be associated with neurotransmitter functions. In fact, Bachelard (1975) has calculated a ratio of energy used for acetylcholine synthesis to that for Na^+ transport of less than 0.001, with a similar value for the total turnover of dopamine, noradrenaline and serotonin.

If such a large proportion of brain energy is expended in ion transport, a question arises as to the costliness of various functions in terms of ion displacement and the relative activity of neurons and glia in the restitution process. In this regard, Creutzfeldt (1975) has calculated the energy consumption due to spike activity alone, based on previously reported values of heat production in action potential firing. It was concluded that less than 3% of cortical energy consumption can be accounted for by spike activity. This parallels the known predominant location of neuronal mitochondria in the dendrites and points to pre- and postsynaptic activities as being most costly. The allocation of energy expenditure for ion transport among different cell types has not been estimated. The acquisition of sodium by activated neurons would be expected to act synergistically with the increased extracellular potassium to stimulate ATP breakdown. Glia are not thought to gain sodium but do appear to gain K^+ after neuronal activity.

The relative activity of the two cell types becomes, therefore, an important question. Neurons contain many more mitochondria than glial cells do. Measurement of mitochondrial volumes in electron microscope plates of serial sections has assigned at least 90% of the total to the neurons, whereas the remainder was mainly unidentifiable in location and only partially of verified glial origin (O'Connor 1977). Thus, the oxidative metabolic supply of the very large fraction of energy used for ion transport must practically be confined to an intraneuronal location and applied mainly in the restoration of the neuronal ion concentrations.

Nevertheless, high Na^+–K^+-stimulated ATPase activity has been reported in glial cells (Medzihradsky *et al.* 1971) and much *in vitro* evidence supports the contention that glia play a role in the regulation of the extracellular ion concentrations in the CNS (see, e.g., Hertz & Schousboe 1975). If so, the role must be quantitatively minor in terms of oxidative metabolism and/or glycolytically generated ATP must make an important contribution. For the latter to be true, evidence in the form of a high titre of lactate in cerebral venous blood should exist. How much of a contribution this makes is best discussed by the following considerations.

ENERGY CONSERVATION

It is well known that cellularly useful free energy derived from the catabolism of all three main categories of ingested foodstuffs (carbohydrates, fats and proteins) can arise at practically any state in their breakdown and the elimination of their molecularly simple waste products. Under normal circumstances, however, the mammalian CNS utilizes predominantly the final oxidative pathways of glucose catabolism. Breakdown and energy conservation can best be divided into three stages: (1) glycolytic conversion to pyruvate, lactate, high energy phosphate and some reducing equivalents; (2) the passing of pyruvate into CO_2, hydrogen in the form of reduced coenzyme moieties and a single high energy phosphate in the operation of the tricarboxylic acid cycle; and (3) the oxidative conversion of these various reducing equivalents to H_2O, with conservation of free energy, again in the form of high energy phosphates. These three steps are shown in Figs. 1–3.

As for an accounting, it is important to realize that the breakdown of glucose to two pyruvate moieties not only yields two ATP molecules but also reduces two molecules of oxidized nicotinamide adenine dinucleotide (NAD^+) to the reduced form (NADH). These coenzyme molecules are not, however, directly available to the mitochondrial enzymes but remain inaccessible in the so-called cytoplasmic compartment. Under aerobic conditions, they are conveyed to the intramitochondrial compartment by the α-glycerophosphate shuttle system shown in Fig. 1. The cost of this is a yield of two rather than the potential three high energy phosphates if cytoplasmic NADH were directly accessible to the mitochondrial respiratory chain and oxidative phosphorylation. In the absence of oxygen or in the absence of a functionally adequate mitochondrial titre or activity, cytoplasmic NADH is reoxidized to NAD^+ in the pyruvate-to-lactate step. Without it, breakdown of glucose would come to a halt through lack of oxidized NAD. The resulting ability to furnish ATP anaerobically is crucially important: glycolysis is the only pathway able to do so.

Drawbacks exist. Each pair of ATP molecules formed from glucose is accompanied by the production of two lactic acid molecules: the problem being not so much a lack of efficiency as one of properly disposing of this waste product. Lactate diffusion out of the cell occurs much more slowly than that of CO_2 and the blood has no binding capacity for it. Thus, the concentration gradient can never be as steep as that of CO_2, and lactate therefore accumulates in the cerebrospinal fluid, with far-reaching pathophysiological consequences.

When O_2 *is* available, pyruvate enters into the mitochondrial tricarboxylic acid (TCA) cycle (Fig. 2). The subsequent dehydrogenation steps produce a

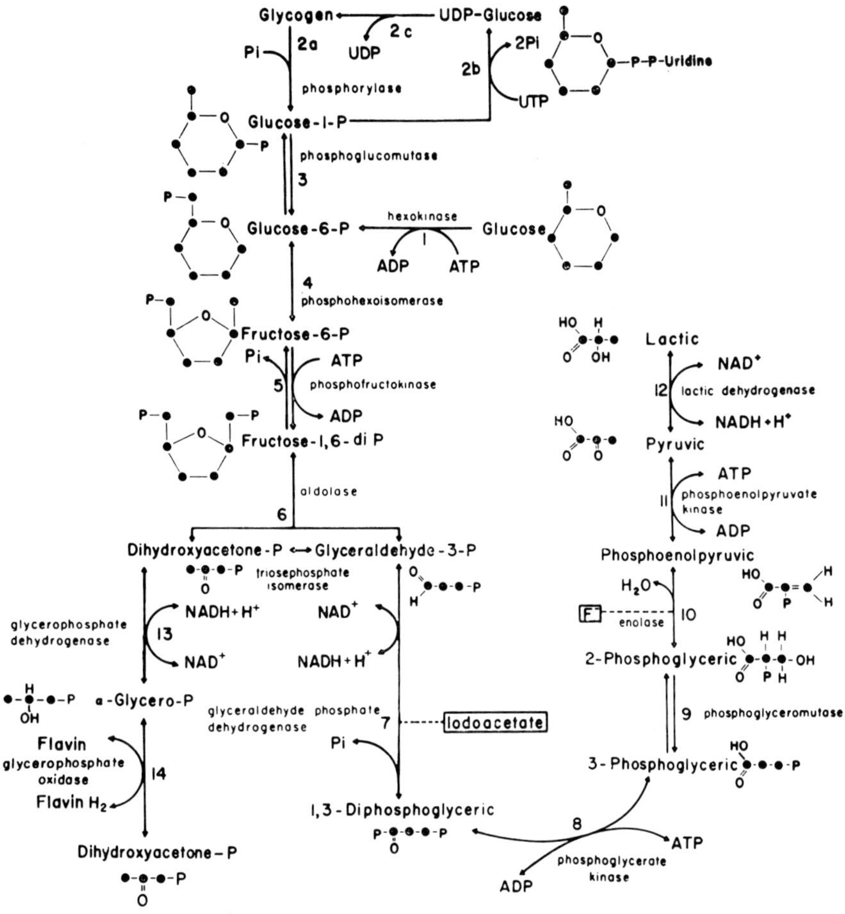

FIG. 1. The Embden-Meyerhoff scheme of glycolysis and the α-glycerophosphate shuttle. The black circles represent carbon atoms; the phosphate (P) groups are shown throughout; O, H and OH groups are only shown if they participate in the reactions of the compound (from Jöbsis 1964).

large complement of reducing equivalents for each pyruvate molecule in the form of four NADH molecules, one reduced flavoprotein (FpH_2) and one NADPH molecule which, with one NAD^+ molecule, can be transhydrogenated to form one more NADH molecule. All these are subsequently oxidized via the respiratory chain with a large yield of high energy phosphates. In contrast, only one high energy phosphate arises in the operation of the cycle, i.e. in the form of guanosine triphosphate (GTP). Otherwise all free energy conservation

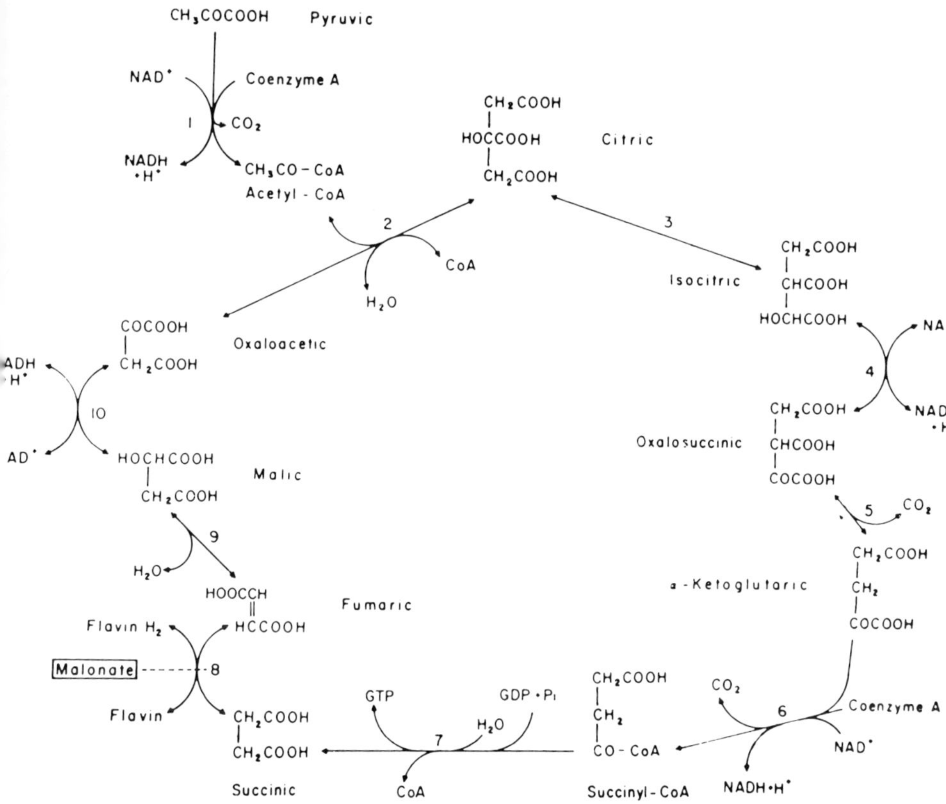

FIG. 2. The mitochondrial tricarboxylic acid (TCA) cycle. This illustrates the entrance of acetyl-coenzyme A derived from pyruvic acid (from Jöbsis 1964).

occurs in the subsequent respiratory chain system. This process provides a continuous reoxidation of the coenzymes, thus allowing the cycle to continue to operate.

Coupled to the redox reactions of the respiratory chain, there occurs the all-important process of oxidative phosphorylation. NADH, flavoproteins, cytochromes and a number of other components form a series of redox couples of ascending redox potentials spanning the potential gap between the hydrogens in the reduced coenzymes and molecular O_2. The usual but now perhaps somewhat limited scheme is shown diagrammatically in Fig. 3. The arrows indicate the flow of reducing equivalents: hydrogen in the NAD and Fp steps, electrons in the subsequent cytochrome reactions. The final reaction is the donation of four electrons to O_2; the combination with four H^+ ions results

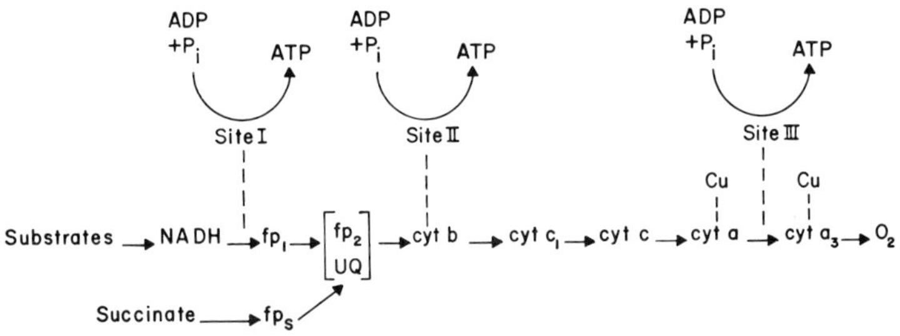

FIG. 3. The respiratory chain and oxidative phosphorylation. The flow of reducing equivalents (hydrogen up to cytochrome *b*, electrons from there on) is indicated by the arrows. This is a representative scheme rather than a complete or universally accepted one. Aside from Mitchell's radically different concept of the coupling mechanism between the phosphorylative and transport steps (see text), differences of opinion exist about the exact location of the free energy conservation sites. (cyt = cytochrome; fp = flavoprotein; Cu = copper; UQ = ubiquinone; P_i = inorganic phosphate.)

in the formation of two H_2O molecules. Along the way, free energy conservation in the form of high energy phosphate bonds takes place (Slater 1953; Chance & Williams 1956).

The redox potentials in this chain of redox reactions are shown better in the somewhat more complete and modern diagram depicted in Fig. 4, from Wilson *et al.* (1974). From these potential differences, free energy yields have been calculated. The best-known energy conservation steps, sites I and II, occur over redox potential spans in which the free energy difference amounts to about 58.6 kJ (14 kcal) each. The third and least understood step, however, is assigned to take place between cytochrome *c* and O_2, i.e. over a redox potential span yielding about 113 kJ (27 kcal). Simple arithmetic shows that the possibility exists for greater energy conservation at this site than is generally considered. We will return later to this intriguing possibility.

Before summing up the net free energy yield of the three phases of glucose catabolism, note that for the scheme of coupling redox reactions to oxidative phosphorylation a very different interpretation exists, in the form of Mitchell's chemiosmotic theory (1966). According to this hypothesis, ion gradients across the mitochondrial membrane are created during the transport of reducing equivalents, thus creating a high potential energy state which is dissipated during the process of ATP formation. At this moment we do not need to await a decision between the two competing hypotheses. It is sufficient to note that the overall free energy difference between NADH and O_2 is considered to yield three ATP molecules, and between FpH_2 and O_2 two ATP molecules, according to either hypothesis. Again it should be pointed out that actually

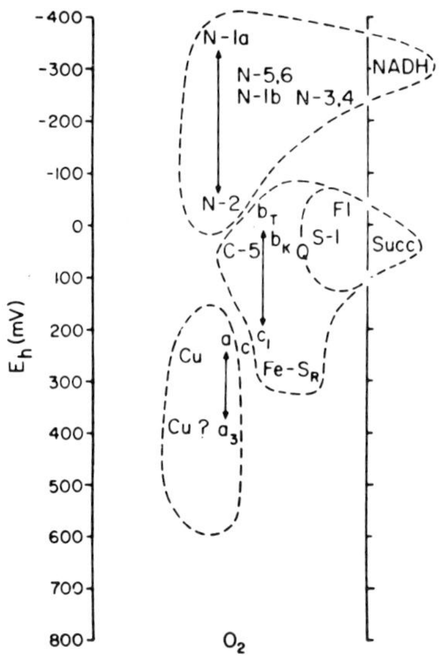

FIG. 4. The oxidation–reduction components of the mitochondrial respiratory chain. Arrows indicate the transfer of reducing equivalents through the three energy transduction sites. Components are enclosed according to the fragment of the respiratory chain in which they are found after fractionation and designated on the ordinate at their half-reduction potentials (from Wilson *et al.* 1974).

a sufficient redox potential difference exists to yield respectively four and three such moieties.

In summary, we should compare the glycolytic yield of two ATP molecules per glucose molecule and 34 molecules by the oxidative phosphorylation steps. The human cerebral uptake of glucose was reported to be about 5 mg (27.8 μM)/(100 g tissue min) whereas the output of lactate under normoxic conditions was about 0.6 mg (6.67 μM)/(100 g tissue min) (Himwich & Himwich 1946). Since 27.8 μM glucose would produce 55.6 μM lactate if all of the glucose were converted along this path, an estimated ratio of 6.67/55.6 or only 12% of the brain glucose normally utilized appears to be converted to lactate. Since production of one molecule of lactate is accompanied by the production of only one molecule of ATP, the rate of ATP production via this pathway should approximate 6.67 μM/(100 g tissue min). If 88% of the 27.8 μM glucose/(100 g tissue min) were utilized in the tricarboxylic acid cycle reactions and mitochondrial oxidative phosphorylation, then the ATP output would equal $(0.88)\times(27.8)\times(36)$ or 880 μM/(100 g tissue min), with a ratio of ATP production via lactate and oxidative phosphorylation approaching 1/132. Thus, even if all lactate production occurred in glial cells, less than 1 % of total brain energy would be produced in this manner. In view of the very large proportion of the energy utilization assigned to active transport, this fraction is insignificant compared to the needs of the brain. The situation may well be different, however, in hypoxic or anoxic conditions. Lactate production rises swiftly to very high levels and it would not be inconceivable that a major part is contributed by the glial components. In this case the glial glycolytic activity might best be considered as an emergency system in situations of respiratory or circulatory stress.

CONCENTRATIONS AND/OR FLUX

From these and well-known previous observations, the evidence points to an overwhelming reliance of cerebral electrophysiological functioning and viability itself on oxidative metabolic activities. This signals the importance of the continuing availability of oxidative energy to the CNS. However, recent evidence demonstrates that even more importance may be ascribed to the maintenance of the flux through the oxidative metabolic pathways or to the maintenance of the capacity of the oxidative metabolic system to conserve energy from the oxidative processes.

Several different viewpoints stress the importance of investigations of the flux rather than the steady state of energy reactions in the central nervous system. First, decreased tissue activity produced by anaesthetics or hypothermia is known to decrease oxygen utilization and slow ATP production, but with no change in ATP, ADP or AMP concentrations (see e.g. Nilsson & Siesjö 1970; Cohen 1973). In contrast, kinetic measurements from intact cerebrum show that intramitochondrial NADH and cytochrome a,a_3 become more reduced with administration of barbiturates or other depressants and the rate of re-reduction of these respiratory chain components after evoked tissue activity is decreased (see, e.g., Rosenthal & La Manna 1975; La Manna *et al.* 1977*a*, *b*). Likewise, in hypoglycaemia, neurological dysfunction and EEG abnormalities have been observed with no alteration in levels of energy metabolites (Ferrendelli & Chang 1973; Lewis *et al.* 1974). Also, in seizures, energy metabolite levels remained unchanged throughout severe alterations in electrographic and behavioural activities (Passonneau 1969), although such activities are accompanied by increased oxygen utilization and a decrease in the ratio of reduced to oxidized intramitochondrial NADH (Jöbsis *et al.* 1971).

Further insight into the relative values of steady state versus flux measurements in the CNS is derived from studies of the rates of decrease of the high energy stores after interruption of the metabolic flux and correlation with physiological function. It is becoming evident that neuronal activity may be altered or curtailed in hypoxia and ischaemia previous to drastic changes in the levels of high energy intermediates. For example, it has been calculated that theoretically the energy stores of the brain will be depleted only after 2–3 min of complete ischaemia although EEG activity has long previously been depressed (Siesjö & Plum 1973). While it is certainly possible that the period of availability of high energy intermediates may be shortened by the unavailability for cellular work of some fraction of these intermediates, nevertheless a clear distinction between depletion of energy stores and the depression of electrophysiological activity is apparent. In fact, just 21 s after a sudden onset of complete ischaemia by myocardial fibrillation in the dog, the EEG became flattened. Yet more than 90% of the high energy phosphate stores was still present at that moment (Woodhall *et al.* 1971). Whether this points towards an anatomically defined small compartment in which the drop may have been much more significant or to a more direct coupling between the oxidative metabolic reactions and excitability is not clear at this time. What is certain, however, is that a continuously maintained oxidative metabolic function, i.e. a flux through the respiratory chain, is required for normal neuronal function.

From an experimental point of view, it therefore becomes less than maximally informative to study the steady-state concentrations of metabolites. Energy demand appears more related to the continuous flux or to the capability of energy production than to steady-state values. What is needed are methods for studying the flux under various physiological conditions, preferably in a manner which does not interfere with these functions. Such studies have classically been performed by means of observations on arteriovenous differences in metabolites, O_2 and CO_2. However, they suffer from drawbacks in lack of localization, time resolution and sensitivity.

A new approach was initiated by the introduction of optical methods for the continuous monitoring of respiratory chain components *in situ*. These methods are based on the fact that many members of the respiratory chain are optically active and that differences exist in the optical properties depending on whether each is in a reduced or an oxidized condition. Thus, each respiratory chain member has relatively narrow light absorption bands which can be used for their identification and measurement as first described in 1925 by Keilin. In addition, the pioneering spectrophotometric techniques of Professor Britton Chance and subsequent biochemical studies showed that the fraction of each respiratory chain species that is reduced or oxidized within a population of these molecules is characteristically related to the rate of oxidative metabolism (Chance & Williams 1956). These measurements were made on isolated

TABLE 1

Metabolic states of mitochondria *in vitro* (based on Chance & Williams 1956)

Characteristics						*Steady-state percentage reduction of components*				
State	$[O_2]$	*ADP level*	*Sub-strate level*	*Res-pira-tion rate*	*Rate-limiting sub-stance*	*a*	*c*	*b*	*Flavo-protein*[a]	$NADH_1$
1	>0	Low	Low	Slow	ADP	0	7	17	21	~ 90
2	>0	High	~0	Slow	Substrate	0	0	0	0	0
3	>0	High	High	Fast	Respiratory chain	4	6	16	20	53
4	>0	Low	High	Slow	ADP	0	14	35	40	99
5	0	High	High	0	Oxygen	~100	~100	~100	~100	~100

[a] These values are based on the amount of flavoprotein of the respiratory chain. Other fractions, reduced by anoxia, are present but disregarded here.

mitochondria *in vitro* but the constraint of the requirement for transillumination hampered and significantly slowed utilization of spectrophotometric techniques in intact tissues. This constraint was subsequently overcome by utilizing the fluorescence of NADH to indicate redox changes of this coenzyme from a single surface and measurements were made on the intact cerebral cortex of cat *in vivo* (Chance *et al.* 1962). Recent evidence has established that spectrophotometric techniques are applicable to intact tissues, and redox changes of cytochromes have been recorded in the cerebral cortex during various physiological states by a reflectance procedure (Jöbsis *et al.* 1975). In addition, some newer techniques are becoming available and will be discussed in the next paper (Jöbsis & Rosenthal, this volume).

The *in vitro* experiments on isolated mitochondria showed that, under maintained rates of oxygen utilization and oxidative phosphorylation, characteristic steady states of balance between oxidation and reduction of several respiratory chain components can be recorded. These are shown in Table 1 for five easily reproducible metabolic conditions or 'states'. For our purposes, the most significant are the state of most rapid oxygen utilization and ATP production, the so-called 'active' state or state 3, and the condition when maximal rates of ATP synthesis are not achieved due to lack of ADP, i.e. the 'resting' state or state 4. It can be seen that the tight coupling of electron transfer to oxidative phosphorylation provides a control mechanism for the entire system and regulates the rate of oxygen uptake by the mitochondria.

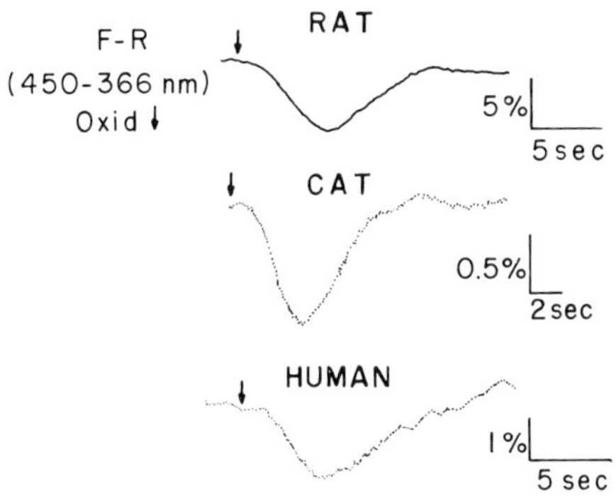

FIG. 5. Responses of NADH to direct cortical stimulation in rat, cat and human measured fluorometrically. One-second trains of pulses (0.5 ms duration, 20 Hz), with intensity in the range of 4–10 V, provoked each of these transient NADH oxidations. The trace from the rat is an original record from a single stimulus presentation. Traces from cat and human are computer-averaged over eight and four sweeps respectively.

Oxidative phosphorylation will not take place if ADP is unavailable, in which case electron transport and oxygen consumption are greatly diminished. If the concentration of ADP increases, oxygen consumption increases, electron transport increases and rephosphorylation of the ADP to ATP occurs. All of this activity alters the oxidation–reduction state of the respiratory chain enzymes in a characteristic manner.

Transposing this concept from isolated mitochondria to intact tissue, we can say that when energy (ATP) is spent in the course of cellular activities (e.g. ionic pumping), the high energy phosphate stores utilized in the process must be restored. Consequently, there is an increased rate of oxidative phosphorylation and oxygen utilization. This 'recovery metabolism' is mediated by increased levels of ADP which initiate transport of reducing equivalents from substrates to molecular oxygen; the over-all result is the production of H_2O and the concomitant rephosphorylation of ADP to ATP. This increased transport rate of reducing equivalents would be expected to be accompanied by new steady-state conditions wherein the ratio of oxidized-to-reduced NADH, Fp, cytochrome *b* and cytochrome *c* is increased, with cytochrome *a* becoming slightly more reduced and cytochrome a_3 remaining almost 100% oxidized. This proved to be the case in the cerebrum when fluorometric methods provided the opportunity to observe the response of NADH to evoked potentials produced by direct cortical stimulation or thalamic stimulation, to spreading depression produced by electrical stimulation or by KCl superfusion, and to seizures produced by a variety of epileptogenic agents (cf. Fig. 5 and

Jöbsis *et al.* 1971; Rosenthal & Jöbsis 1971; Jöbsis *et al.* 1972; Rosenthal & Somjen 1973). Each of these responses is a transient one: after a period of time, the ADP has been rephosphorylated to ATP and the system returns to the previous steady state.

To repeat, these observations are in full agreement with expectations from extrapolation of the data from mitochondria *in vitro*. These transient responses provide information on the transition between states as a tool for the study of intracellular energy metabolism. In addition, these responses have been used to study the effects of various agents or conditions on the energy-utilizing system (e.g. LaManna *et al.* 1976), to indicate the rate of breakdown of ATP to ADP via Na^+–K^+-ATPase (Rosenthal & LaManna 1975; LaManna & Rosenthal 1975), to denote the mitochondrial state for biopsy sampling (Sylvia *et al.* 1977), and to indicate the capability of the respiratory chain to respond to increased energy demand after ischaemic insult (Rosenthal *et al.* 1976). And although modifications of the *in vitro* scheme now appear warranted from recent data based on reflection spectrophotometry of cytochromes (see Jöbsis & Rosenthal, this volume), nevertheless many basic premises from mitochondrial studies still apply to the intact CNS.

In conclusion, it is important to understand and to emphasize the close interactions between energy-utilizing and energy-providing systems. Because of the great rapidity of action of both systems, little change occurs in the steady-state concentrations of intermediary metabolites. Only at intensely exhausting levels of activity are important changes found. The study of fluxes or the transition from one steady state to the next appears to be an important conceptual tool for the understanding of the metabolic activity of tissues *in situ*.

ACKNOWLEDGEMENTS

This work was supported by PHS grants HL 17391, NS 06233 (to FFJ) and NS 10384 and NS 13319 (to MR).

References

BACHELARD, H. S. (1975) Energy utilized by neurotransmitters, in *Brain Work* (Ingvar, D. H. & Lassen, N. A., eds.) *(Alfred Benzon Symp. 8)*, pp. 79–81, Munksgaard, Copenhagen

CALDWELL, P. C., HODGKIN, A. L., KEYNES, R. D. & SHAW, T. I. (1960) The effect of injecting 'energy rich' phosphate compounds on the active transport of ions in the giant axons of *Loligo*. *J. Physiol. (Lond.) 152*, 561–590

CHANCE, B. & WILLIAMS, G. R. (1956) The respiratory chain and oxidative phosphorylation. *Adv. Enzymol. Relat. Areas Mol. Biol. 17*, 65–134

CHANCE, B., COHEN, P., JÖBSIS, F. F. & SCHOENER, B. (1962) Intracellular oxidation-reduction states *in vivo*. *Science (Wash. D.C.) 137*, 499–508

COHEN, P. J. (1973) Effect of anesthetics on mitochondrial function. *Anesthesiology 39*, 153–164

CREUTZFELDT, O. D. (1975) Neurophysiological correlates of different functional states of the brain, in *Brain Work* (Ingvar, D. H. & Lassen, N. A., eds.) *(Alfred Benzon Symp. 8)*, pp. 21–46, Munksgaard, Copenhagen

FERRENDELLI, J. A. & CHANG, M. M. (1973) Brain metabolism during hypoglycemia. *Arch. Neurol. 28*, 173–177

HERTZ, L. & SCHOUSBOE, A. (1975) Ion and energy metabolism of the brain at the cellular level. *Int. Rev. Neurobiol. 18*, 141–211

HIMWICH, W. A. & HIMWICH, H. E. (1946) Pyruvic acid exchange of the brain. *J. Neurophysiol. 9*, 133–136

JÖBSIS, F. F. (1964) Basic processes in cellular respiration, in *Handb. Physiol.* Sect. 3: *Respiration*, vol. 1 (Fenn, W. O. & Rahn, H., eds.), pp. 63–124, American Physiological Society, Washington, D.C.

JÖBSIS, F. F., O'CONNOR, M. J., VITALE, A. & VREMAN, H. (1971) Intracellular redox changes in functioning cerebral cortex. 1. Metabolic effects of epileptiform activity. *J. Neurophysiol. 34*, 735–749

JÖBSIS, F. F., O'CONNOR, M. J., ROSENTHAL, M. & VANBUREN, J. M. (1972) Fluorometric monitoring of metabolic activity in the intact cerebral cortex, in *Neurophysiology Studied in Man* (Somjen, G., ed.), pp. 18–27, ICS 253, Excerpta Medica, Amsterdam

JÖBSIS, F. F., ROSENTHAL, M., LAMANNA, J. C., LOTHMAN, E., CORDINGLEY, G. & SOMJEN, G. (1975) Metabolic activity in epileptic seizures, in *Brain Work* (Ingvar, D. H. & Lassen, N. A., eds.) *(Alfred Benzon Symp. 8)*, pp. 185–196, Munksgaard, Copenhagen

KEILIN, D. (1925) On cytochrome, a respiratory pigment, common to animals, yeast and higher plants. *Proc. R. Soc. Lond. B Biol. Sci. 98*, 312–339

LAMANNA, J. C. & ROSENTHAL, M. (1975) Effect of ouabain and phenobarbital on oxidative metabolic activity associated with spreading cortical depression in cats. *Brain Res. 88*, 145–149

LAMANNA, J. C., SYLVIA, A. L., MARTEL, D. & ROSENTHAL, M. (1976) Fluorometric monitoring of the effects of adrenergic agents on oxidative metabolism in intact cerebral cortex. *Neuropharmacology 15*, 17–24

LAMANNA, J. C., CORDINGLEY, G. & ROSENTHAL, M. (1977*a*) Phenobarbital actions *in vivo:* effects on extracellular potassium activity and oxidative metabolism in cat cerebral cortex. *J. Pharmacol. Exp. Ther. 200*, 560–569

LAMANNA, J. C., YOUNTS, B. W. & ROSENTHAL, M. (1977*b*) The cerebral oxidative metabolic response to acute ethanol administration in rats and cats. *Neuropharmacology 6*, 283–288

LEWIS, D. V. & SCHUETTE, W. H. (1975) NADH fluorescence and [K^+] changes during hippocampal stimulation. *J. Neurophysiol. 38*, 405–417

LEWIS, L. D., LJUNGGREN, B., RATHCHESON, R. A. & SIESJÖ, B. K. (1974) Cerebral energy state in insulin-induced hypoglycemia, related to blood glucose and to EEG. *J. Neurochem. 23*, 673–679

LOTHMAN, E., LAMANNA, J. C., CORDINGLEY, G., ROSENTHAL, M. & SOMJEN, G. (1975) Responses of electrical potential, potassium levels and oxidative metabolic activity of the cerebral neocortex of cats. *Brain Res. 88*, 15–36

MEDZIHRADSKY, F., NANDHASRI, P. S., IDOYAGA-VARGAS, V. & SELLINGER, O. Z. (1971) A comparison of the ATPase activity of the glial cell fraction and the neuronal perikaryal fraction isolated in bulk from rat cerebral cortex. *J. Neurochem. 18*, 1599–1603

MITCHELL, P. (1966) Chemiosmotic coupling in oxidative and photosynthetic phosphorylation. *Biol. Rev. (Camb.) 41*, 445–502

MORRIS, M. E. (1974) Hypoxia and extracellular potassium activity in the guinea-pig cortex. *Can. J. Physiol. Pharmacol. 52*, 872–882

NAIR, V., PALM, D. & ROTH, L. J. (1960) Relative vascularity of certain anatomical areas of the brain and other organs of the rat. *Nature (Lond.) 155*, 497–498

NILSSON, L. & SIESJÖ, B. K. (1970) The effect of anesthetics upon labile phosphates and upon extra- and intracellular lactate, pyruvate and bicarbonate concentrations in the rat brain. *Acta Physiol. Scand. 80*, 235–248

O'CONNOR, M. J. (1977) Origin of labile NADH tissue fluorescence, in *Oxygen and Physiological Function* (Jöbsis, F. F., ed.), pp. 90–99, Professional Information Library, Dallas

PASSONNEAU, J. V. (1969) Energy metabolites in experimental seizures, in *Basic Mechanisms of the Epilepsies* (Jasper, H. H. *et al.*, eds.), pp. 98–103, Little, Brown, Boston

RANG, H. P. & RITCHIE, J. M. (1968) On the electronic sodium pump in mammalian non-myelinated nerve fibres and its activation by various external cations. *J. Physiol. (Lond.) 196*, 183–221

RITCHIE, J. M. (1967) The oxygen consumption of mammalian non-myelinated nerve fibres at rest and during activity. *J. Physiol. (Lond.) 188*, 309–329

ROSENTHAL, M. & JÖBSIS, F. F. (1971) Intracellular redox changes in functioning cerebral cortex. II. Effects of direct cortical stimulation. *J. Neurophysiol. 34*, 750–761

ROSENTHAL, M. & LAMANNA, J. C. (1975) Effect of ouabain and phenobarbital on the kinetics of cortical metabolic transients associated with evoked potentials. *J. Neurochem. 24*, 111–116

ROSENTHAL, M. & SOMJEN, G. (1973) Spreading depression, sustained potential shifts and metabolic activity of cerebral cortex of cats. *J. Neurophysiol. 36*, 739–749

ROSENTHAL, M., MARTEL, D. L. & LAMANNA, J. C. (1976) Effects of incomplete and complete ischemia on mitochondrial functioning measured in intact cerebral cortex of cats. *Exp. Neurol. 52*, 433–446

SCHMIDT, C. F. (1964) The measurement of Po_2 in tissues, in *Oxygen in the Animal Organism*, vol. 31 (Dickens, F. & Neil, E., eds.), pp. 239–246, Pergamon Press, London

SIESJÖ, B. K. & PLUM, F. (1973) Pathophysiology of anoxic brain damage, in *Biology of Brain Dysfunction*, vol. 1 (Gaull, G. E., ed.), pp. 319–372, Plenum Press, New York

SLATER, E. C. (1953) Mechanism of phosphorylation in the respiratory chain. *Nature (Lond.) 172*, 975–978

SYLVIA, A. L., LAMANNA, J. C., ROSENTHAL, M. & JÖBSIS, F. F. (1977) Metabolite studies of methamphetamine effects based upon mitochondrial respiratory state in rat brain. *J. Pharmacol. Exp. Ther. 201*, 117–125

WHITTAM, R. (1961) Active cation transport as a pace-maker of respiration. *Nature (Lond.) 191*, 603–604

WILSON, D. F., ERECINSKA, M. & DUTTON, P. L. (1974) Thermodynamic relationships in mitochondrial oxidative phosphorylation, in *Annual Review of Biophysics and Bioengineering*, vol. 3 (Mullins, L. J. *et al.*, eds.), pp. 203–230, Annual Reviews, Inc., Palo Alto, California

WOODHALL, B., KRAMER, R. S., CURRIE, W. D. & SANDERS, A. P. (1971) Brain energetics and neurosurgery, *J. Neurosurg. 34*, 3–13

YAMADA, S., LAMANNA, J., YOUNTS, B., ROSENTHAL, M. & SOMJEN, G. (1977) Responses of oxidative metabolism and extracellular potassium to afferent stimulation of the cat spinal cord. *Fed. Proc. 36*, 516

Discussion

Plum: By the terms of your clear presentation, there is in brain an overwhelming commitment of energy metabolism to ion transport. You imply that a tiny amount of energy goes to axoplasmic or structural synthesis and perhaps to enzyme synthesis for detoxification of the extracellular fluids. On the other hand, as Kety suggested, could it be that these gross distributions mask the functional vulnerability of the tissues to energy lack? A tiny change in oxidative metabolism, so small as to be unmeasurable, may influence critical enzymes and the synthesis of transmitters. This could happen without any interference with resting membrane potentials or even the spike potentials. If so, it would require that one look in exactly the opposite way to understand why, for example, during hypoglycaemia or hypoxia, crucial changes in brain function precede any measurable change in ATP, ADP or other high energy reserves.

Jöbsis: There is an argument related to the need for oxygen for other neurotransmitter functions or synthesis. Some oxidative steps involved in these reactions are commonly considered to need much higher oxygen concentrations than cytochrome *a*,*a*3 and therefore oxidative phosphorylation, as determined by *in vitro* determinations after isolation from the cell.

Plum: I was not speaking about the use of molecular oxygen for synthesis but about the energetics required to run enzymes whose consumption is too small to be reflected in whole tissue measurements but may be the most vulnerable initial point for failure.

Jöbsis: Candidates for such enzymes are for instance MAO or catecholamine synthesis. These oxidases and oxygenases need high oxygen concentrations. If we are going to lower the oxygen concentration of the brain they ought to be affected first. They are mostly enzymes for synthesis and they would be affected. For these effects to become noticeable, though, the hypoxia will have to last some time. Here I was emphasizing the very rapid reactions, leaving the others to our next paper. However, as will become clear from that paper, I am not sure that there is such a large difference in the oxygen affinity of the other oxidases and of cytochrome *a*,*a*3 while in the intact tissue.

Siesjö: Bachelard (1975) calculated that the amount of ATP used for acetylcholine synthesis could be at most 1% of that utilized in ion transport, while amine synthesis requires a very small fraction of the oxygen taken up by the tissue. However, although these figures suggest that transmitter metabolism does not consume much energy, the recovery events may be more energy-requiring.

Jöbsis: I think the figure was 0.1%.

Siesjö: Do we really know that a relatively substantial part of the energy doesn't go into renewal of cell constituents? Weiss (1969) recalled that an axon will grow at a speed of about 1–2 mm/day, and estimated that the neuron has to renew its whole macromolecular population once a day. Mitochondria and vesicles may turn over very quickly. There is also axonal transport which requires ATP and GTP, so possibly a relatively substantial part of the energy may go into renewal of cell constituents by the synthetic apparatus.

Sokoloff: From studies with protein synthesis inhibitors, it would appear that less than 10% of the body's energy consumption is used for protein synthesis (Weiss & Sokoloff 1963), and that includes the energy consumption of the liver which is a much more important protein-synthesizing organ than the brain. I don't think, therefore, that biosynthetic processes account for very much of the high energy metabolism of brain. One would think that most would go to active transport—50% or even 75–80%. Neurotransmitters need molecular oxygen for the hydroxylation reactions in their synthesis but these are not energy-consuming reactions.

Lübbers: The direct oxidative pathway of glucose (pentose shunt) has been much discussed. Isn't this a very important part of brain metabolism? There are different figures for this.

Sokoloff: The best current estimate in mature brain is that no more than 8% of the glucose consumption goes through the pentose phosphate shunt pathway (Maker *et al.* 1976). In the developing brain, particularly during myelination, it is probably higher.

Siesjö: There are new estimates that the hexose monophosphate shunt may consume 15–20% of the glucose utilized by the brain (Hakim & Moss 1972; Hakim *et al.* 1976).

Jöbsis: That particular pathway is especially concerned with synthetic reactions, rather than with free energy, i.e. high energy phosphate-providing reactions. It is logical that in the young animal with a high rate of growth there would be emphasis on that particular pathway.

Lübbers: If ambient P_{O_2} is reduced the membrane potential of brain cells usually changes if the oxygen pressure goes down to 10–20 mmHg. This is completely against what we would assume if the cytochrome oxidase from the respiratory chain was involved.

Siesjö: Does it depolarize?

Lübbers: Yes. There is a characteristic behaviour of the membrane potential. It depends also on the CO_2. So what is the sensor for this reaction? I was looking for another oxidase which must be immediately involved in membrane processes. What kind of candidate is there for this oxidative process?

Jöbsis: I shall be talking about that next.

Siesjö: Kerkut & York (1971) speculated that there might be an electrogenic component to the membrane potential. If the electrogenic sodium transport is inhibited that may lead to rapid depolarization.

Sokoloff: Are we prematurely ruling out a loss in energy reserves as being responsible for the functional deficiencies in hypoxia? In brain more than in any other tissue there is the terrible problem of compartmentation. When we measure the energy reserves of the brain as a whole, we are probably measuring mainly large pools that may be turning over slowly. There may be some small pools that are turning over rapidly and are observed when we measure the energy reserves of the brain as a whole.

Jöbsis: There is a problem there, because nobody has been able to measure the high energy phosphate concentrations in sufficiently small volumes, i.e. cells or parts of cells.

Lübbers: This doesn't hold for measurements with local Po_2 electrodes. These electrodes monitor from single cells. They monitor the balance of oxygen, the Po_2, as it comes in and is used up by the cell.

Siesjö: But Dr Sokoloff is talking about changes in ATP, ADP and AMP in the vicinity of the membrane-bound ATPase.

Lübbers: But if there is enough oxygen for the cytochrome oxidase then there should not be a loss of ATP.

Sokoloff: Later I shall provide evidence that the highest rates of oxygen metabolism are in regions with dense axo-dendritic connections, i.e. the synaptic-rich regions. The ATP in the cell bodies may not be so important as the ATP in the synaptic elements.

Jöbsis: At this point we can only say that further evidence is needed before we can either exclude or include high energy phosphate changes as the mechanism of vulnerability to ischaemia or hypoxia. It is very difficult even to estimate the total volume of those particular areas that might be affected first. We don't know what the concentrations of ATP are. Another way of going about it is to do what Professor Lübbers is suggesting, that is make local measurements of Po_2 balance or rate of disappearance during a sudden ischaemic episode, and try to work back from there. Even then we should carefully consider from how large a volume the O_2 consumed by the electrode is drawn. It may well be much larger than the synaptic structure. We cannot solve the problem at this point.

References

BACHELARD, H. S. (1975) Energy utilized by neurotransmitters, in *Brain Work* (Ingvar, D. H. & Lassen, N. A., eds.) *(Alfred Benzon Symposium 8)*, pp. 79–81, Munksgaard, Copenhagen.

HAKIM, A. M. & MOSS, G. (1972) Direct *in vivo* quantitation of the pentose phosphate pathway in brain. *Trans. N.Y. Acad. Sci. Series II 34*, 473–484

HAKIM, A. M., MOSS, G. & GOLLOMP, S. M. (1976) The effect of hypoxia on the pentose phosphate pathway in brain. *J. Neurochem. 26*, 683–688

KERKUT, G. A. & YORK, B. (1971) *The Electrogenic Sodium Pump*, Scientechnica, Bristol

MAKER, H. S., CLARKE, D. D. & LAJTHA, A. L. (1976) Intermediary metabolism of carbohydrates and amino acids, in *Basic Neurochemistry* (Siegel, G. J. *et al.*, eds.), 2nd edn., pp. 279–307, Little, Brown, Boston

WEISS, P. A. (1969) Neuronal dynamics and neuroplasmic ('axonal') flow, in *Cellular Dynamics of the Neuron* (Barondes, S. H., eds.), pp. 3–34, Academic Press, New York

WEISS, W. P. & SOKOLOFF, L. (1963) Reversal of thyroxine-induced hypermetabolism by puromycin. *Science (Wash. D.C.) 140*, 1324–1326

Behaviour of the mitochondrial respiratory chain in vivo

FRANS F. JÖBSIS* and MYRON ROSENTHAL+

* *Department of Physiology, Duke, University, Durham, North Carolina and*
\+ *Departments of Neurology and Physiology, University of Miami, Miami, Florida*

Abstract The interrelation of neuronal function and oxidative metabolism of the brain is most incisively studied by optical techniques *in vivo*. When O_2 becomes limited the respiratory chain becomes reduced, extracellular potassium activity is increased, the EEG is depressed and excitability declines, all as expected. Under mildly hyperoxic conditions however, the opposite responses occur, which indicate an absence of a critical tissue Po_2 and a continuum of dependence on the O_2 concentration, including levels well above the limits for maximal activity of the respiratory chain in isolated mitochondria *in vivo*. The unexpectedly high steady state of reduction of cytochrome a,a_3 provides the basis for a new hypothesis of an extra energy conservation site between cytochrome a_3 and O_2 and leads to a consideration of a reaction mechanism of O_2 with four electrons and four H^+ ions occurring at an enzymically active centre of cytochrome a,a_3. A special function of the cytochrome a,a_3 complex is implied in regulating cellular K^+ transport and thus excitability.

For many years, the main effort in our laboratories has been the investigation of the interrelations between functional activity and oxidative metabolism recorded *in situ* by means of non-invasive optical and electrophysiological techniques. The primary focus has been the study of optical signals arising from the disturbance of the normal redox steady state of the mitochondrial respiratory chain in response to imposed stresses. These so-called 'forcing functions' can either be in the biochemical realm aimed at metabolic parameters, e.g. changes in blood gases, administration of substrates, inhibitors and the like, or in the physiological realm, i.e. changes in functional activity of the tissue (see, e.g., Jöbsis *et al.* 1975; Jöbsis & LaManna 1977; Rosenthal & LaManna 1977). In the central nervous system (CNS), the latter range from the production of evoked potentials to the more pathological conditions of spreading depression and seizures, but it should be emphasized that the minimal stress producing a useful, i.e. measurable, disturbance of a steady state provides the most telling information. Therefore, evoked potentials are ultimately preferred. Pharmacological agents have been used either as a tool when their mode of action is well known and highly specific (Rosenthal & LaManna 1975; LaManna & Rosenthal 1975) or as the subject of the investigation when their mechanisms of action need clarification (LaManna *et al.* 1976, 1977*a*, *b*).

In addition to signals arising from the respiratory chain, we have also expended much effort in establishing non-invasive methods for other tissue parameters. By optical means, it is possible to monitor changes in blood volume, the steady state between haemoglobin (Hb) and oxyhaemoglobin (HbO_2), local blood flow, the intracellular oxygen concentration and changes in pH (Mitnick & Jöbsis 1976; Macdonald *et al.* 1977; Jöbsis *et al.* 1977; LaManna *et al.* 1978). Initial experiments in intact CNS were confined to measurements of redox changes of intramitochondrial NAD by fluorometry, a procedure which required the exposure of only a single tissue surface. The constraint of the requirement for transillumination in spectrophotometry, however, was more recently overcome by a reflectance procedure which also allows continuous monitoring from a single surface. For measurements in the infrared range, spectrophotometry by transillumination of the entire brain has now been achieved (Jöbsis 1977).

Measurement of the redox state of cytochromes and of the oxygenation state of haemoglobin rests on the optical properties of these molecules. Each of these has relatively narrow light absorption bands which can be used for their identification and measurement. These absorption peaks are shifted characteristically when the compound is oxidized or reduced (oxygenated or disoxygenated for Hb) which allows monitoring of the redox state or of the balance between arterial and venous blood. The procedure developed for the CNS measures the difference in intensity of two or three narrow 'monochromatic' bands of light scattered back out of the solid tissues on which they impinge. During passage into and out of the tissue light absorption takes place and this absorption differs depending on the redox state of the components.

Since all of these optical procedures can be used continuously, they do not require biopsy sampling and they leave the tissue in a continuously functioning state; in addition, electrophysiological recordings can be made within the areas being monitored for metabolic activities. Semi-microelectrode recordings of extracellular potassium, voltage changes of the extracellular fluid and electrocorticogram (ECoG) have been made and these various signals enhance the reach and grasp of our understanding of the complex interactions between metabolism and physiological activity. In this regard, it might not be superfluous to stress that the functional parameters of the tissue and of the experimental subject must be measured accurately to the best standards of physiology. And conversely, the patterns of energy metabolites in various steady states must be ascertained by reverting to biopsy or to killing the animal and doing a biochemical analysis (Sylvia *et al.* 1977). Only then can new signals arising from shifts in these physiological and biochemical steady states be interpreted meaningfully.

The interpretation of data thus obtained has rested largely on biochemical information derived by standard techniques. In the previous presentation (Jöbsis & Rosenthal, this volume) we showed by fluorometry that a transient oxidation of NADH occurs in response to a brief series of stimuli of sufficient strength to produce evoked potentials. This is in good agreement with expectations from studies of the reactions of NADH in isolated mitochondria *in vitro* upon the addition of ADP, i.e. for a transition from state 4 to state 3. Extension of these observations to cytochrome a,a_3, however, produced results at variance with expectations from the biochemical literature. Of the cytochrome absorption peaks, the one at 603–605 nm proved to be the most easily measured in the presence of haemoglobin by reflection spectrophotometry. It is ascribed to the final redox members of the respiratory chain, cytochrome *c* oxidase (EC 1.9.3.1) or cytochromes *a* and a_3, but predominantly cytochrome *a* (Lemberg 1969). When the cerebral cortex or spinal cord was provoked to activity, cytochrome a,a_3 became transiently more oxidized with a time course of response similar to that of NADH recorded by fluorometry (Fig. 1 and Jöbsis *et al.* 1975; Yamada *et al.* 1977; Peretsman & Rosenthal 1977). In contrast, cytochrome a,a_3 in isolated mitochondria *in vitro* is highly oxidized in all states except the anaerobic one. In addition, during state 4 to 3 transitions, the steady-state redox levels show a small increase in the direction of reduction. The observation of oxidative responses to increased functional activity *in vivo* was, therefore, most unexpected.

In order to rule out the possibility that local vascular reactions to the increased neuronal activity might produce the cytochrome a,a_3 oxidation by a temporary local increase in P_{O_2}, we did experiments on the excised toad brain. In this preparation O_2 was supplied by diffusion from the surface. Transient oxidative responses of cytochromes *a* and a_3 were observed, thus ruling out this possibility (Moffett & Jöbsis 1976).

These data, as well as many others discussed later, have made it clear that the respiratory chain *in vivo* is in a different (i.e. more reduced) steady state under normoxic conditions than in isolated mitochondria *in vitro*. This has produced a need to analyse carefully the entire biochemical background of respiratory chain activity and oxidative phosphorylation. It also documents

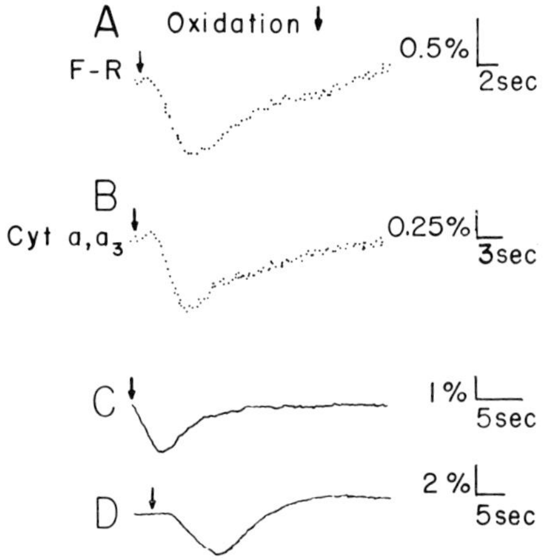

FIG. 1. Typical oxidative responses recorded optically for NADH (labelled F–R for fluorometry) and cytochrome a,a_3 (at 605–590 nm by reflection spectrophotometry). Traces A and B are each averages recorded from cerebral cortex of acute cat preparations (cerveau isolé); C is an average of four responses from an awake cat with a chronically implanted window over a cranial aperture; and D is the response recorded from cat spinal cord provoked by stimulation of a dorsal nerve root.

the necessity for *in situ* studies of oxidative metabolism for an understanding of the functioning of the central nervous system.

THE STEADY STATE IN VIVO

Logical first questions for the *in vivo* system are: how reduced is cytochrome a,a_3 at 'rest', and can the redox ratio be altered by oxygen availability? To approach this, the inspired oxygen level was varied from anoxia to 100% in acutely prepared cats and in awake rabbits with chronically implanted cranial windows (Rosenthal *et al.* 1976*a*). This produced a change in the level of oxidation–reduction, as shown in Fig. 2. Bringing oxygen levels to below room air levels produced a change towards reduction, as expected from a state 4–5 transition of isolated mitochondria. However, increased oxygen levels produced an oxidation of cytochrome a,a_3, again at variance with the concept of a fully oxidized cytochrome oxidase and a critical P_{O_2} for brain. When 5% CO_2 was added to the inspired gas, increased oxidation occurred no matter what the level of oxygen. Similar effects have been reported in cat spinal cord (Yamada *et al.* 1976) and in human neurosurgical patients (Austin *et al.* 1977).

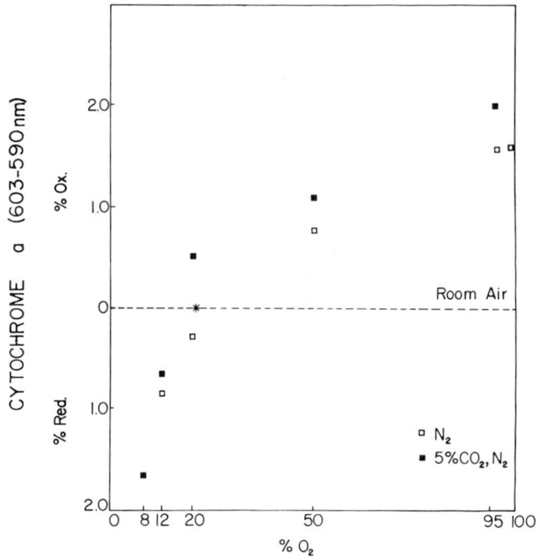

FIG. 2. Redox state of cytochrome a,a_3 expressed as percentage changes from 'rest' or full-scale level as a function of changes in the percentage of inspired oxygen with and without 5% CO_2. (From Rosenthal *et al.* 1976*c*.)

By comparing the redox ratio of cytochrome a,a_3 in the unstimulated, unperturbed control state to that during respiration of 100% O_2 and then of N_2, one can calculate an approximate value for the 'resting' percentage of reduced cytochrome a,a_3. This value was consistently near 30% in both cats and rats and was shown not to vary with the age of the rat preparations (Sylvia & Rosenthal 1978). This ratio changed, however, when rats showed signs of chronic lung disease (it was decreased) and when they exhibited both acute and chronic respiratory distress (it was increased, indicative of cellular hypoxia). Preliminary studies show that this value is also altered in cortical tumours (A. L. Sylvia *et al.*, personal communication, 1977). Both astrocytoma and neuroblastoma tumours, when inoculated under the cortical surface and allowed to grow to a visible extent, exhibited nearly fully oxidized cytochrome a,a_3. This is in contrast to adjacent, non-tumour areas from which near 30% levels of cytochrome reduction were recorded.

The 30% value of the resting level of reduced cytochrome a,a_3, based on respiration of 100% O_2 or 95% O_2 with 5% CO_2, is an experimentally useful parameter. Higher levels of inspired oxygen obtained by exposure of cats to hyperbaric pressures and increased levels of CO_2 produced further oxidation of this cytochrome, well beyond any expected range. This is shown in Figs. 3

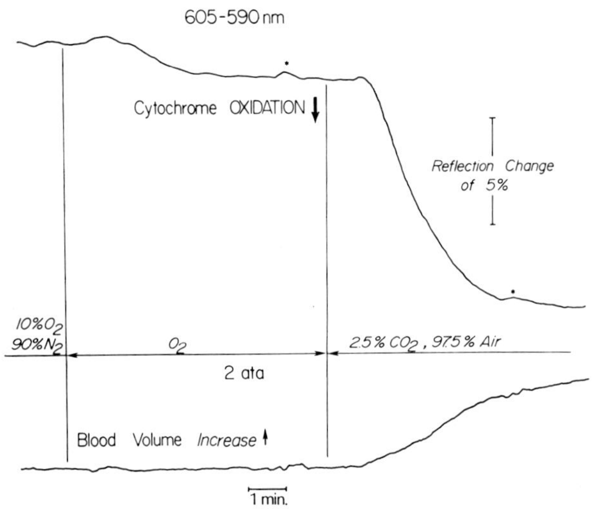

FIG. 3. Effect of hyperbaric O_2 (2 atmospheres) and of hyperbaric O_2 + hypercapnia on the redox state of cytochrome a,a_3 in the cat cerebral artery.

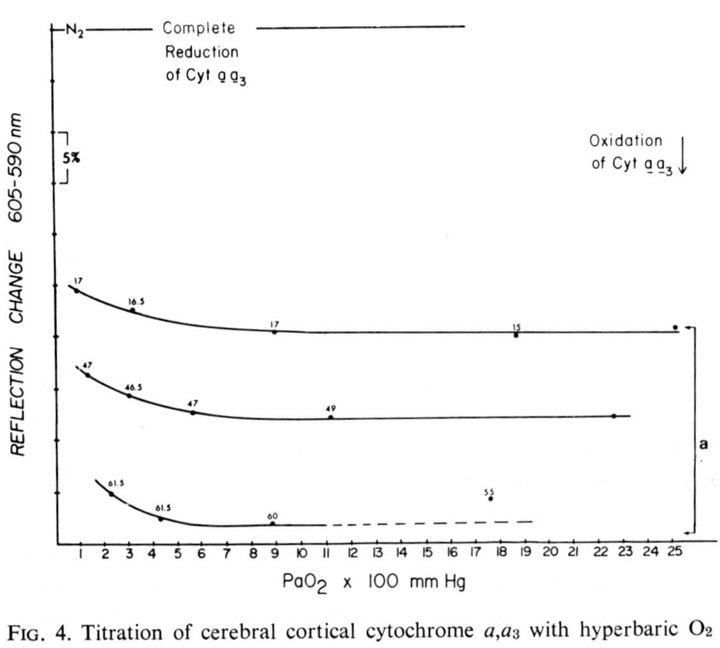

FIG. 4. Titration of cerebral cortical cytochrome a,a_3 with hyperbaric O_2 at three ranges of Pa_{CO_2}.

and 4 from which it is clear that increases in O_2 levels of up to four atmospheres of O_2, producing maximally a Pa_{O_2} of 2500 mmHg, are only partially effective in oxidizing cytochrome *a,a*$_3$. The much larger effect occurs when CO_2 is added to the inhalation mixture. In the lower Pa_{CO_2} ranges a definite increase in cerebral blood volume (see Fig. 3) points to an increased local O_2 delivery as a probable cause. However at Pa_{CO_2} levels beyond 75 mmHg little or no further effect on the vasculature is evident and a more direct effect on respiratory chain reactions must be assumed. Two possibilities exist. High levels of CO_2 and the concomitant increases in tissue H^+ concentration may well interfere with the glycolytic and tricarboxylic acid (TCA) cycle pathways. Inhibition of their operation would decrease the availability of reducing equivalents, thus resulting in a 'starved' state (state 2) of the respiratory chain signified by a general oxidation. Fluorometric observations on the steady-state reduction level of NAD do show an oxidation but the effect is slower and smaller than expected for a transition to state 2. The second possibility is that the increased availability of H^+ ions directly furthers the reaction of reduced cytochrome *a,a*$_3$ with O_2. In this reaction the final reduction of O_2 to H_2O requires four H^+ ions. Higher concentrations of the reactant would, therefore, lead to an increased rate of the final step with a concomitant change of cytochrome *a,a*$_3$ towards a more oxidized steady state as discussed in more detail in the last section of this article. Although we favour the second explanation on both experimental and theoretical grounds, both mechanisms would explain the effectiveness of high CO_2 levels in oxidizing cytochrome *a,a*$_3$ *in vivo*.

In this manner, it was estimated that in the cerebral cortex *in vivo*, cytochrome *a,a*$_3$ is 85% reduced under normoxic conditions (Hempel *et al.* 1977). This compares with the value of about 1% expected from observations on isolated mitochondria. This discrepancy is of extreme interest not only in terms of the mechanism by which the high reduction level originates in the normal intracellular environment, but also in regard to the extra energy available for the reaction of cytochrome *a,a*$_3$ with oxygen. It is important to point out that the free energy available at sites I and II of ATP production is about 58.6 kJ (14 kcal), depending somewhat on the redox steady state assumed for the reaction. The free energy available from cytochrome *c* to O_2, in which only one energy conservation site has been identified *in vitro*, is 113 kJ (27 kcal). This latter value is certainly sufficient for one additional energy conservation step besides the site III reaction.

The questions then arise of how the differences between *in vivo* and *in vitro* metabolism influence the relations between function and oxygen utilization and whether electrophysiological functioning is related to the redox state of cytochrome *a,a*$_3$. The concept has always been that electrophysiological activity was the determinant of oxygen utilization and metabolic turnover except in conditions limiting metabolism itself. Thus, correlations between EEG and metabolism have been demonstrated in a variety of cerebral disorders characterized by reduced metabolism and slow waves in the EEG (Kety 1950), and in anoxia a plateau of NADH (full reduction) was quickly reached and EEG depression soon followed (Chance & Schoener 1962). Conversely, stimulation of reticular formation produced EEG desynchronization accompanied by increased cerebral blood flow (CBF) and oxygen metabolism (CMR_{O_2}) (Meyer *et al.* 1969).

However, when the ECoG integral of the cat (*cerveau isolé* preparation) was used as a crude measure of tissue activity, both hyperoxia and hypoxia were characterized by decreases. ECoG frequency analysis showed that the former was due to high frequency activity with decreased amplitude, while the latter was due to a frequency decline (Rosenthal & LaManna 1977). These data demonstrate that ECoG activity, like the redox level of cytochrome a,a_3, varies with O_2 availability. The changes in ECoG and cytochrome oxidase are each magnified (hypercapnia) or attenuated (hypocapnia) by CO_2, but they are readily seen with oxygen alone, suggesting that increased ECoG frequency in hyperoxia is the result of oxygen directly or the oxygen effect on tissue metabolism rather than an effect of CO_2.

Another line of investigation further demonstrates the complexity of the relationship between electrophysiological activity and oxidative metabolism. In earlier observations, Morris (1974) reported a correlation between inspired O_2 and the activity of extracellular potassium in guinea-pig cerebral cortex. As expected, hypoxia was accompanied by an increase in the concentration of extracellular potassium, $[K^+]_o$, but hyperoxic conditions were sometimes accompanied by a decrease in $[K^+]_o$. Similar findings have recently been reported in cat spinal cord, i.e. respiration of 100% O_2 produced a slight but consistent decrease in the level of extracellular potassium and an oxidation of cytochrome a,a_3 (Rosenthal *et al.* 1977). Each of these changes was greatly magnified, and blood volume was markedly increased, by respiration of 95% O_2 with 5% CO_2.

These findings call into question the concept that function determines metabolism at oxygen levels above a 'critical P_{O_2}'. In fact, there is a continuum of oxygen dependency of both oxidative reactions and electrophysiological functioning throughout the hypoxic and hyperoxic range. Physiological function and the cytochrome a,a_3 reduction level vary continuously with oxygen provision, rather than a threshold existing, as would be expected from extrapolation of the data from isolated mitochondria. It is of marginal interest, perhaps, that this continuum invalidates the concept of a 'critical P_{O_2}' but, more importantly, it provides a basis for understanding the observations of effects on higher mental functions by relatively minor manipulations of the Po_2 of the inspired air. It also necessitates amendment of the generally held unidirectional idea that physiological function of an organ determines its metabolic rate. The issue appears to be more complicated. What we have demonstrated is a mutual interdependence: subtle changes in metabolism appear to have effects on function as well.

ACTIVITY-RELATED METABOLISM IN VIVO

As already considered, stimulation of cortex or spinal cord is accompanied by increases in the ratios of oxidation/reduction of the respiratory chain components. Such stimulation is, as expected, accompanied by transiently increased concentrations of extracellular potassium and negative shifts in the voltage of the extracellular fluid (steady potential). The tight coupling between electrophysiological activity and metabolism was demonstrated in reports showing the linear correlation among the peak amplitudes of these responses (Lewis & Schuette 1975; Lothman *et al.* 1975). This suggests strongly that much of the oxidative energy of the CNS and certainly the major portion of activity-related metabolism is expended in the maintenance and restoration of ion concentration gradients (see also Somjen *et al.* 1976).

The changes in oxidative metabolism associated with the recovery from the more pathological conditions of spreading depression and seizures show an increased complexity. In both of these conditions, NADH became more oxidized, but the extent of this oxidation is greater than expected from extrapolation of the relationship of extracellular potassium load and NADH oxidation provoked by mild stimulation. It was speculated that normal regulatory mechanisms of metabolic activity fail or that extraordinary demands other than ion transport are placed on tissue respiration by these pathological conditions (Lothman *et al.* 1975).

The cytochrome response in spreading depression and seizures differed significantly from that of NADH. In both conditions, preliminary studies indicate that cytochromes *b* and *c* became more oxidized, as did cytochrome a,a_3 in spreading depression. However, cytochrome a,a_3 became more reduced during seizure activity provoked by either intense stimulation, pentylenetetrazole or strychnine. The fact that other members of the respiratory chain became more oxidized in seizures is an indication that lack of O_2 is not the reason for the reduction of cytochrome a,a_3. Although in seizures this cytochrome reacts in the direction predicted from isolated mitochondria, it is only qualitatively correct since the large extent of reduction is inconsistent with a state 4–3 transition. The increased reduction level of cytochrome a,a_3 in seizures may be an intrinsic response within the mitochondrial system, or it may be related to hypoxia associated with decreases in the haemoglobin oxygenation observed concurrently in the tissue.

Recent preliminary investigations indicate that this is not the only aspect of cytochrome a,a_3 functioning that does not fit an easily discerned pattern. Age-related differences in cytochrome a,a_3 activity were found in response to evoked potentials and spreading depression in rat cerebral cortex (Sylvia & Rosenthal 1977). In young animals (4–5 months), both evoked potentials and spreading depression were accompanied by an expected oxidation of cytochrome a,a_3. However, in aged rats (24–26 months), evoked potentials produced an oxidation but spreading depression was accompanied by an increased level of reduced cytochrome a,a_3 together with an increase in blood volume and an oxygenation of haemoglobin. We speculate that the aged brain may lose the capacity to metabolically sustain energy needs accompanying recovery processes after extreme functional demands and that the mitochondrial respiratory chain itself may provide a rate limitation to energy conservation under highly active conditions in the aged central nervous system.

These investigations again provide support for the conclusion that the study of ongoing activities of the oxidative metabolic apparatus may be more conclusive than indications of the steady-state levels of the reactants (see Jöbsis & Rosenthal, this volume). This is apparent since, as shown, 'resting' redox levels of cytochrome a,a_3 in young and aged rats are approximately equal. In another line of study, a similar dichotomy of 'resting' and 'active' metabolism is also presented. It has previously been shown that, after short periods of transient cortical ischaemia, the rates of recovery to initial ratios of reduction/oxidation of the mitochondrial components indicate an uncoupling of oxidative phosphorylation (Rosenthal *et al.* 1976*b*). Thus, although pre-ischaemia redox levels are achieved when circulation is restored, it was expected that activity-related metabolism would be impaired. This proved to be the case, since the rate of re-reduction of NADH after evoked potential activity was retarded increasingly with increasing ischaemic episodes, yet all responses were recorded at the same baseline level of NAD reduction (see Fig. 5 and Rosenthal *et al.* 1976*c*).

Thus, the study of the changes in mitochondrial reactions during and in relation to activity provides us with a unique opportunity to improve our understanding of the functioning of the central nervous system. As is now evident, the questions are multiple and complex. Nevertheless, a basis for these studies will be provided by a better understanding of the unexpected reactions of cytochrome a,a_3 in the intact intracellular environment in nervous

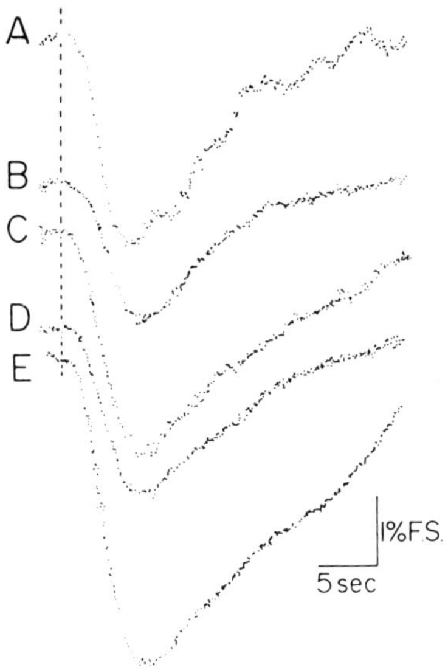

% Control

Trace	T_{Pmax}	$T_{\frac{1}{2}}$-$T_{Stim\ on}$	$T_{\frac{1}{2}}$-T_{Pmax}
A	100	100	100
B	115	96	80
C	110	125	137
D	110	115	120
E	108	158	196

FIG. 5. Cortical NADH responses to electrical stimulation before and after complete ischaemic insults. Values in table are presented as percentages of control rates. T_{Pmax} = time from stimulation to peak decrease of fluorescence; $T_{\frac{1}{2}} - T_{stim}$ = time from onset of stimulation until the response returns to half of its baseline value; $T_{\frac{1}{2}} - T_{Pmax}$ = time from peak decrease of fluorescence until this signal returns halfway to baseline. Trace A = control; B = 3 min after the first 1-min ischaemic insult; C and D = after a second and third 1-min ischaemic period and E = 10 min after D. (From Rosenthal *et al.* 1976*b*.)
(F.S. = full-scale fluorometric signal at rest during normoxia.)

tissue. For this reason, we have extended our enquiries to the absorption bands of the two copper ions which are part of the cytochrome a,a_3 enzyme complex.

CYTOCHROME a,a_3 IN VIVO

The two copper ions of the cytochrome oxidase complex also act as redox components and have been relatively neglected until recently. The absorption bands of these ions provide a means of considering their activities *in vivo*; since they are close together they form a general weak reduction peak in the 820 to 830 nm range. They can be observed in mitochondrial suspensions as depicted in Fig. 6 (Chance 1966). It should be noted that in this case oxidized cytochrome a,a_3 absorbs light while the reduced form does not exhibit the band.

Because of the greatly increased penetrating power of radiation in the

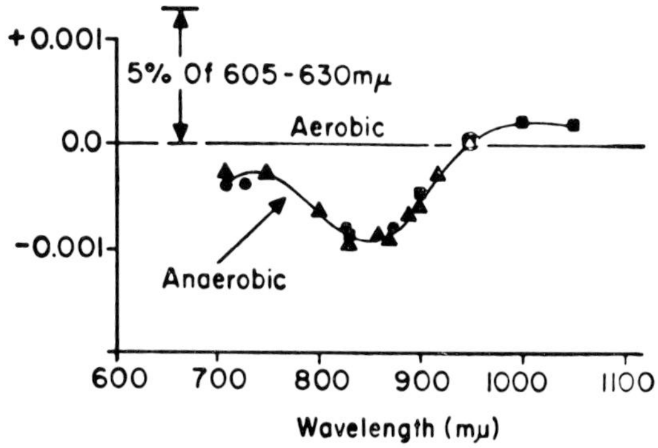

FIG. 6. Aerobic–anaerobic transition changes in pigeon heart mitochondria measured by infrared absorption (from Chance 1966).

near-infrared region of the spectrum, it was not necessary to expose the cerebral cortex in our studies. Measurements were made by transillumination of the head of cats at the level of temples. A difference spectrum of the 700 to 900 nm region is shown in Fig. 7 (Jöbsis 1977). In this case, the spectrum obtained from the normoxic, anaesthetized animal was subtracted from the one recorded after asphyxiation. The small peak at 760 nm is identified with the deoxygenated haemoglobin, and by normalization of the spectrum at 740 and 780 nm to the Hb minus HbO_2 difference spectrum obtained *in vitro*, a good concurrence with the expected spectrum of haemoglobin is obtained (broken line). The solid line indicates the trend of the data in the region of cytochrome a,a_3 absorption. What is notable is a trough centring at 840 nm. By subtraction of the known spectrum of purified cytochrome a,a_3, as is shown in the second panel of Fig. 7, it becomes clear that one absorption peak is missing. This lower wavelength band, which apparently is already nearly fully reduced in normoxia, is identified with the copper most closely associated with the a_3 haem. The one that does show, centred at 840 nm, is identified with the copper closely related to cytochrome *a*. Thus, it appears that the copper with the higher redox potential, i.e. most closely approaching that of oxygen, is nearly fully reduced in normoxia.

From these findings, it is concluded that a relative insensitivity of cytochrome a,a_3 in the reduced state exists for the reaction with oxygen. In other words, the K_m is considerably greater *in vivo* than the value of < 0.1 mmHg found for mitochondria *in vitro*. This is further emphasized by tissue Po_2 determinations using pyrenebutyric acid, an intracellular fluorescent probe for O_2, which show

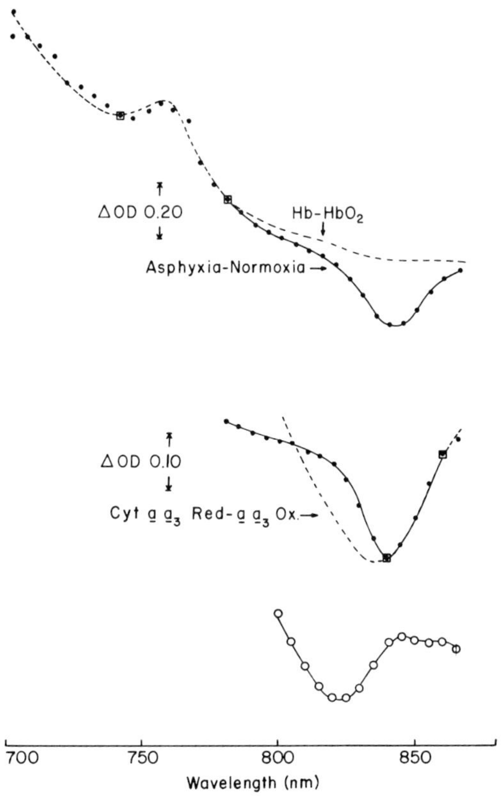

FIG. 7. Transillumination spectrophotometry applied to a cat's head. Top trace shows difference spectrum between anoxia after asphyxiation and normoxia. The data points (dots) conform to the difference spectrum of Hb minus HbO_2 (broken line) normalized at 740 and 780 nm (squared points) except in the region above 780 nm. Middle trace shows the 780 to 865 nm range after subtraction of the Hb–HbO_2 curve; drawn on a scale twice as large as top trace. The broken line shows the *in vitro* difference spectrum of purified reduced minus oxidized cytochrome a,a_3, normalized at 840 and 865 nm. Bottom trace is the 800 to 865 nm region of purified cytochrome a,a_3 after subtraction of the purified enzyme difference spectrum. (From Jöbsis 1977.)

a mean level of 42 mmHg (Mitnick & Jöbsis 1976). If the *in vitro* K_m applied *in vivo*, our present results on cytochrome a,a_3 would mean that 85% of the cortex would have a Po_2 of $\ll 0.1$ mmHg whereas the remaining 15% has a Po_2 of 240 mmHg in normoxia. This is patently impossible.

Some additional aspects of these studies should be reported in this symposium on the control of cerebral vascular smooth muscle. The novel method of

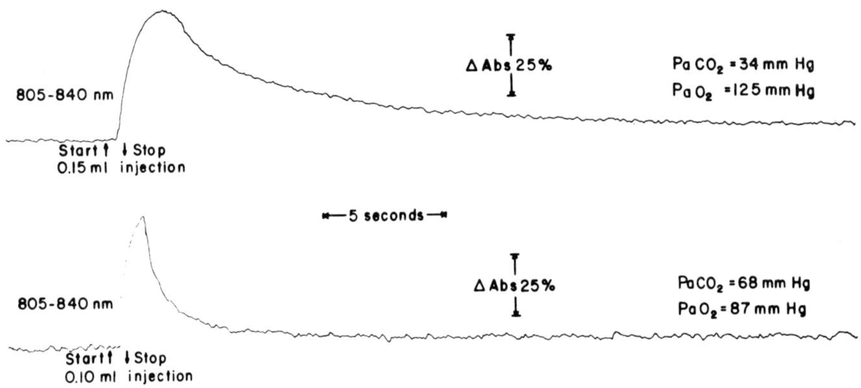

FIG. 8. Measurement of cerebral blood flow by transillumination of a duck's head. Depicted are traces of absorption changes in response to a close arterial injection of Cardio-Green dye. The animal was maintained by artificial respiration with 30% O_2, 3% CO_2, balance N_2. For the hypercapnic episode, the animal was breathing 21% O_2, 10% CO_2, balance N_2. (Experiment of Dr J. Colacino & Dr B. Grubb.)

non-invasive, infrared monitoring of oxidative metabolic events related to the redox state of cytochrome a,a_3 is also applicable to recording of the steady state between venous and arterial blood in the transilluminated tissue. This is done by monitoring in the region of the absorption peak of haemoglobin at 760 nm. Similarly, the cerebral blood volume can be studied by measurements at the 815 nm isobestic point of Hb–HbO_2. In addition, we have been able to measure the cerebral blood flow rate by clearance techniques using either the rapid injection of a small bolus of Cardio-Green dye or by a single-breath carbon monoxide technique. This is shown in Fig. 8 by transillumination across a duck's head. Using the height-over-area method, a mean blood flow rate of 32 ml/(100 g tissue min) was calculated in normocapnia. In the hypercapnic conditions, the rate became 109 ml/(100 g tissue min). These calculations were based on the assumption of 3 ml blood/100 g tissue. Comparison with ^{133}Xe clearance techniques can be made since the small size of the head and the delicacy of the bone structure allow radioactivity measurements from the same brain volume as observed by transillumination. These studies are now under way, with results that are highly encouraging in their reproducibility between the two techniques.

Thus, a number of important parameters can be measured in animal experimentation. Recently, successful monitoring has been performed in human volunteers by the atraumatic infrared method (Jöbsis 1977). It is hoped that measurement of circulatory parameters and oxygen sufficiency for cytochrome *a*,a_3 function may contribute to our better understanding of the role of the cerebral vasculature in the regulation of cerebral blood flow and thus of oxygen sufficiency for neuronal function.

THE REDUCTION OF O_2 TO H_2O

Let us now consider the requirements and possible mechanism of the reduction of O_2 to H_2O in the final step(s) of respiratory chain function. The first and most striking feature of this reaction is the fact that no less than nine reactants are involved: four electrons, four H^+ ions and one O_2 molecule. For such a complex reaction to take place, the reactants must bind close to each other if the (entirely improbable) likelihood that all reactants will collide simultaneously is to be raised. Otherwise, a series of sequential steps must be proposed which lead directly to the second important consideration: if the reduction of O_2 occurred in single electron transfer steps, biochemically highly destructive oxygen radicals would arise. In addition, because of their high reactivity with various intracellular compounds, their lifetime would be curtailed below the expected requirement for additional electrons to become available. Again in the reaction of a hypothetical $O^=$ ion with H^+ ions, lifetime considerations make it highly improbable that bimolecular reaction mechanisms occur. We propose, therefore, that the cytochrome *c* oxidase complex provides the binding site for the reactants and thus fulfils its catalytic role.

Because of the almost complete reduction of the copper atom more closely associated with haem a_3, whereas the other three redox components are less strongly reduced, we consider that the following schedule of events takes place. The first electron arriving at the completely oxidized cytochrome *a*,a_3 enzyme complex occupies the place of highest redox potential, i.e. the copper associated with the a_3 haem. Thus in a population of cytochrome *a*,a_3 molecules the a_3 copper is found to be mostly reduced at any one time. The next three electrons sequentially fill haem a_3 and *a* and the second copper. At this time, the enzyme reacts in one step with oxygen, donating the four electrons to produce two $O^=$ ions. Their very high reactivity with hydrogen ions of the environment or associated directly with the enzyme complex produces water in an immediate further step. The high sensitivity of the reduction level of intracellular cytochrome *a*,a_3 to the P_{CO_2} suggests that the availability of H^+ ions affects the rate of transfer of electrons to O_2. The following tentative scheme is proposed. Cytochrome *a*,a_3 cannot reduce oxygen until all four electrons are present at the redox centres and until four H^+ ions are available by being adsorbed at nearby locations. When these eight reactants are in place, transfer occurs in one step to an oxygen molecule which is probably adsorbed to the enzyme complex, i.e. producing the oxygenated form (cf. Lemberg 1969). This scheme provides a good qualitative explanation for our observations. It also avoids the postulation of the formation of highly reactive oxygen free radicals if electron transfer took place in sequential steps.

The inability of electrons to react with oxygen, which is shown by the high reduction level of cytochrome a,a_3 *in vivo*, can be informally expressed as a block existing between cytochrome a_3 and oxygen. This block apparently disappears or is lost during the isolation of mitochondria for *in vitro* studies. In a variety of tissues specialized for ion transport functions, such as gastric mucosa, intestinal mucosa, heart muscle and now the cerebral cortex, higher levels of cytochrome a,a_3 reduction exist than in other tissues such as skeletal muscle. In addition, when transport is stimulated, an oxidation of the cytochromes, including cytochrome a,a_3, is observed (Hersey & Jöbsis 1969; Hassinen & Hiltunen 1975; Mandel *et al.* 1975; Moffett & Jöbsis 1976).

We speculate that a close relation may exist between the final step of oxygen reduction and the transport function of the tissues. This could even be related to a concomitant reaction of H^+ exchange for a transported cation. The additional free energy available between site III and O_2 may fuel this reaction. The actual reaction imparting a direction to such a transport reaction is not difficult to visualize qualitatively in view of the fact that the cytochrome a,a_3 complex spans the inner mitochondrial membrane, haem a_3 being on the inside surface and a on the outer surface. Thus, a functional displacement of reactants or products can speculatively be assigned to an asymmetrical system much in the same spirit as Mitchell's reactions scheme. As for transport from the intracellular to the extracellular space, it should be realized that in tissues specialized for ion transport a dense network of invaginations of the cellular reticular system envelops the mitochondria. Thus mitochondrial ion transport may well produce intense concentration differences in the spaces delineated by this reticular maze, so that passive entry from or exit to the extracellular space is accomplished.

The conditions setting up the high K_m for O_2 are apparently easily lost during mitochondrial isolation. We speculate that at least the first uncoupling reaction observed after temporary ischaemia or anoxia takes place at this location. This is in agreement with the difficulty in showing uncoupling *in vitro* with mitochondria isolated after cerebral anoxia or ischaemia (cf. Rosenthal *et al.* 1976*b*, *c*). The new concept of an early uncoupling of cytochrome a,a_3 function also leads to implications concerning the malfunction of ion transport and normal ion and water balance relations resulting in oedema after such insults.

ACKNOWLEDGEMENTS

It is a pleasure to express our gratitude to the Durham Instrument Laboratory (DILINC) for aid in designing and modifying much of the optical instrumentation used in these studies. These investigations were supported by PHS grants HL 17391 and NS 06233 (to FFJ) and NS 13319 and NS 10384 (to MR).

References

AUSTIN, G., HAUGEN, G. & LAMANNA, J. (1977) Cortical oxidative metabolism following microanastomosis for brain ischemia, in *Oxygen and Physiological Function* (Jöbsis, F. F., ed.), pp. 531–544, Professional Information Library, Dallas

CHANCE, B. (1966) Spectrophotometric observations of absorbance changes in the infrared region in suspensions of mitochondria and in submitochrondrial particules, in *The Biochemistry of Copper* (Peisach, J. *et al.*, eds.), pp. 293–300, Academic Press, New York

CHANCE, B. & SCHOENER, B. (1962) Correlation of oxidation-reduction changes of intracellular reduced pyridine nucleotide and changes in electroencephalogram of the rat in anoxia. *Nature (Lond.) 185*, 956–958

HASSINEN, I. E. & HILTUNEN, K. (1975) Respiratory control in isolated perfused rat heart. Role of the equilibrium relations between the mitochondrial electron carriers and the adenylate system. *Biochem. Biophys. Acta 408*, 319–330

HEMPEL, F. G., JÖBSIS, F. F., LAMANNA, J. C., ROSENTHAL, M. & SALTZMAN, H. A. (1977) Oxidation of cerebral cytochrome a,a_3 by oxygen plus carbon dioxide at hyperbaric pressures. *J. Appl. Physiol. 43*, 873–879

HERSEY, S. J. & JÖBSIS, F. F. (1969) Redox changes in the respiratory chain related to acid secretion by the intact gastric mucosa. *Biochem. Biophys. Res. Commun. 36*, 243–250

JÖBSIS, F. F. (1977) Non-invasive, infra-red monitoring of cerebral and myocardial oxygen sufficiency and circulatory parameters. *Science (Wash D.C.), 198*, 1264–1267

JÖBSIS, F. F. & LAMANNA, J. (1977) Kinetic aspects of intracellular reactions. In vivo effects during and after hypoxia and ischemia, in *Extrapulmonary Manifestations of Respiratory Disease* (Robin, E. D., ed.), pp. 63–106, Dekker, New York

JÖBSIS, F. F. & ROSENTHAL, M. (1978) Cerebral energy consumption and provision: the predominance of neuronal and oxidative metabolic processes, in this volume

JÖBSIS, F. F., ROSENTHAL, M., LAMANNA, J. C., LOTHMAN, E., CORDINGLEY, G. & SOMJEN, G. (1975) Metabolic activity in epileptic seizures, in *Brain Work* (Ingvar, D. H. & Lassen, N. A., eds.) *(Alfred Benzon Symp. 8)*, pp. 185–196, Munksgaard, Copenhagen

JÖBSIS, F. F., KEIZER, J., LAMANNA, J. C. & ROSENTHAL, M. (1977) Reflectance spectrophotometry of cytochrome a,a_3 in vivo. *J. Appl. Physiol. 43*, 858–872

KETY, S. S. (1950) Circulation and metabolism of the human brain in health and disease. *Am. J. Med. 8*, 205–217

LAMANNA, J. C. & ROSENTHAL, M. (1975) Effect of ouabain and phenobarbital on oxidative metabolic activity associated with spreading cortical depression in cats. *Brain Res. 88*, 145–149

LAMANNA, J. C., SYLVIA, A. L., MARTEL, D. & ROSENTHAL, M. (1976) Fluorometric monitoring of the effects of adrenergic agents on oxidative metabolism in intact cerebral cortex. *Neuropharmacology 15*, 17–24

LAMANNA, J. C., CORDINGLEY, G. & ROSENTHAL, M. (1977*a*) Phenobarbital actions *in vivo:* effects on extracellular potassium activity and oxidative metabolism in cat cerebral cortex. *J. Pharmacol. Exp. Ther. 200*, 560–569

LAMANNA, J. C., YOUNTS, B. W. & ROSENTHAL, M. (1977*b*) The cerebral oxidative metabolic response to acute ethanol administration in rats and cats. *Neuropharmacology 6*, 283–288

LAMANNA, J. C., SAIVE, J.-J., MACDONALD, V. W. & JÖBSIS, F. F. (1978) Simultaneous monitoring by optical techniques of respiratory chain and intracellular pH in toad 'ventricle strip., *Experientia (Basel)*, in press

LEMBERG, M. R. (1969) Cytochrome oxidase. *Physiol. Rev. 49*, 48–111

LEWIS, D. V. & SCHUETTE, W. H. (1975) NADH fluorescence and [K^+] changes during hippocampal stimulation. *J. Neurophysiol. 38*, 405–417

LOTHMAN, E., LAMANNA, J. C., CORDINGLEY, G., ROSENTHAL, M. & SOMJEN, G. (1975) Responses of electrical potential, potassium levels and oxidative metabolic activity of the cerebral neocortex of cats. *Brain Res. 88*, 15–36

MACDONALD, V. M., KEIZER, J. H. & JÖBSIS, F. F. (1977) Spectrophotometric measurements of metabolically induced pH changes in frog skeletal muscle. *Arch. Biochem. Biophys., 184*, 423–430

MANDEL, L. J., MOFFETT, D. F. & JÖBSIS, F. F. (1975) Redox state of respiratory chain enzymes and potassium transport in silkworm mid-gut. *Biochim. Biophys. Acta 408*, 123–134

MEYER, J. S., NOMURA, F., SAKAMOTO, K. & KONDO, A. (1969) Effect of stimulation of the brain-stem reticular formation on cerebral blood flow and oxygen consumption. *Electroencephalogr. Clin. Neurophysiol. 26*, 125–132

MITNICK, M. H. & JÖBSIS, F. F. (1976) Pyrenebutyric acid as an optical oxygen probe in the intact cerebral cortex. *J. Appl. Physiol. 41*, 593–596

MOFFETT, D. F. & JÖBSIS, F. F. (1976) Response of toad brain respiratory chain enzymes to ouabain, elevated potassium and electrical stimulus. *Brain Res. 117*, 239–255

MORRIS, M. E. (1974) Hypoxia and extracellular potassium activity in the guinea-pig cortex. *Can. J. Physiol. Pharmacol. 52*, 872–882

PERETSMAN, S. J. & ROSENTHAL, M. (1977) Brain cytochrome a,a_3 redox states measured *in situ* in chronic cat preparations: effects of hyperoxia and direct cortical stimulation. *Brain Res., 128*, 553–558

ROSENTHAL, M. & LAMANNA, J. C. (1975) Effect of ouabain and phenobarbital on the kinetics of cortical metabolic transients associated with evoked potentials. *J. Neurochem. 24*, 111–116

ROSENTHAL, M. & LAMANNA, J. C. (1977) Oxidative metabolism and electrophysiological activity in intact central nervous system, in *Oxygen and Physiological Function* (Jöbsis, F. F., ed.), pp. 515–530, Professional Information Library, Dallas

ROSENTHAL, M., LAMANNA, J. C., JÖBSIS, F. F., LEVASSUER, J., KONTOS, H. & PATTERSON, J. (1976*a*) Effects of respiratory gases on cytochrome *a* in intact cerebral cortex; is there a critical P_{O_2}? *Brain Res. 108*, 143–154

ROSENTHAL, M., MARTEL, D., LAMANNA, J. C. & JÖBSIS, F. F. (1976*b*) Oxidative energy metabolism *in situ* during and following short periods of transient cortical ischemia in cats. *Exp. Neurol. 50*, 477–494

ROSENTHAL, M., MARTEL, D. L. & LAMANNA, J. C. (1976*c*) Effects of incomplete and complete ischemia on mitochondrial functioning measured in intact cerebral cortex of cats. *Exp. Neurol. 52*, 433–446

ROSENTHAL, M., YOUNTS, B., LAMANNA, J., YAMADA, S. & SOMJEN, G. (1977) Inspired gas mixtures and changes in redox level of cytochrome a,a_3 and extracellular potassium in cat spinal cord. *Fed. Proc. 36*, 431

SOMJEN, G., ROSENTHAL, M., CORDINGLEY, G., LAMANNA, J. & LOTHMAN, E. (1976) Potassium, neuroglia and oxidative metabolism in central gray matter. *Fed. Proc. 35*, 1266–1271

SYLVIA, A. L. & ROSENTHAL, M. (1978) Age-dependent differences in cytochrome a,a_3 redox activities associated with evoked potentials and spreading cortical depression. *Physiologist, 20* (4), 93

SYLVIA, A. L. & ROSENTHAL, M. (1978) The effect of age and lung pathology and cytochrome a,a_3 redox in rat cerebral cortex. *Brain Res.*, in press

Sylvia, A. L., LaManna, J. C., Rosenthal, M. & Jöbsis, F. F. (1977) Metabolite studies of methamphetamine effects based upon mitochondrial respiratory state in rat brain. *J. Pharmacol. Exp. Ther. 201*, 117–125

Yamada, S., Sanders, D. & Haugen, G. (1976) Functional and metabolic responses of the spinal cord to anoxia and asphyxia, in *Contemporary Aspects of Cerebrovascular Disease* (Austin, G., ed.), pp. 239–246, Professional Information Library, Dallas

Yamada, S., LaManna, J. C., Younts, W. B., Rosenthal, M. & Somjen, G. (1977) Responses of oxidative metabolism and extracellular potassium to afferent stimulation of the cat spinal cord. *Fed. Proc. 36*, 516

Discussion

Siesjö: You get oxidation by increasing O_2 and CO_2 so we should discuss the possible effects of CO_2, apart from increasing oxygen tension and H^+ concentration. Fanestil *et al.* (1963) postulated that, at least in liver tissue, CO_2 may uncouple oxidative phosphorylation. In a later paper Kasbekar (1966) suggested there might be inhibition of succinate oxidation. If that were the case in the brain how would it affect your interpretation of the redox state of cytochrome a,a_3 when you give more oxygen and increase CO_2?

Jöbsis: Taking out the proof of the step from $4H^+$ to H_2O would not jeopardize our interpretation of the finding of the high reduction level of cytochrome a,a_3 in normoxia and normocapnia.

Siesjö: If, by electrical stimulation, you increase flux in the electron transport chain and deliver more electrons to the terminal carriers, how could cytochrome a,a_3 get oxidized?

Jöbsis: In the classical *in vitro* observations (cf. Chance & Williams 1956) when the flux is increased by increased levels of ADP there is oxidation of NADH, flavoprotein and cytochrome *b*, and reduction of cytochrome *c* and of cytochrome a,a_3.

Siesjö: I agree, but what about the electrons?

Jöbsis: They would tend to accumulate at the cytochrome a,a_3 end of the respiratory chain. These blocks are strong blocks, well-coupled reactions. As soon as flow is allowed to take place it depletes the NADH and flavoprotein and tends to accumulate very slightly at the a,a_3 site. My proposition is that there is another coupling point between a_3 and oxygen which forms another final block for the cytochrome interaction. Electrons accumulate there. If this block is relieved there will be a sudden outpouring of reducing equivalents from all members of the chain. This we observed in the toad brain (Moffett & Jöbsis 1976).

Siesjö: So the interpretation of the changes in cytochrome a,a_3 rests on the assumption that there is a fourth coupling site between a_3 and oxygen?

Jöbsis: Not quite the *assumption*, but the *interpretation* of our observation. In the toad brain experiment, for example, all the members become more oxidized upon increased neuronal activity, and we have similar indications from the cat cortex too.

Siesjö: If there is a fourth coupling point there will be a relatively small overall ΔG for the whole process. As many people have emphasized (e.g. Newsholme & Start 1973), the loss of energy when only three ATP molecules are made from one NADH is the price nature has to pay to make the process irreversible under all circumstances. That is, the cell has to be able to make ATP even if the ADP and P_i concentrations change. So with four coupling points, especially if there is a ΔG of about 50–54 kJ/mol (12 or 13 kcal/mol), the system is approaching an equilibrium system.

Jöbsis: That is not an equilibrium system. There is an irreversible step but it is the last one. There is a total of about 230 kJ (55 kcal).

Lübbers: With four or five cells with 200 kJ (48 kcal) there are still 29 kJ (7 kcal) left for fun. This is what you get for ATP without using any tricks to make it higher. The normal potential is between 7 and 8 kcal.

Jöbsis: It depends on the ATP/ADP concentration. There is a difference between the synthesis and the hydrolysis. There is already built into it an efficiency factor of only 50%.

Siesjö: My point is that if a fourth coupling point is added the overall ΔG is so small that under certain intracellular conditions it could well be insufficient to drive ATP production.

Jöbsis: The calculations are complicated by the need to know the exact concentrations of a number of components and there is now a lot of leeway in them. It is much more convenient to consider not the entire chain but just the points around each site. They can be made to function by themselves. When sites I and II are making ATP from ADP there is a free energy change of about 50 kJ/mol (12 kcal/mol). Then one can compare that with the last site between cytochrome *c* and oxygen, which is about 113 kJ (27 kcal), with only a single ATP production site identified at present.

Astrup: How much light can you get through the intact head?

Jöbsis: I used my own head first, because it is particularly large and dense, providing the worst conditions for this experiment! It is difficult to translate individual photon counts to fluxes. It is an extrapolation backwards to different densities and different sizes of heads. We estimate that somewhere between 1 in 10 million to one in 100 million photons come through.

Astrup: Where is all this absorbed?

Jöbsis: There are losses upon entry and then there are losses by scattering and absorption. Once the photons have entered the tissue about 90% is lost for each 2 cm of soft tissue.

For fresh moist bone it is about 1.5–1.6 cm. If the bone is dry it becomes a very bad scatterer, so if you want to do an experiment buy an American steak with the bone left in and start work on it immediately. In the human head we have to use photon counting in order to get enough resolution. In the experiments on cats and ducks we can use analogue techniques since the rate of photons entering the photomultiplier is sufficient to produce a constant current which can be measured by the usual electronics.

Rubio: When you illuminate the cortex how thick is the layer of brain tissue that you see?

Jöbsis: I don't know. Since the grey matter has most of the mitochondria we might expect most of the signal to come from the cortex. But there may be considerable bouncing around inside the skull. A very tortuous path may have been followed by those photons that we pick up on the other side. They may not have crossed the cortex at a 90° angle but may have been guided in the longitudinal direction, i.e. grazing the white matter. Incidentally, the great advantage of using women rather than men as experimental subjects is that we gain a factor of about 10, because the intertemple distance is smaller and the bone is a bit lighter.

References

CHANCE, B. & WILLIAMS, G. R. (1956) The respiratory chain and oxidative phosphorylation. *Adv. Enzymol. Relat. Areas Mol. Biol. 17*, 65–134

FANESTIL, D. D., HASTINGS, A. B. & MAHOWALD, T. A. (1963) Environmental CO_2 stimulation of mitochondrial adenosine triphosphatase activity. *J. Biol. Chem. 238*, 836–842

KASBEKAR, D. K. (1966) Effect of carbon dioxide-bicarbonate mixtures on rat liver mitochondrial oxidative phosphorylation. *Biochim. Biophys. Acta 128*, 205–208

MOFFETT, D. F. & JÖBSIS, F. F. (1976) Response of toad brain respiratory chain enzymes to ouabain, elevated potassium, and electrical stimulus. *Brain Res. 117*, 239–255

NEWSHOLME, E. A. & START, C. (1973) *Regulation in Metabolism*, Wiley, Chichester

Local cerebral energy metabolism: its relationships to local functional activity and blood flow

LOUIS SOKOLOFF

Laboratory of Cerebral Metabolism, National Institute of Mental Health, Bethesda, Maryland, USA

Abstract The results of studies with the [^{14}C]deoxyglucose technique unequivocally establish that local functional activity in cerebral tissues is, as in other tissues, closely coupled to the local rate of energy metabolism. Stimulation of local functional activity increases the local rate of glucose utilization; reduced functional activity depresses it. Local cerebral blood flow is normally distributed among the cerebral structures in almost exact proportion to their rates of glucose utilization and it changes together with local glucose consumption in response to altered local functional activity. These results demonstrate that the level of functional activity in the structural and functional components of the central nervous system regulates the local rate of energy metabolism, and local blood flow is adjusted to the local metabolic demand.

The concept that the regulation of the cerebral circulation is at least in part mediated by the products of cerebral metabolism and that cerebral blood flow is adjusted to local cerebral metabolism and functional activity is almost a century old. In a classic paper published in 1890, Roy & Sherrington (1890) stated 'the chemical products of cerebral metabolism contained in the lymph which bathes the walls of the arterioles of the brain can cause variations of the calibre of the cerebral vessels . . .in this re-action the brain possesses an intrinsic mechanism by which its vascular supply can be varied locally in correspondence with local variations of functional activity'. The validity of this hypothesis has been generally assumed, and it has been the basis of many of our current ideas about the regulation of the cerebral circulation. Direct experimental evidence in support of it, however, has awaited the development of methods for the measurement of blood flow and energy metabolism in discrete structural components of the brain exhibiting alterations in functional activity.

Methods for the determination of local cerebral blood flow in conscious laboratory animals have been available for at least 20 years. The autoradiographic inert gas technique was originally designed for use with the radioactive inert gas, [^{131}I]trifluoroiodomethane (Landau *et al.* 1955; Kety 1960); this method provided the means of measuring the rates of blood flow simultaneously in all the macroscopic structures of the brain visible on autoradiographs (Landau *et al.* 1955; Freygang & Sokoloff 1958). In order to avoid the technical difficulties associated with the use of a volatile tracer, the method was modified for use with the non-volatile tracer, [^{14}C]antipyrine (Reivich *et al.* 1969). The diffusion of [^{14}C]antipyrine across the blood–brain barrier has been found, however, to be sufficiently restricted to limit its uptake by the cerebral tissues, and its use leads to underestimates of local cerebral blood flow (Eckman *et al.* 1975). This limitation has recently been overcome by the use of [^{14}C]iodoantipyrine, an analogue with far more rapid diffusion through the blood–brain barrier, which provides values for local cerebral blood flow essentially the same as those obtained originally with the [^{131}I]-trifluoroiodomethane (Sakurada *et al.* 1978).

These autoradiographic methods have been used to demonstrate that local blood flow in the brain is indeed altered in response to changes in local functional activity. For example, retinal stimulation by light has been found to increase blood flow in discrete regions of the central visual pathways of the cat, such as the lateral geniculate ganglion, superior colliculus and visual cortex (Sokoloff 1961). Because the cerebral circulatory response was slow, it was presumed that the mechanism of the regulation was chemical, possibly mediated by the products of metabolism. There was, however, no demonstration that local energy metabolism is coupled to local functional activity in the brain as it is in other tissues.

The recently developed [^{14}C]deoxyglucose method has provided the last link needed to study the relationships among local functional activity, energy metabolism and blood flow in the brain. This method can be used to measure the local rates of glucose utilization simultaneously in all the macroscopically visible structures of the brain. It can be applied to normal conscious animals as well as those in experimentally altered states of cerebral activity. Furthermore, the [^{14}C]deoxyglucose method also employs an autoradiographic technique which provides pictorial representations of the relative rates of glucose utilization throughout the various components of the brain; even without quantification these autoradiographs provide clearly visible markers that map cerebral regions with increased or decreased rates of energy metabolism in altered physiological, pharmacological and pathological states. This method has provided unequivocal evidence of a close relationship between functional activity and energy metabolism in discrete structural and/or functional units of the nervous system. Together with the techniques for measuring local blood flow, this method has also demonstrated the remarkably close correlation between local blood flow and energy metabolism.

METHODOLOGY

A detailed and comprehensive description of the theoretical basis of the [^{14}C]deoxyglucose method has recently been published (Sokoloff *et al.* 1977). A brief summary of its essential principles is necessary, however, to clarify the salient features of its design, its rigid procedural requirements, and the limitations on its applications.

The method was designed to take advantage of the extraordinary spatial resolution afforded by the quantitative autoradiographic technique that was originally developed for the measurement of local cerebral blood flow (Landau *et al.* 1955; Reivich *et al.* 1969). The dependence on autoradiography prescribed the use of radioactive substrates for energy metabolism, the labelled products of which could be assayed in the tissues by the autoradiographic technique. Although oxygen consumption is the most direct measure of energy metabolism, the volatility of oxygen and the short physical half-life of its radioactive isotopes precluded measurement of oxidative metabolism by the autoradiographic technique. In most circumstances glucose is almost the sole substrate for cerebral oxidative metabolism, and its utilization is stoichiometrically related to oxygen consumption (Kety 1957; Sokoloff 1976). Radioactive glucose is, however, not fully satisfactory because its labelled products have too short a biological half-life and are lost too rapidly from the cerebral tissues. The labelled analogue of glucose, 2-deoxy-D-[1-^{14}C]glucose, was therefore selected because it has some special biochemical properties that make it particularly appropriate for tracing glucose metabolism and for measuring the local rates of cerebral utilization of glucose by the autoradiographic technique.

Theory

The method is derived from a model based on the biochemical properties of 2-deoxyglucose (Sokoloff *et al.* 1977). 2-Deoxyglucose (2-deoxy-D-glucose; 2-DG) is transported bi-directionally between blood and brain by the same carrier that transports glucose across the blood–brain barrier (Bidder 1968; Oldendorf 1971). In the cerebral tissues it is phosphorylated by hexokinase

(EC 2.7.1.1) to 2-deoxyglucose-6-phosphate (2-DG-6-P) (Sols & Crane 1954). Deoxyglucose and glucose are therefore competitive substrates for both blood–brain transport and hexokinase-catalysed phosphorylation. Unlike glucose-6-phosphate, however, which is metabolized further via the glycolytic and tricarboxylic acid cycle pathways or the hexosemonophosphate shunt, deoxyglucose-6-phosphate cannot be converted to fructose-6-phosphate and is not a substrate for glucose-6-phosphate dehydrogenase (Sols & Crane 1954). There is very little glucose-6-phosphatase activity in brain (Hers 1957) and even less deoxyglucose-6-phosphatase activity (Sokoloff *et al.* 1977). Deoxyglucose-6-phosphate, once formed, is therefore essentially trapped in the cerebral tissues, at least long enough for the duration of the measurement. The half-lives of [^{14}C]deoxyglucose-6-phosphate in the various cerebral tissues have been experimentally estimated; the average half-lives are 7.7 (S.D. = $\pm$ 1.6) and 9.7 (S.D. = $\pm$ 2.6) hours in grey and white matter, respectively (Sokoloff *et al.* 1977). The shortest half-life is 6.1 h in the inferior colliculus (Sokoloff *et al.* 1977).

If the interval is kept short enough, for example less than one hour, to allow the assumption of negligible loss of [^{14}C]DG-6-P from the tissues, then the quantity of [^{14}C]DG-6-P accumulated in any cerebral tissue at any given time after the introduction of [^{14}C]DG into the circulation is equal to the integral of the rate of [^{14}C]DG phosphorylation by hexokinase in that tissue during that interval of time. This integral is in turn related to the amount of glucose that has been phosphorylated over the same interval, depending on the time courses of the relative concentrations of [^{14}C]DG and glucose in the precursor pools and the Michaelis–Menten kinetic constants for hexokinase with respect to both [^{14}C]DG and glucose. With cerebral glucose consumption in a steady state, the amount of glucose phosphorylated during the interval of time equals the steady-state flux of glucose through the hexokinase-catalysed step times the duration of the interval, and the net rate of flux of glucose through this step equals the rate of glucose utilization.

These relationships can be mathematically defined and an operational equation derived if the following assumptions are made: (1) a steady state for glucose (i.e. a constant concentration of plasma glucose and a constant rate of glucose consumption) throughout the period of the procedure; (2) a homogeneous tissue compartment within which the concentrations of [^{14}C]DG and glucose are uniform and exchange with the plasma; and (3) tracer concentrations of [^{14}C]DG (i.e. molecular concentrations of free [^{14}C]DG essentially equal to zero). The operational equation which defines R_i, the rate of glucose consumption per unit mass of tissue, i, in terms of measurable variables is as follows:

$$R_i = \frac{C_i^*\ (T) - k_1^*\ e^{-(k_2^* + k_3^*)T} \int_0^T C_P^*\ e^{(k_2^* + k_3^*)t}\, dt}{\left(\dfrac{\lambda\ V_m^*\ K_m}{\phi\ V_m\ K_m^*}\right)\left[\int_0^T (C_P^*/C_P)dt - e^{-(k_2^* + k_3^*)T} \int_0^T (C_P^*/C_P)\, e^{(k_2^* + k_3^*)t}\, dt\right]} \qquad [1]$$

where $C_i^*\ (T)$ equals the combined concentrations of [^{14}C]DG and [^{14}C]DG-6-P in the tissue, i, at time, T, determined by quantitative autoradiography; C_P^* and C_P equal the arterial plasma concentrations of [^{14}C]DG and glucose, respectively; k_1^*, k_2^*, and k_3^* are the rate constants for the transport from the plasma to the tissue precursor pool, for the transport back from tissue to plasma, and for the phosphorylation of free [^{14}C]DG in the tissue, respectively; λ equals the ratio of the distribution volume of [^{14}C]DG in the tissue to that of glucose; ϕ equals the fraction of glucose which once phosphorylated continues down the glycolytic pathway; and K_m^*, V_{max}^*, K_m and V_{max} are the familiar Michaelis–Menten kinetic constants of hexokinase for [^{14}C]DG and glucose, respectively.

The rate constants are determined in a separate group of animals by a non-linear, iterative process which provides the least squares best-fit of an equation which defines the time course of the total ^{14}C concentration in tissue in terms of the time, the history of the plasma concentration, and the rate constants to the experimentally determined time courses of tissue and plasma concentrations of ^{14}C (Sokoloff *et al.* 1977). The rate constants have thus far been determined only in normal conscious albino rats; the mean values $\pm$ S.E.M. obtained for k_1^*, k_2^*, and k_3^* are 0.189 $\pm$ 0.012, 0.245 $\pm$ 0.040, and 0.052 $\pm$ 0.010 per minute in grey matter and 0.079 $\pm$ 0.008, 0.133 $\pm$ 0.046, 0.020 $\pm$ 0.020 per minute in white matter, respectively (Sokoloff *et al.* 1977). Preliminary estimates indicate that the values are quite similar in the conscious monkey (C. Kennedy, O. Sakurada, M. Shinohara & L. Sokoloff, unpublished observations).

The λ, ϕ, and the enzyme kinetic constants are grouped together to constitute a single, lumped constant (see Equation [1]). It can be shown mathematically that this lumped constant is equal to the asymptotic value of the product of the ratio of the cerebral extraction ratios of [^{14}C]DG and glucose and the ratio of the arterial blood to plasma specific activities when the [^{14}C]DG concentration in arterial plasma is maintained constant. The lumped constant is also determined in a separate group of animals from arterial and cerebral venous blood samples drawn during a programmed intravenous infusion which produces and maintains a constant [^{14}C]DG concentration in arterial plasma (Sokoloff *et al.* 1977). Thus far this constant has been determined only in the albino rat and the monkey. Values are 0.483 (S.E.M. = $\pm$ 0.022) in the rat (Sokoloff *et al.* 1977) and 0.344 (S.E.M. = $\pm$ 0.036) in the monkey

(C. Kennedy *et al.*, unpublished observations). The lumped constant appears to be characteristic of the species and does not appear to change significantly in a wide range of conditions (Sokoloff *et al.* 1977).

Despite its complex appearance, Equation [1] is really nothing more than a general statement of the standard relationship by which rates of enzyme-catalysed reactions are determined from measurements made with radioactive tracers. The numerator of the equation represents the amount of radioactive product formed in a given interval of time; it is equal to C_i^*, the combined concentrations of [^{14}C]DG and [^{14}C]DG-6-P in the tissue at time, T, measured by the quantitative autoradiographic technique, less a term that represents the free unmetabolized [^{14}C]DG still remaining in the tissue. The denominator represents the integrated specific activity of the precursor pool times a factor, the lumped constant, which is equivalent to a correction factor for an isotope effect. The term with the exponential factor in the denominator takes into account the lag in the equilibration of the tissue precursor pool with the plasma.

Procedure

Because local rates of cerebral glucose utilization are calculated by means of Equation [1], this equation dictates the variables to be measured. The specific procedure employed is designed to evaluate these variables and to minimize potential errors that might occur in the actual application of the method. If the rate constants, k_1^*, k_2^*, and k_3^*, are precisely known, then Equation [1] is generally applicable with any mode of administration of [^{14}C]DG and for a wide range of time intervals. At present the rate constants have been determined only in the normal conscious rat. These rate constants can be expected to vary with the condition of the animal, however, and for the most accurate results they should be re-determined for each condition studied. The structure of Equation [1] suggests a more practicable alternative. All the terms in the equation that contain the rate constants approach zero with increasing time if the [^{14}C]DG is so administered that the plasma [^{14}C]DG concentration also approaches zero. From the values of the rate constants determined in normal animals and the usual time course of the clearance of [^{14}C]DG from the arterial plasma after a single intravenous pulse at zero time, an interval of 30–45 min is adequate for these terms to become sufficiently small for a considerable latitude in inaccuracies of the rate constants to be permissible without appreciably increased error in the estimates of local glucose consumption (Sokoloff *et al.* 1977). An additional advantage derived from the use of a single pulse of [^{14}C]DG, followed by a relatively long interval before the animal is killed for measurement of the concentration of ^{14}C in local tissue, is that by then most of the free [^{14}C]DG in the tissues has been either converted to [^{14}C]DG-6-P or transported back to the plasma; the optical densities in the autoradiographs then represent mainly the concentrations of [^{14}C]DG-6-P and, therefore, reflect directly the relative rates of glucose utilization in the various cerebral tissues.

The experimental procedure is to inject a pulse of [^{14}C]DG intravenously at zero time and to decapitate the animal at a measured time, T, 30–45 min later; in the interval timed arterial samples are taken for the measurement of plasma [^{14}C]DG and glucose concentrations. Tissue concentrations of ^{14}C, C_i^*, are measured at time, T, by the quantitative autoradiographic technique. Local cerebral glucose utilization is calculated by Equation [1] (Sokoloff *et al.* 1977).

LOCAL RATES OF GLUCOSE UTILIZATION IN THE RAT BRAIN

Thus far quantitative measurements of the local rates of cerebral utilization of glucose have been completed only in the albino rat. These values are presented in Table 1. The local rates of utilization of glucose in the normal conscious rat vary widely throughout the brain. The values in white structures tend to group together and are always considerably below those of grey structures. The average value in grey matter is about three times that of white matter, but the individual values vary from about 50 to 200 μmol glucose/(100 g min). The highest values are in the structures involved in auditory functions, with the inferior colliculus clearly the most metabolically active structure in the brain.

Local cerebral utilization of glucose in the normal conscious monkey is now being quantitatively determined in this laboratory, and the values will be reported soon. The results thus far indicate similar heterogeneity in the monkey brain to that in the rat, but the values are considerably lower, about one-third to one-half those in the rat, probably because of the lower cellular packing density and greater amounts of white matter (C. Kennedy *et al.*, unpublished observations).

In the albino rat thiopental (thiopentone sodium) anaesthesia reduces the rates of glucose utilization in all structures of the brain (Table 1). The effects are not uniform; the percentage effects in white matter are relatively small compared to those in most grey structures. Anaesthesia also markedly reduces the heterogeneity normally present within grey matter, an effect clearly visible in the autoradiographs (Sokoloff *et al.* 1977). These results are in agreement with those of previous studies in which anaesthesia has been found to decrease the cerebral metabolic rate of the brain as a whole (Kety 1950; Lassen 1959; Sokoloff 1976).

TABLE 1

Normal values for local cerebral utilization of glucose in the conscious and thiopental-anaesthetized albino rat* (from Sokoloff *et al.* 1977)

Structure	*Local cerebral utilization of glucose ($\mu mol\ 100\ g^{-1}\ min^{-1}$)*		*% Effect*
	Control (6)[a]	*Anaesthetized (8)*[a]	
	Grey matter		
Visual cortex	111 ± 5	64 ± 3	− 42
Auditory cortex	157 ± 5	81 ± 3	− 48
Parietal cortex	107 ± 3	65 ± 2	− 39
Sensory-motor cortex	118 ± 3	67 ± 2	− 43
Lateral geniculate body	92 ± 2	53 ± 3	− 42
Medial geniculate body	126 ± 6	63 ± 3	− 50
Thalamus: lateral nucleus	108 ± 3	58 ± 2	− 46
Thalamus: ventral nucleus	98 ± 3	55 ± 1	− 44
Hypothalamus	63 ± 3	43 ± 2	− 32
Caudate-putamen	111 ± 4	72 ± 3	− 35
Hippocampus: Ammon's horn	79 ± 1	56 ± 1	− 29
Amygdala	56 ± 4	41 ± 2	− 27
Cochlear nucleus	124 ± 7	79 ± 5	− 36
Lateral lemniscus	114 ± 7	75 ± 4	− 34
Inferior colliculus	198 ± 7	131 ± 8	− 34
Superior olivary nucleus	141 ± 5	104 ± 7	− 26
Superior colliculus	99 ± 3	59 ± 3	− 40
Vestibular nucleus	133 ± 4	81 ± 4	− 39
Pontine grey matter	69 ± 3	46 ± 3	− 33
Cerebellar cortex	66 ± 2	44 ± 2	− 33
Cerebellar nucleus	106 ± 4	75 ± 4	− 29
	White matter		
Corpus callosum	42 ± 2	30 ± 2	− 29
Genu of corpus callosum	35 ± 5	30 ± 2	− 14
Internal capsule	35 ± 2	29 ± 2	− 17
Cerebellar white matter	38 ± 2	29 ± 2	− 24

*Determined 30 min after pulse of [^{14}C]deoxyglucose.

[a]The values are the means ± standard errors obtained in the number of animals indicated in parentheses. All the differences are statistically significant at the $P < 0.05$ level.

RELATION BETWEEN LOCAL FUNCTIONAL ACTIVITY AND ENERGY METABOLISM

The results of a variety of applications of the method demonstrate a clear relationship between local functional activity and glucose consumption in the brain. The most striking demonstrations of the close coupling between function and energy metabolism are seen with experimentally induced local alterations in functional activity that are restricted to a few specific areas in the brain. The effects on local glucose consumption are then so pronounced that they are not only observed in the quantitative results but can also be seen directly on the autoradiographs which are really pictorial representations of the relative rates of glucose utilization in the various structural components of the brain.

Effects of increased functional activity

Effects of sciatic nerve stimulation. Electrical stimulation of one sciatic nerve in the rat under barbiturate anaesthesia causes pronounced increases in glucose

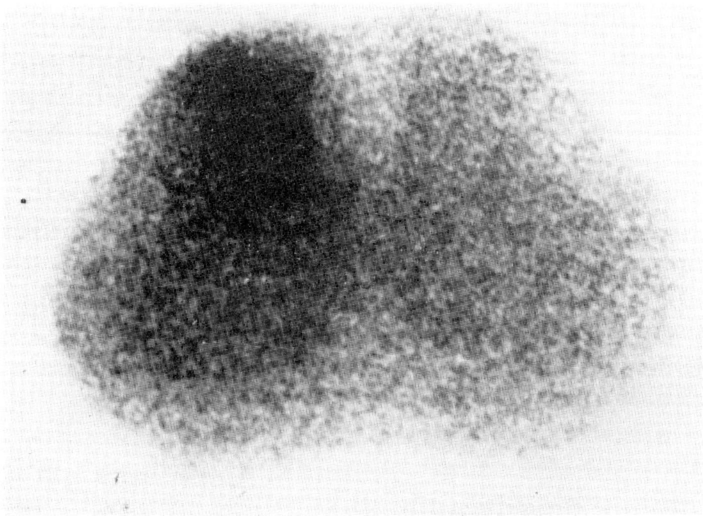

FIG. 1. Effects of unilateral electrical stimulation of the sciatic nerve on local utilization of glucose in the lumbar spinal cord of the anaesthetized rat. The illustration is an autoradiograph of a section of the lumbar spinal cord, which provides a pictorial representation of the relative rates of local glucose utilization in the tissues: the greater the optical density, the greater the rate of glucose utilization. Note the asymmetrical increased density in the region of the dorsal horn on the side ipsilateral to the stimulated nerve (from Kennedy *et al.* 1975.)

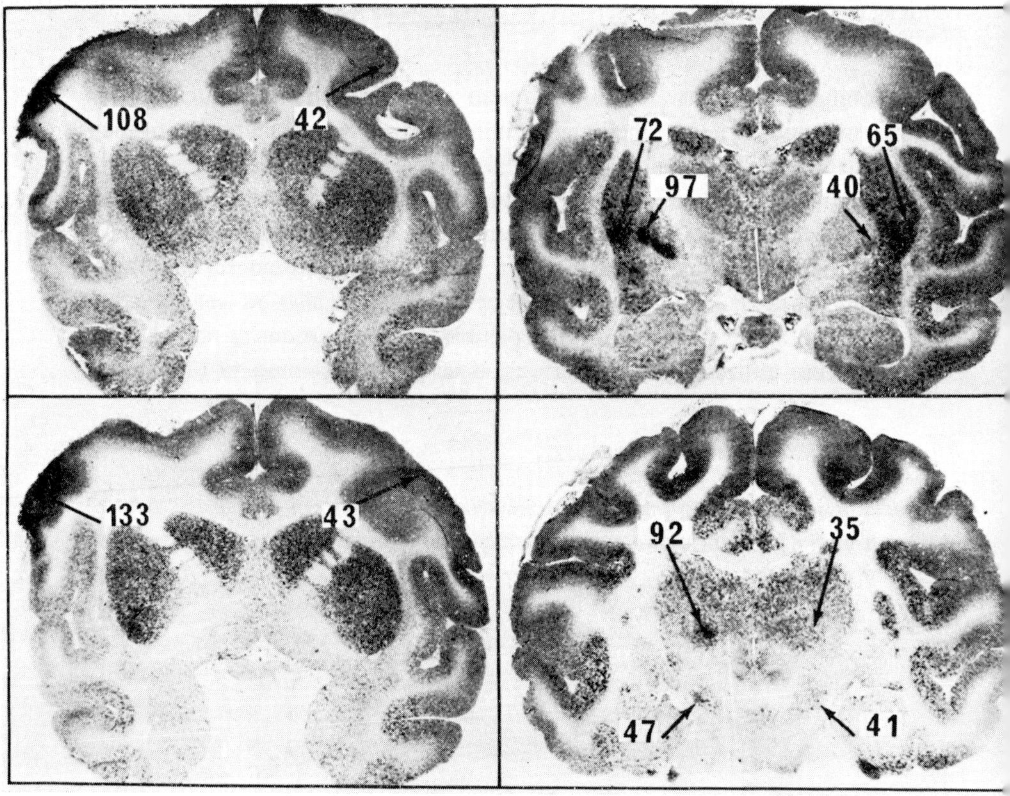

FIG. 2. Effects of local seizures produced by local application of penicillin to motor cortex on local cerebral utilization of glucose in the rhesus monkey. The penicillin was applied to the hand and face area of the left motor cortex. The left side of the brain is on the left in each of the autoradiographs in the figure. The numbers are the rates of local cerebral utilization of glucose in μmol (100 g tissue)$^{-1}$ min^{-1}. Note the following: *upper left*, motor cortex in region of penicillin application and corresponding region of contralateral motor cortex; *lower left*, ipsilateral and contralateral motor cortical regions remote from area of penicillin applications; *upper right*, ipsilateral and contralateral putamen and globus pallidus; *lower right*, ipsilateral and contralateral thalamic nuclei and substantia nigra. (From Kennedy *et al.* 1975.)

consumption (i.e. increased optical density in the autoradiographs) in the ipsilateral dorsal horn of the lumbar spinal cord (Fig. 1) (Kennedy *et al.* 1975).

Effects of experimental focal seizures. The local injection of penicillin into the hand–face area of the motor cortex of the rhesus monkey has been shown to induce electrical discharges in the adjacent cortex and to result in recurrent focal seizures involving the face, arm and hand on the contralateral side (Caveness 1969). Such seizure activity causes selective increases in glucose consumption in areas of motor cortex adjacent to the penicillin locus and in small discrete regions of the putamen, globus pallidus, caudate nucleus, thalamus and substantia nigra of the same side (Fig. 2) (Kennedy *et al.* 1975). Similar studies in the rat have led to comparable results and provided evidence on the basis of an evoked metabolic response of a 'mirror' focus in the motor cortex contralateral to the penicillin-induced epileptogenic focus (Collins *et al.* 1976).

Effects of decreased functional activity

Decrements in functional activity result in reduced rates of glucose utilization. These effects are particularly striking in the auditory and visual systems of the rat and the visual system of the monkey.

Effects of auditory deprivation. In the albino rat some of the highest rates of local cerebral utilization of glucose are found in components of the auditory system, i.e. auditory cortex, medial geniculate ganglion, inferior colliculus, lateral lemniscus, superior olive and cochlear nucleus (Table 1). The high metabolic activities of some of these structures are clearly visible in the autoradiographs (Fig. 3). Bilateral auditory deprivation by occlusion of both external auditory canals with wax markedly depresses the metabolic activity in all of these areas symmetrically on both sides (Fig. 3) (M. H. Des Rosiers, C. Kennedy & L. Sokoloff, unpublished observations). Unilateral auditory deprivation also depresses the glucose consumption of these structures but to a lesser degree, and some of the structures are asymmetrically affected. For example, it is the metabolic activity of the ipsilateral cochlear nucleus that is predominantly affected whereas the metabolic activity of the lateral lemniscus, superior olive and medial geniculate ganglion is reduced slightly more on the contralateral side. The contralateral inferior colliculus is markedly lower in metabolic activity than the ipsilateral structure (Fig. 3). These results demonstrate that there is some degree of lateralization and crossing of auditory pathways in the rat.

Visual deprivation in the rat. In the rat, the visual system is 80 to 85% crossed at the optic chiasma (Lashley 1934; Montero & Guillery 1968), and unilateral enucleation removes most of the visual input to the central visual structures of the contralateral side. In the conscious rat studied 24 h after unilateral enucleation, there are marked decrements in glucose utilization in

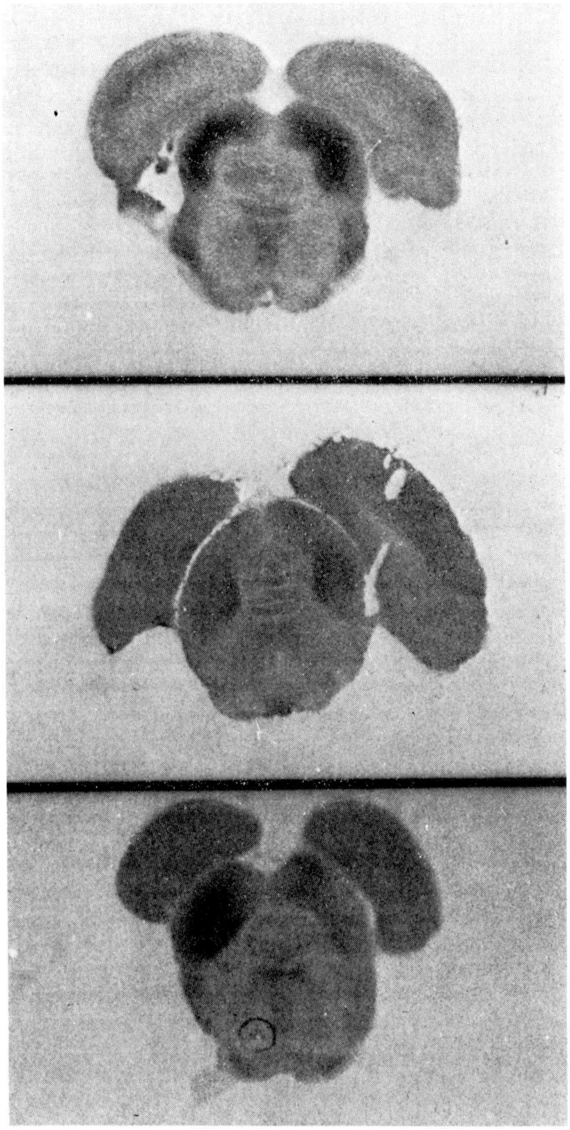

FIG. 3. Effects of auditory deprivation on cerebral glucose utilization of some components of the auditory system of the albino rat. *Upper*, autoradiograph of section of brain from normal conscious rat with intact bilateral hearing in ambient noise of laboratory. The autoradiograph shows the inferior colliculi, the lateral lemnisci and the superior olives, all of which exhibit bilateral symmetry of optical densities. *Middle*, autoradiograph of comparable section of brain from rat with external auditory canals bilaterally occluded with wax and kept in sound-proof room. Note the virtual disappearance of the inferior colliculi, lateral lemnisci and superior olives. *Lower*, autoradiograph of comparable section of brain from rat with one external auditory canal blocked. Note the asymmetry of the inferior colliculi, and the almost symmetrical intermediate reductions of densities in the lateral lemnisci and superior olives. The ear that was blocked was contralateral to the inferior colliculus that was markedly depressed. (From M. H. Des Rosiers, C. Kennedy & L. Sokoloff, unpublished observations.)

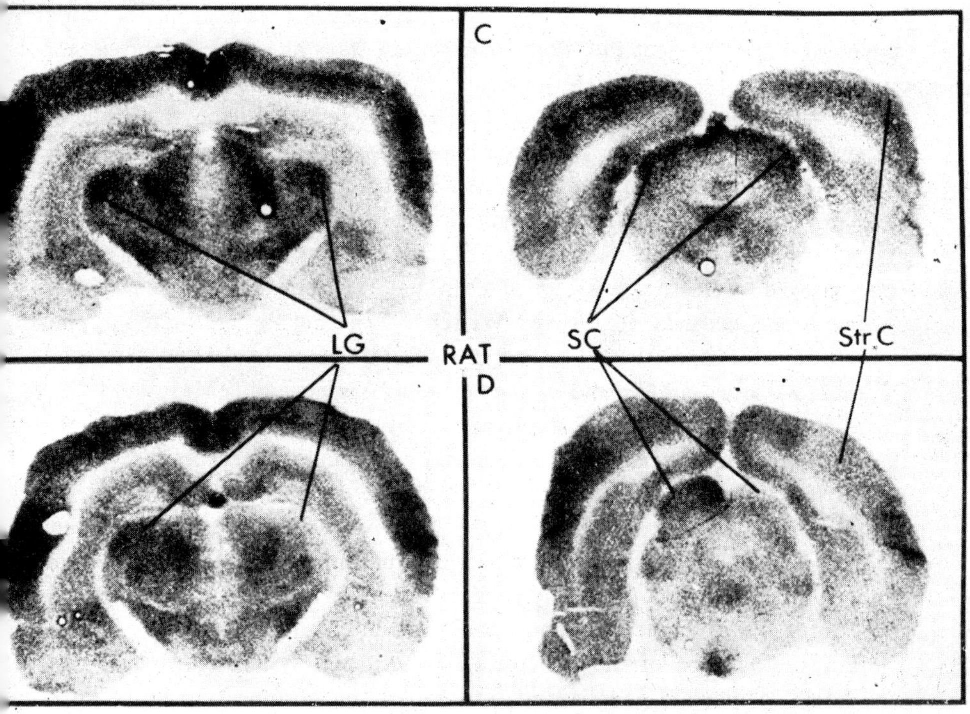

FIG. 4. Effects of unilateral enucleation on [^{14}C]deoxyglucose uptake in components of the visual system in the rat. In the normal rat with both eyes intact the uptakes in the lateral geniculate bodies (LG), superior colliculi (SC) and striate cortex (Str C) are approximately equal on both sides (A and C). In the unilaterally enucleated rat there are marked decreases in optical densities in the areas corresponding to these structures on the side contralateral to the enucleation (B and D). (From Kennedy *et al.* 1975.)

the contralateral superior colliculus, lateral geniculate ganglion and visual cortex as compared to the ipsilateral side (Fig. 4) (Kennedy *et al.* 1975). In the rat with both eyes intact, no asymmetry in the autoradiographs is observed (Fig. 4).

Visual deprivation in the monkey. In animals with binocular visual systems, such as the rhesus monkey, there is only about 50% crossing of the visual pathways, and the structures of the visual system on each side of the brain receive equal inputs from both retinas. Although each retina projects more or less equally to both hemispheres, their projections remain segregated and terminate in six well-defined laminae in the lateral geniculate ganglia, three each for the ipsilateral and contralateral eyes (Hubel & Wiesel 1968, 1972;

Wiesel *et al.* 1974; Rakic 1976). This segregation is preserved in the optic radiations which project the monocular representations of the two eyes for any segment of the visual field to adjacent regions of Layer IV of the striate cortex (Hubel & Wiesel 1968, 1972). The cells responding to the input of each monocular terminal zone are distributed transversely through the thickness of the striate cortex, resulting in a mosaic of columns, 0.3–0.5 mm in width, alternately representing the monocular inputs of the two eyes. The nature and distribution of these ocular dominance columns have previously been characterized by electrophysiological techniques (Hubel & Wiesel 1968), Nauta degeneration methods (Hubel & Wiesel 1972), and by autoradiographic visualization of axonal and transneuronal transport of [^{3}H]proline- and [^{3}H]fucose-labelled protein and/or glycoprotein (Wiesel *et al.* 1974; Rakic 1976). Bilateral or unilateral visual deprivation, either by enucleation or by the insertion of opaque plastic discs, produces consistent changes in the pattern of distribution of the rates of glucose consumption, all clearly visible in the autoradiographs; these changes coincide closely with the changes in functional activity expected from known physiological and anatomical properties of the binocular visual system (Kennedy *et al.* 1976).

In animals with intact binocular vision no bilateral asymmetry is seen in the autoradiographs of the structures of the visual system (Figs. 5A, 6A). The lateral geniculate ganglia and oculomotor nuclei appear to be of fairly uniform density and essentially the same on both sides (Fig. 5A). The visual cortex is also the same on both sides (Fig. 6A), but throughout all of Area 17 there is heterogeneous density distributed in a characteristic laminar pattern. These observations indicate that in animals with binocular visual input the rates of glucose consumption in the visual pathways are essentially equal on both sides of the brain and relatively uniform in the oculomotor nuclei and lateral geniculate ganglia, but markedly different in the various layers of the striate cortex.

Autoradiographs from animals with both eyes occluded exhibit generally decreased labelling of all components of the visual system, but the bilateral symmetry is fully retained (Figs. 5B, 6B), and the density within each lateral geniculate body is for the most part fairly uniform (Fig. 5B). In the striate cortex, however, the marked differences in the densities of the various layers seen in the animals with intact bilateral vision (Fig. 6A) are virtually absent so that, except for a faint delineation of a band within Layer IV, the concentration of the label is essentially homogeneous throughout the striate cortex (Fig. 6B).

Autoradiographs from monkeys with only monocular input (one eye occluded) exhibit markedly different patterns from those described above. Both lateral geniculate bodies exhibit exactly inverse patterns of alternating

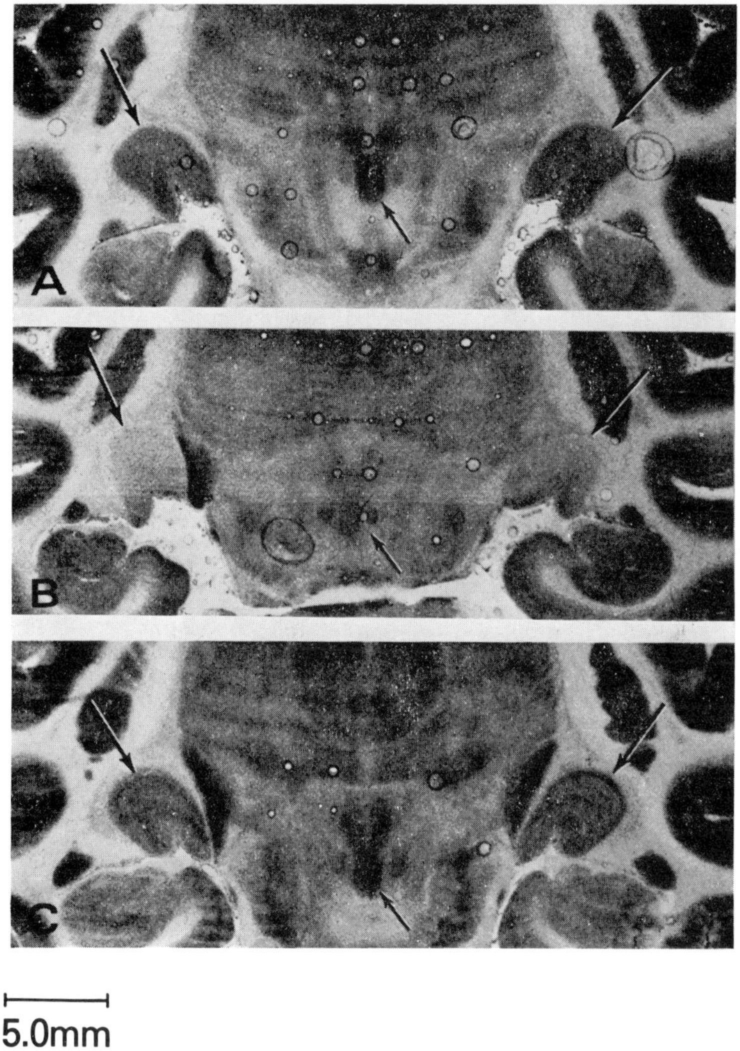

FIG. 5. Autoradiographs of coronal brain sections from rhesus monkeys at the level of the lateral geniculate bodies. Large arrows point to the lateral geniculate bodies; small arrows point to oculomotor nuclear complex. (A) *Animal with intact binocular vision.* Note the bilateral symmetry and relative homogeneity of the lateral geniculate bodies and oculomotor nuclei. (B) *Animal with bilateral visual occlusion.* Note the reduced relative densities, the relative homogeneity, and the bilateral symmetry of the lateral geniculate bodies and oculomotor nuclei. (C) *Animal with right eye occluded.* The left side of the brain is on the left side of the photograph. Note the laminae and the inverse order of the dark and light bands in the two lateral geniculate bodies. Note also the lesser density of the oculomotor nuclear complex on the side contralateral to the occluded eye. (From Kennedy *et al.* 1976.)

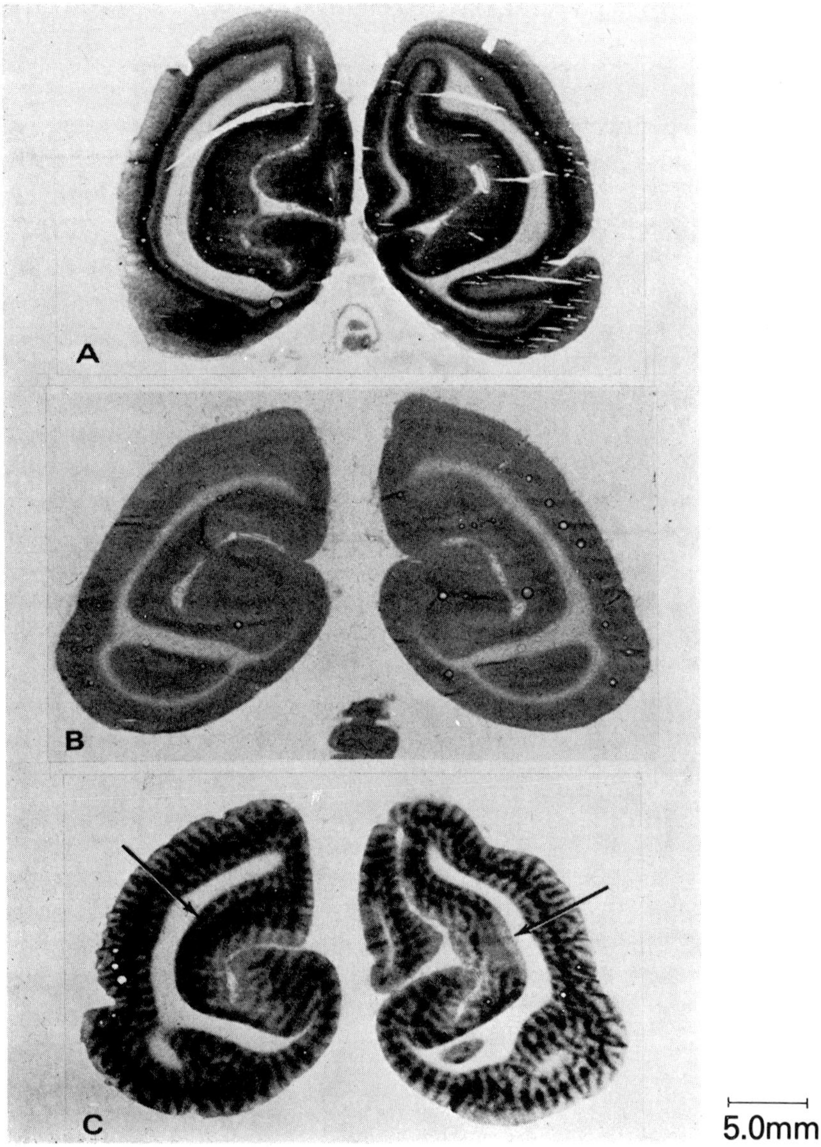

FIG. 6. Autoradiographs of coronal brain sections from rhesus monkeys at the level of the striate cortex. (A) *Animal with normal binocular vision.* Note the laminar distribution of the density; the dark band corresponds to Layer IV. (B) *Animal with bilateral visual deprivation.* Note the almost uniform and reduced relative density, especially the virtual disappearance of the dark band corresponding to Layer IV. (C) *Animal with right eye occluded.* The half-brain on the left side of the photograph represents the left hemisphere contralateral to the occluded eye. Note the alternate dark and light striations, each about 0.3 to 0.4 mm in width, representing the ocular dominance columns. These columns are most apparent in the dark lamina corresponding to Layer IV but extend through the entire thickness of the cortex. The arrows point to regions of bilateral asymmetry where the ocular dominance columns are absent. These are presumably areas with normally only monocular input. The one on the left, contralateral to the occluded eye, has a continuous dark lamina corresponding to Layer IV which is completely absent on the side ipsilateral to the occluded eye. These regions are believed to be the loci of the cortical representations of the blind spots. (From Kennedy *et al.* 1976.)

dark and light bands corresponding to the known laminae representing the regions receiving the different inputs from the retinas of the intact and occluded eyes (Fig. 5C). Bilateral asymmetry is also seen in the oculomotor nuclear complex; a lower density is apparent in the nuclear complex contralateral to the occluded eye (Fig. 5C). In the striate cortex the pattern of distribution of the [14C]DG-6-P appears to be a composite of the patterns seen in the animals with intact and bilaterally occluded visual input. The pattern in the former regularly alternates with that of the latter in columns oriented perpendicularly to the cortical surface (Fig. 6C). The dimensions, arrangement and distribution of these columns are identical to those of the ocular dominance columns described by Hubel and Wiesel (Hubel & Wiesel 1968, 1972; Wiesel *et al.* 1974). These columns reflect the interdigitation of the representations of the two retinas in the visual cortex. Each element in the visual fields is represented by a pair of contiguous bands in the visual cortex, one for each of the two retinas or their portions that correspond to the given point in the visual fields. With symmetrical visual input bilaterally, the columns representing the two eyes are equally active and, therefore, not visualized in the autoradiographs (Fig. 6A). When one eye is blocked, however, only those columns representing the blocked eye become metabolically less active, and the autoradiographs then display the alternate bands of normal and depressed activities corresponding to the regions of visual cortical representation of the two eyes (Fig. 6C).

In the autoradiographs from the animals with unilateral visual deprivation a pair of regions can be seen in the folded calcarine cortex that exhibit bilateral asymmetry (Fig. 6C). The ocular dominance columns are absent on both sides, but on the side contralateral to the occluded eye this region has the appearance of visual cortex from an animal with normal bilateral vision, and on the ipsilateral side this region looks like cortex from an animal with both eyes occluded (Fig. 6A, B). These regions are the loci of the cortical representation of the blind spots of the visual fields and normally have only monocular input (Kennedy *et al.* 1975, 1976). The area of the optic disc in the nasal half of each retina cannot transmit to this region of the contralateral striate cortex, which therefore receives its sole input from an area in the temporal half of the ipsilateral retina. Occlusion of one eye deprives this region of the ipsilateral striate cortex of all input while the corresponding region of the contralateral striate cortex retains uninterrupted input from the intact eye. The metabolic reflection of this ipsilateral monocular input is seen in the autoradiograph in Fig. 6C.

The results of these studies with the [14C]deoxyglucose method in the binocular visual system of the monkey demonstrate most dramatically the close

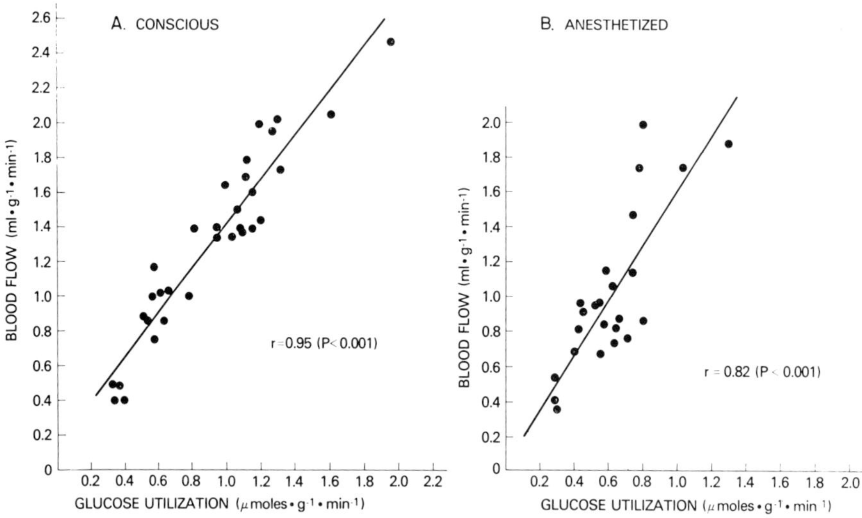

FIG. 7. Correlation between local cerebral blood flow, measured with the [^{14}C]iodoantipyrine technique (Sakurada *et al.* 1978), and local cerebral utilization of glucose, measured with the [^{14}C]deoxyglucose technique (Sokoloff *et al.* 1977). Each point represents a different structure in the brain. (A) *Normal conscious rat.* Each point represents the mean local glucose utilization obtained from 10 rats and the mean local blood flow obtained from 6 rats. (B) *Thiopental anaesthesia.* Each point represents the mean values of local glucose utilization and blood flow obtained from 8 animals and 6 animals, respectively. (From M. H. Des Rosiers, O. Sakurada, M. Shinohara, C. Kennedy, and L. Sokoloff, unpublished observations.)

relationship between physiological changes in functional activity and the rate of energy metabolism in specific components of the central nervous system.

RELATIONSHIP BETWEEN LOCAL ENERGY METABOLISM AND LOCAL BLOOD FLOW IN THE BRAIN

The availability of methods for measuring both glucose utilization and blood flow in individual discrete structural components of the brain has made it possible to examine directly the relationship between them. The results demonstrate that they are indeed closely related (Des Rosiers *et al.* 1974). In the normal conscious rat the coefficient of correlation between the rates of glucose utilization and blood flow in the various cerebral structures is equal to 0.95 ($P < 0.001$) (Fig. 7A). Thiopental anaesthesia reduces the rates of both metabolism and blood flow in almost all the structures, but the correlation, though reduced, still remains quite close ($r = 0.80$, $P < 0.001$) (Fig. 7B).

These results confirm that the individual cerebral structures are normally perfused more or less in proportion to their metabolic demands.

Not only do the rates of blood flow in the various structural components of the brain normally parallel the local rates of glucose consumption, but local blood flow is generally altered, just as local energy metabolism is, in response to changes in local functional activity. Local blood flow is measured with an autoradiographic technique like that of the [^{14}C]deoxyglucose technique that demonstrates the relative rates of blood flow in the various cerebral structures. These autoradiographs demonstrate that the same structures that exhibit changes in glucose utilization also exhibit comparable changes in blood flow in altered physiological states. For example, retinal stimulation with a photoflash produces increased blood flow in discrete regions of the visual cortex, lateral geniculate body and superior colliculus of the conscious cat (Sokoloff 1961). Unilateral enucleation in the rat reduces blood flow and glucose utilization contralaterally in these structures (Fig. 4); indeed the autoradiographs obtained with [^{14}C]antipyrine are then almost indistinguishable from those obtained with [^{14}C]deoxyglucose (M. H. Des Rosiers, unpublished observations). Focal seizures produced by the application of penicillin to the motor cortex in the monkey result in local increases in blood flow in the same structures that exhibit increased glucose consumption (Fig. 2) (Caveness *et al.* 1975).

It is clear from the results of the studies of local cerebral blood flow and glucose utilization that energy metabolism and functional activity are closely coupled in the nervous system and that local blood flow is distributed and adjusted in the cerebral tissues to local metabolic demand and thereby to local functional activity. The results fully confirm this hypothesis of Roy & Sherrington (1890), but the mechanisms responsible for the close coupling of these vital functions remain unknown.

ACKNOWLEDGEMENTS

The author wishes to express his appreciation to Mrs Ruth Bower for her excellent editorial and bibliographic assistance.

References

Bidder, T. G. (1968) Hexose translocation across the blood-brain interface: configurational aspects. *J. Neurochem. 15*, 867–874

Caveness, W. F. (1969) Ontogeny of focal seizures, in *Basic Mechanisms of the Epilepsies* (Jasper, H. H. *et al.*, eds.), pp. 517–534, Little, Brown, Boston

CAVENESS, W. F., UENO, H. & KEMPER, T. L. (1975) Subcortical factors in experimental Jacksonian seizures, in *Proc. 7th Int. Congr. Neuropathol.*, vol. 2 (Kornyey, S. *et al.*, eds.), pp. 29–34, I.C.S. No. 362, Excerpta Medica, Amsterdam

COLLINS, R. C., KENNEDY, C., SOKOLOFF, L. & PLUM, F. (1976) Metabolic anatomy of focal motor seizures. *Arch. Neurol. 33*, 536–542

DES ROSIERS, M. H., KENNEDY, C., PATLAK, C. S., PETTIGREW, K. D., SOKOLOFF, L. & REIVICH, M. (1974) Relationship between local cerebral blood flow and glucose utilization in the rat. *Neurology 24*, 389

ECKMAN, W. W., PHAIR, R. D., FENSTERMACHER, J. D., PATLAK, C. S., KENNEDY, C. & SOKOLOFF, L. (1975) Permeability limitation in estimation of local brain blood flow with [^{14}C]antipyrine. *Am. J. Physiol. 229*, 215–221

FREYGANG, W. H. Jr. & SOKOLOFF, L. (1958) Quantitative measurement of regional circulation in the central nervous system by the use of radioactive inert gas. *Adv. Biol. Med. Phys. 6*, 263–279

HERS, H. G. (1957) *Le Métabolisme du Fructose*, p. 102, Editions Arscia, Bruxelles

HUBEL, D. H. & WIESEL, T. N. (1968) Receptive fields and functional architecture of monkey striate cortex. *J. Physiol. (Lond.) 195*, 215–243

HUBEL, D. H. & WIESEL, T. N. (1972) Laminar and columnar distribution of geniculo-cortical fibers in the Macaque monkey. *J. Comp. Neurol. 146*, 421–450

KENNEDY, C., DES ROSIERS, M., JEHLE, J. W., REIVICH, M., SHARP, F. & SOKOLOFF, L. (1975) Mapping of functional neural pathways by autoradiographic survey of local metabolic rate with [^{14}C]deoxyglucose. *Science (Wash. D.C.) 187*, 850–853

KENNEDY, C., DES ROSIERS, M. H., SAKURADA, O., SHINOHARA, M., REIVICH, M., JEHLE, J. W. & SOKOLOFF, L. (1976) Metabolic mapping of the primary visual system of the monkey by means of the autoradiographic [^{14}C]deoxyglucose technique. *Proc. Natl. Acad. Sci. U.S.A. 73*, 4230–4234

KETY, S. S. (1950) Circulation and metabolism of the human brain in health and disease. *Am. J. Med. 8*, 205–217

KETY, S. S. (1957) The general metabolism of the brain *in vivo*, in *The Metabolism of the Nervous System* (Richter, D., ed.), pp. 221–237, Pergamon Press, London

KETY, S. S. (1960) Measurement of local blood flow by the exchange of an inert, diffusible substance. *Methods Med. Res. 8*, 228–236

LANDAU, W. M., FREYGANG, W. H. JR., ROWLAND, L. P., SOKOLOFF, L. & KETY, S. S. (1955) The local circulation of the living brain; values in the unanesthetized and anesthetized cat. *Trans. Am. Neurol. Assoc. 80*, 125–129

LASHLEY, K. S. (1934) The mechanism of vision. VII. The projection of the retina upon the primary optic centers of the rat. *J. Comp. Neurol. 59*, 341–373

LASSEN, N. A. (1959) Cerebral blood flow and oxygen consumption in man. *Physiol. Rev 39*, 183–238

MONTERO, V. M. & GUILLERY, R. W. (1968) Degeneration in the dorsal lateral geniculate nucleus of the rat following interruption of the retinal or cortical connections. *J. Comp. Neurol. 134*, 211–242

OLDENDORF, W. M. (1971) Brain uptake of radiolabeled amino acids, amines, and hexoses after arterial injection. *Am. J. Physiol. 221*, 1629–1638

RAKIC, P. (1976) Prenatal genesis of connections subserving ocular dominance in the rhesus monkey. *Nature (Lond.) 261*, 467–471

REIVICH, M., JEHLE, J., SOKOLOFF, L. & KETY, S. S. (1969) Measurement of regional cerebral blood flow with antipyrine-^{14}C in awake cats. *J. Appl. Physiol. 27*, 296–300

ROY, C. S. & SHERRINGTON, C. S. (1890) On the regulation of the blood supply of the brain *J. Physiol. (Lond.) 11*, 85–108

SAKURADA, O., KENNEDY, C., JEHLE, J., BROWN, J. D., CARBIN, G. L. & SOKOLOFF, L. (1978) Measurement of local cerebral blood flow with [^{14}C]iodoantipyrine, *Am. J. Physiol. 234*, H59–H66

SOKOLOFF, (1961) Local cerebral circulation at rest and during altered cerebral activity induced by anesthesia or visual stimulation, in *The Regional Chemistry, Physiology and Pharmacology of the Nervous System* (Kety, S. S. & Elkes, J., eds.), pp. 107–117, Pergamon Press, Oxford

SOKOLOFF, L. (1976) Circulation and energy metabolism of the brain, in *Basic Neurochemistry* (Siegel, G. J. *et al.*, eds.), 2nd edn., pp. 388–413, Little, Brown, Boston

SOKOLOFF, L., REIVICH, M., KENNEDY, C., DES ROSIERS, M. H., PATLAK, C. S., PETTIGREW, K. D., SAKURADA, O. & SHINOHARA, M. (1977) The [^{14}C]deoxyglucose method for the measurement of local cerebral glucose utilization: theory, procedure, and normal values in the conscious and anesthetized albino rat. *J. Neurochem. 28*, 897–916

SOLS, A. & CRANE, R. K. (1954) Substrate specificity of brain hexokinase. *J. Biol. Chem. 210*, 581–595

WIESEL, T. N., HUBEL, D. H. & LAM, D. M. K. (1974) Autoradiographic demonstration of ocular dominance columns in the monkey striate cortex by means of transneuronal transport. *Brain Res. 79*, 273–279

Discussion

Meldrum: What is the evidence that hexokinase activity consistently correlates with oxygen consumption?

Sokoloff: One of the requirements of the method is that the glucose metabolism be in a steady state. The net rate of each individual step of the glycolytic pathway is then equal to the rate of the overall pathway. In a steady state the net rate of the hexokinase-catalysed reaction is then equal to the rate of glucose consumption. In most circumstances oxygen and glucose are consumed in almost stoichiometric proportions and, therefore, their rates of utilization are very closely correlated. In starvation or other conditions associated with ketosis, the brain can use ketone bodies, at least in part, in place of glucose, and glucose consumption may then be reduced, even though oxygen consumption remains at a normal level. In most circumstances, however, there is adequate glucose in the blood and no ketosis. The correlation between oxygen consumption and glucose utilization (i.e. hexokinase-catalysed glucose phosphorylation) is then very close.

Meldrum: In a physiologically stable situation there will be a correlation. But during seizures or spreading depression one cannot assume that there is a close correlation between cerebral metabolic rate and hexokinase measurements.

Sokoloff: In the absence of a steady state the relationships among oxygen consumption, glucose utilization and glucose phosphorylation by hexokinase may be very loose and, perhaps, even non-existent transiently over short intervals of time. Over long periods of time, however, increased oxygen consumption will almost certainly reflect an average increase in the rate of glucose consumption and the average rate of glucose phosphorylation by hexokinase. This is what we see in seizures and in spreading depression, even though there is clearly no steady state in those conditions.

Siesjö: You mentioned the problems with the turnover of the free glucose pool, also that under normal conditions one can reduce the time after injection to 20 min. What would be the effect of decreasing or increasing glucose flux and of changing glucose concentration in the tissue; i.e., what times could be used then?

Sokoloff: Changes in the concentrations of free glucose in the plasma and tissues, whether caused by hyperglycaemia, hypoglycaemia, or changes in the rates of flux of glucose through the brain, can be expected to alter the rate constants for the turnover of the free glucose and [^{14}C]deoxyglucose pools in the brain tissue. The influence of the rate constants on the final result decreases progressively with increasing time after a pulse of [^{14}C]deoxyglucose. The rate constant for turnover and the half-life of the free pool are related by dividing either one into the natural logarithm of 2 to get the other. In the grey matter of the normal conscious rat, the half-life of the free [^{14}C]deoxyglucose pools equals approximately 2.5 min. We cannot, however, measure the half-life in each animal in which we are measuring local cerebral glucose utilization and must use a best estimate of its value. If we use 2.5 min as our best estimate and allow 45 min after the pulse of [^{14}C]deoxyglucose, then our values for local glucose utilization fall within $\pm$ 5% of the true value for actual half-lives of 0 to 5 min. We have determined this by means of simulation analyses. At 30 min the error is somewhat greater; the result then falls within $\pm$ 10% of the true value for the same range of half-lives. With increasing plasma and brain glucose concentrations, the rate constants should all decrease. We have, however, been unable to detect any systematic effects of plasma glucose concentration for the calculated rate of glucose utilization for plasma concentrations between 100 and 300 mg glucose/100 ml plasma. Above 330 mg/100 ml there is an effect, indicating that the rate constants have decreased too far from our best estimates and will have to be determined for the higher glucose concentrations.

Siesjö: What happens if you reduce the time to 20 min?

Sokoloff: If we know the rate constants accurately, then we can work just as well at 20 min. If we use the estimated pool half-life of 2.5 min then we may have errors of 10–20% for actual half-lives between 0 and 5 min.

Siesjö: If you decrease or increase glucose flux would you still be able to use 20 min instead of 45 min?

Sokoloff: Yes, if we have accurate values for the rate constants. If not, and we use the value of 2.5 min as the pool half-life, then there will be errors, the magnitude depending on how different the true half-life is from the 2.5 min. We can tolerate reduced half-lives better; the maximum reduction is from

2.5 min to 0 min, and the error at 20 min would then be close to 20%. Lengthening of the half-life can occur without limit, and the potential errors are then greater.

Siesjö: You got a beautiful correlation between metabolic rate and blood flow. Where there was high activity in layer 4 in the cortex what happened to the correlation with blood flow?

Sokoloff: We can't measure blood flow to layer 4 in the cortex. The resolution is not good enough. [^{14}C]Deoxyglucose gives better resolution than [^{14}C]iodoantipyrine because metabolism is a function of individual cells whereas blood flow supplies a whole region, not single cells. Theoretically it is not possible to get the same kind of resolution with a blood flow method as with a metabolism method.

Lübbers: We made flow measurements in rat brain which agree with what you found.

Raichle: The problem of timing is always an issue. One has to wait a long time to capture these events. You are giving a pulse of a tracer, so the major deposition of the tracer is in the early minutes. To what extent is your measurement really a weighted average towards that early time?

Sokoloff: It is weighted very heavily for the early times. Most of the [^{14}C]deoxyglucose-6-phosphate that is formed is accumulated in the first 15–20 min. It is for accurate quantification that the long interval is required, i.e. to allow unmetabolized [^{14}C]deoxyglucose to clear from the tissues and mainly to minimize the effects of any inaccuracies in the estimated value for the free pool half-life. In the first 15 min we can find most of the autoradiographic resolution.

Plum: It would be helpful if you could calculate, at several different rates of metabolism, the error per unit time. That is, the error is a log declining error per unit time, with a pulse injection. So would the error be about 30% in 5 min?

Sokoloff: At 5 min the error can be several hundred per cent. The shorter the time, the more critical it is to have accurate values for the rate constants and the pool half-life.

Siesjö: Could you calculate error against time at different metabolic rates and at different glucose concentrations? That would provide very useful information to all of us who want to use the method.

Sokoloff: If we only use a short time, the half-life of the pool becomes a critical factor. If we know the half-life of the pool precisely, then we could use as short a time as one might want. But we don't know the half-life in the particular animal that we are studying and, therefore, we prefer to allow enough time to minimize the influence of the half-life on the final results.

The shorter the time, the greater the error, because of the greater effect of any discrepancy between the estimated and true precursor pool half-lives. That is why we prefer the longer times, because the influence of the pool half-life declines with increasing time. If one uses an estimated pool half-life of 2.5 min and the true half-life is between 0 and 5 min, then the error can be estimated to be within about 5% at 45 min, 10% at 30 min, and 20% at 20 min. If this error is too great, or if the pool half-life is expected to increase beyond 5 min, then the error can be reduced by experimental redetermination of the pool half-life in another series of experiments. At any time the errors can be expected to be higher the lower the metabolic rate, merely because the lower the amount of product accumulated, the greater the measurement errors (e.g. densitometric measurement of tissue concentration).

Purves: Are you reasonably certain that at 30 min you are going to get adequate bunching under all conditions that you might meet?

Sokoloff: No. I am certain that there are conditions for which the rate constants will have to be redetermined. Those that we use are for rats in or near the normal state.

Raichle: To what extent does the half-life vary with changing levels of blood glucose? Would you expect it to deviate substantially, as you have shown here?

Sokoloff: Yes, I would expect it to vary with the plasma glucose level. If the plasma glucose level is increased, and the rate of glucose consumption remains the same, then the half-life is going to be increased more or less proportionately, depending on the exact change in the size of the free tissue pool itself. Although we determined the rate constants for normal conscious animals, we are not compelled to use those values for all conditions. For half-lives remaining within the range of 0 to 5 min, we can use the 45-min, or even the 30-min interval, with tolerable errors. For greater changes in half-lives, we can always redetermine the rate constants for the condition of interest.

Purves: What would happen if you changed the plasma volume, for example in hypoxia, where your tissue pool might remain relatively constant?

Sokoloff: The k_1 and k_2 values incorporate within them the effects of blood flow, and so if we changed the blood flow, we could also change the values for these constants and the half-life of the pool.

Purves: Would you still be able to make the same kind of prediction that you ought to be able to make at 20 min plus?

Sokoloff: Yes, with increases in blood flow. I am not certain how much of a decrease in blood flow can be tolerated. We haven't really tested the extremes. In the non-pathological states that we have been studying, 0.5 to

5 min for the pool half-life is a realistic range, and the error limits are as I described previously. I don't know what would happen in pathological states, for example in an infarcted region or something like that.

McDowall: You showed us that with thiopentone there was a reduction in overall activity. But the sort of stimulation you were using is rather resistant to anaesthesia. In your anaesthetized animals did you look at glucose metabolism, with stimulation, and does it still relate to flow or is there some breakdown of the relationship?

Sokoloff: I don't know whether it is still related to flow. However, D. Hubel & T. Wiesel (personal communication, 1977), who are now using the method, are using various stimulations of the visual system in lightly anaesthetized animals. Their autoradiographs show the effects of the stimulation as well as or probably even better than ours.

McDowall: So there is still the same activation of these local cortical areas related to the pattern of afferent input under thiopentone anaesthesia?

Sokoloff: Yes.

Rosendorff: You showed the relationship between glucose utilization and blood flow in conscious and anaesthetized animals. Glucose consumption in the anaesthetized animals seemed somewhat higher than in the conscious animals. Are these slopes statistically significantly different?

Sokoloff: The slopes probably are different. The effects of anaesthesia on blood flow were less than the effect on glucose utilization, possibly because of changes in the arterial P_{CO_2}.

Purves: What limit of resolution has been reached with this method? Can you identify a hypercomplex cell?

Sokoloff: No. In theory this method could be used to measure the glucose consumption of a single cell. But there is a large gap between theory and practice. The main problem is that deoxyglucose-6-phosphate is water-soluble. At present we section the brains in a frozen state, and during freezing there is some distortion with some movement of the water-soluble molecules. There is not enough distortion to bother us seriously at the present level of resolution, but even now not all of our autoradiographs are equally good. The distortion is probably serious enough, however, to allow some movement of the deoxyglucose-6-phosphate over a distance of several microns. That is enough to prevent us from identifying the origin of radioactivity from particular cell bodies. The solution, we think, is to find some means of perfusing the brain with a chemical agent that will chemically bond the deoxyglucose-6-phosphate to a protein. Then we could go ahead with dehydration, fixation and staining procedures without moving the label from the cells. It is a technical problem but one that might be soluble.

Owman: Let me remind you of an interesting aspect related to the studies on visual activation, cerebral blood flow and its neurogenic control. In the rat, at least, there is a direct connection between the eye and the superior cervical sympathetic ganglion by a neural pathway running via an accessory optical tract and the median forebrain bundle to the brain-stem and upper thoracic spinal cord, from which preganglionic neurons reach the superior cervical. This ganglion innervates the pineal (Ariëns Kappers 1960), and it is the pathway through which external lighting conditions influence certain rhythmic biochemical changes in the gland (Wurtman *et al.* 1968). This is also precisely the ganglion which innervates the brain vessels. There is thus an anatomical possibility that the brain vessels could also be influenced by light stimuli through this neural pathway. It would be interesting to see whether interruption of the pathway interferes with the pattern of changed metabolism and flow in regions related to the visual system. In any event, this neuronal link has not been sufficiently taken into account in discussions of reflex mechanisms influencing the brain circulation: the superior cervical ganglion is unique among the sympathetic ganglia in that it directly receives external light impulses, and it happens to be the ganglion which alone supplies the brain circulation with its extrinsic adrenergic innervation. There is a very clear diurnal rhythmicity in cerebral haemodynamics (Edvinsson *et al.* 1973).

Sokoloff: Is the suprachiasmatic nucleus involved in this pathway?

Owman: Yes, it is.

Sokoloff: Dr William Schwartz (personal communication, 1977) has found a diurnal rhythm in the glucose utilization of the suprachiasmatic nucleus which appears to be entrained by light. This may be related to your observations.

Moskowitz: The superior cervical ganglion also innervates iris muscle and can thereby regulate the diameter of the pupil. This ganglion controls the amount of light that strikes the retina and can influence activity within the occipital cortex and pineal organ; it ultimately feeds back on itself via the sympathetic nerve system.

Rubio: You see incorporation of label into brain cells with increased function—is this due strictly to the increased supply of deoxyglucose?

Sokoloff: There is increased phosphorylation of [^{14}C]deoxyglucose which in turn reflects an increased rate of glucose consumption.

Purves: But is it flow-independent?

Sokoloff: Yes, at 45 min it is largely flow-independent but if we used short times, then we wouldn't be able to separate out the effects of blood flow and metabolism.

Reis: In the functional studies you must maintain the stimulus for 45 min. How long do you flash the light?

Sokoloff: In the monkey studies we stimulated by means of an illuminated, rotating, geometric black and white pattern around the monkey's head. We started the illumination and rotation about 5 min before the pulse of [^{14}C]-deoxyglucose, and continued them throughout the study.

Reis: So for any pathway mapping you have to give a very prolonged stimulation?

Sokoloff: It is only for accurate quantification that we use a long time. If we just wanted to see the autoradiograph, we could probably get away with a much shorter time. Most of the deoxyglucose-6-phosphate is formed in the first 15 min. The rest of the time we are waiting for the unmetabolized deoxyglucose to disappear.

Plum: To study this problem, Collins (1976) used quantitative histochemistry of the epileptic and the mirror focus coupled with relatively short-term radio-autographs of 2-deoxyglucose. During the repetitive spike discharge induced by focal injection of penicillin into rat cortex, Collins observed increased uptake of 2-deoxyglucose in both the seizure focus and the mirror focus. ATP decreased in both the seizure focus and, to a lesser extent, the mirror focus. During the appearance of spikes with after-discharge, lactate rose even more in the seizure focus and in the homotypic mirror focus as well.

Sokoloff: I have been talking about an autoradiographic method which doesn't discriminate between [^{14}C]deoxyglucose-6-phosphate and free [^{14}C]-deoxyglucose. We could dissect out pieces of the brain and separate and measure the [^{14}C]deoxyglucose-6-phosphate and free deoxyglucose chemically. This might allow some shortening of the time period.

References

Ariëns Kappers, J. (1960) The development, topographical relations and innervation of the epiphysis cerebri in the albino rat. *Z. Zellforsch. 52*, 163–215

Collins, R. C. (1976) Metabolic response to focal penicillin seizures in rat: spike discharge vs. afterdischarge. *J. Neurochem. 27*, 1473–1482

Edvinsson, L., Nielsen, K. C. & Owman, Ch. (1973) Diurnal rhythm in cerebral blood volume of mice. *Experientia (Basel) 29*, 432–433

Wurtman, R. J., Axelrod, J. & Kelly, D. E. (1968) *The Pineal*, Academic Press, New York

Coupling of cerebral metabolism and blood flow in epileptic seizures, hypoxia and hypoglycaemia

B. NILSSON, S. REHNCRONA and B. K. SIESJÖ

MRC Cerebral Metabolism Group and Departments of Neurology and Neurosurgery, University of Lund, Lund

Abstract This study examines the possibility that changes of cerebral extracellular pH (pH_e) or adenosine concentration may provide coupling mechanisms of a general nature, adjusting cerebral blood flow (CBF) to metabolic demands.

Although there is considerable indirect evidence that CBF varies inversely with pH_e, results obtained during the last few years indicate that large increases in flow may occur in the absence of a fall in pH_e. Thus, induction of hypoxia or epileptic seizures leads to maximal increase in CBF before pH_e falls or even when there is initial alkalosis due to concomitant hypocapnia. Furthermore, CBF increases in hypoglycaemia and after administration of amphetamine, two conditions unassociated with tissue acidosis.

The possibility that adenosine may be a coupling factor was examined in hypoxia and during epileptic seizures in rats. In both conditions a four- to fivefold increase in CBF occurs in spite of the fact that tissue adenosine concentrations remain at or below 1 μmol kg^{-1}. It is concluded that adenosine accumulates first when there is a perturbation of cerebral energy state with a rise in AMP concentration. It seems unlikely that adenosine, formed by breakdown of AMP, acts as a general coupling factor.

In spite of considerable investigative effort there is little precise information on factors that couple cerebral metabolism and blood flow. It has been assumed that the homeostatic regulation of cerebral blood flow (CBF) in various states of cerebral activity or in conditions of reduced oxygen or substrate availability generally occurs by feedback control, with the appropriate signals emanating from a perturbation of cellular metabolism. Among the possible coupling factors involved the extracellular activities of H^+, K^+ and adenosine have attracted the largest attention.

There is much evidence that the extracellular pH is an important regulator of CBF (see Lassen 1968; Betz 1972). First, the fact that hypercapnia promptly dilates cerebral vessels, while non-respiratory plasma acidosis does not, suggests that H^+ ions released at the tissue side of the blood-brain barrier have an effect. Supportive evidence is provided by the vasodilatation occurring in hypoxia or ischaemia, both conditions being accompanied by tissue lactic acidosis. Second, continuous measurements of extracellular pH and regional CBF demonstrate a parallelism between a fall in pH and increase in CBF (e.g. Betz & Heuser 1967). Third, microapplication of solutions with varying pH to pial vessels demonstrates an inverse relationship between pH and vessel dilatation (Kuchinsky *et al.* 1972).

The hypothesis that the extracellular K^+ activity acts as a coupling factor is supported by microapplication studies. It is also of interest that enhanced neuronal activity is accompanied by release of K^+. Inherent in this hypothesis is the assumption that Na^+–K^+-ATPase activity is insufficient to keep K^+ ions within the cells during hypoxia and ischaemia, a compensatory vasodilatation thus being elicited by an increase of extracellular K^+ activity (see Betz 1972).

Recently, evidence has been presented that adenosine is a potent vasodilator in the brain. Again, this evidence appears from the results of microapplication studies (Wahl & Kuchinsky 1976). However, it has also been reported that tissue adenosine concentrations are increased in hypoxia and during electrical stimulation of the cerebral cortex, both conditions being accompanied by marked vasodilatation (Rubio *et al.* 1975). It is implied that increased metabolic activity or reduced oxygen supply leads to enhanced dephosphorylation of AMP to adenosine, and to translocation of adenosine to the extracellular fluid.

The objective of the present studies was to explore the possibility that extracellular H^+ or adenosine activities provide coupling mechanisms of a more general nature, thus explaining the increase of CBF during states of increased metabolic rate or when there is reduced supply to the brain of oxygen or substrate. Another paper (Astrup *et al.*, this volume) will give further details of extracellular pH, and of the extracellular K^+ activity, in these conditions.

MEASUREMENTS OF CBF AND CEREBRAL METABOLIC RATE

The experiments to be reported here were performed on male Wistar rats that were initially anaesthetized with 2–3% halothane and later maintained artificially ventilated on 30% O_2/70% N_2O with control of body temperature, blood pressure and arterial P_{O_2}, P_{CO_2} and pH. For measurements of cerebral metabolites by means of enzymic, fluorometric analyses, the tissue was frozen *in situ* (see Norberg & Siesjö 1975, 1976). Adenosine was measured in perchloric acid extracts using high-pressure liquid chromatography (Nordström *et al.* 1977).

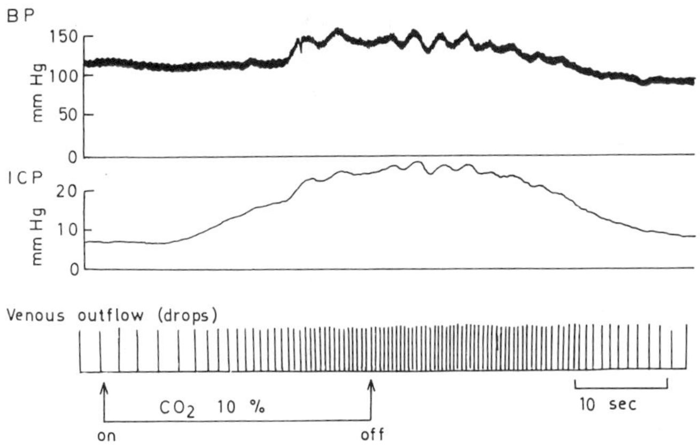

FIG. 1. Responses of blood pressure (BP), cisterna magna pressure (ICP) and cerebral venous outflow in male Wistar rats to inhalation of 10% CO_2 for 30 s. The on–off markings denote the period of admixture of CO_2 to the gas mixture delivered to the respirator, involving a time lag of 5–10 s before actual inhalation of CO_2. Arterial P_{CO_2} at 'on', 32 mmHg; at 'off' 58 mmHg.

Values for CBF and cerebral oxygen consumption (CMR_{O_2}) were obtained with a ^{133}Xe modification of the Kety & Schmidt (1948) technique, using either the superior sagittal sinus or one retroglenoid vein for sampling of cerebral venous blood (Norberg & Siesjö 1974; Nilsson & Siesjö 1976). These methods give values representing cerebral cortex and whole brain, respectively. The CBF was calculated from the arterial and venous ^{133}Xe desaturation curves. Measurements of arterial and cerebral venous oxygen contents allowed CMR_{O_2} to be calculated. A third CBF method allowed transient changes in CBF (and CMR_{O_2}) to be estimated. In this method the outflow of cerebral venous blood from one retroglenoid vein was monitored with a drop recorder in a closed circuit where blood was returned via the external jugular vein. During the measurements the contralateral retroglenoid vein was occluded but no other venous collaterals were interfered with. The characteristics of the method are illustrated in Fig. 1, which shows arterial blood pressure and cisterna magna pressure (ICP) as well as venous outflow during a short-lasting period of hypercapnia. Methodological studies (Nilsson & Siesjö 1978) show that the 'CMR_{O_2}' calculated from the venous outflow volume and the arteriovenous differences of oxygen content (AVD_{O_2}) (venous samples taken from the outflow cannula) remains essentially constant during changes of up to 10-fold in CBF induced by variations in arterial P_{CO_2}. This indicates that the venous drainage recorded in the individual preparation represents a relatively constant mass of tissue despite wide variations in CBF. Furthermore, the CBF response during variations in arterial blood pressure was compatible with normal autoregulation. Fig. 1 further demonstrates that changes in ICP occur in parallel with the changes in CBF, indicating the possibility of using ICP measurements to follow the time course of rapid cerebral vasomotor changes. From the venous outflow recording, and AVD_{O_2} determinations, CBF, cerebrovascular resistance (CVR) and CMR_{O_2} can be expressed in conventional terms according to the following procedure. (1) Using an experimentally derived diagram, relating number of drops/min to venous outflow in ml/min, the outflow volume is calculated. (2) Steady-state measurements of CBF and CMR_{O_2}, using the ^{133}Xe technique with the retroglenoid vein for sampling, show that CMR_{O_2} under control conditions is 7.6 ml 100 g^{-1} min^{-1} (Nilsson & Siesjö 1976). If this figure applies to the individual animal, and if AVD_{O_2} is known, a control CBF value can be calculated ($7.6/AVD_{O_2}$) which corresponds to the actual venous outflow volume calculated according to (1) at the time of AVD_{O_2} determination. (3) From the CBF value, and the cerebral perfusion pressure (CPP=mean arterial blood pressure — ICP), CVR can be conventionally derived.

GENERAL RELATIONSHIP BETWEEN METABOLIC RATE AND CBF

In general there is a tight correlation between metabolic rate and CBF. Fig. 2 illustrates steady-state data obtained in rats that were normocapnic or (in hyperthermia and hypothermia) maintained at constant arterial pH. A decrease in CMR_{O_2} during anaesthesia or hypothermia is accompanied by a fall in CBF, while hyperthermia, immobilization stress, and epileptic seizures induce an increase in CMR_{O_2} and CBF. In contrast, CBF increases with little or no change in CMR_{O_2} during hypercapnia, hypoxia and pronounced insulin-induced hypoglycaemia (Norberg & Siesjö 1974, 1976; Jóhannsson & Siesjö 1975; Nilsson & Siesjö 1976).

In the present studies we have analysed the relationship between cerebral metabolism and CBF in one condition of vasodilatation coupled to a high metabolic rate (epileptic seizures), and in another two without a corresponding rise in metabolic rate (hypoxia and hypoglycaemia). Fig. 2 shows that various types of epileptic seizures have different influences on the metabolic and circulatory response. The present studies mainly deal with seizures induced by intravenous injection of bicuculline (Meldrum & Nilsson 1976; Borgström *et al.* 1976; Chapman *et al.* 1977).

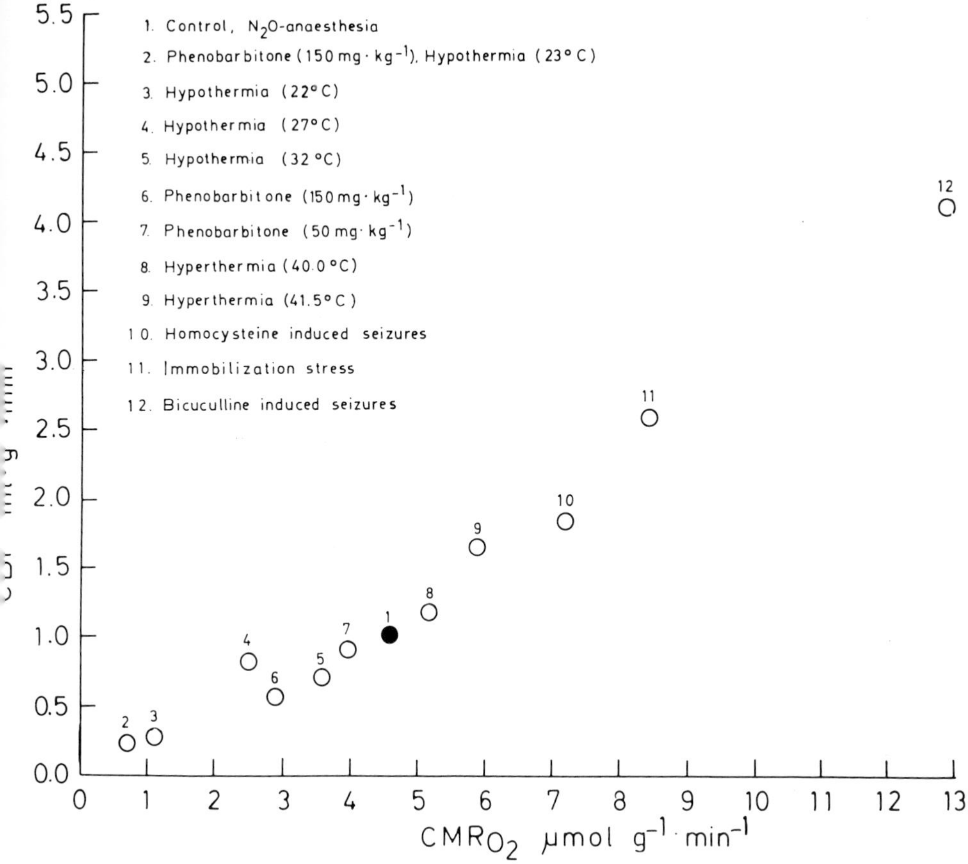

FIG. 2. Cerebral blood flow (CBF) in relation to cerebral metabolic rate for oxygen ($CMRo_2$) in various situations with different $CMRo_2$ values (steady state). The data were obtained from: 1, Norberg & Siesjö 1974; 2, Nordström & Rehncrona 1977; 3, 4, 5, Hägerdal *et al.* 1975; 6, 7, Nilsson & Siesjö 1975; 8, 9, Carlsson *et al.* 1976; 10, Blennow *et al.* 1976; 11, Carlsson *et al.* 1977; and 12, Meldrum & Nilsson 1976.

CEREBRAL BLOOD FLOW AND METABOLISM IN EPILEPTIC SEIZURES

Measurements of CBF and $CMRo_2$ during steady-state and transient changes of bicuculline-induced status epilepticus have been reported previously (Meldrum & Nilsson 1976). Further measurements have been made to analyse cerebrovascular changes in more detail, and to study flow and metabolic rate under conditions in which the seizure response was modified by hypoglycaemia, hypoxia or ischaemia (see Nilsson *et al.* 1977; Blennow *et al.* 1977).

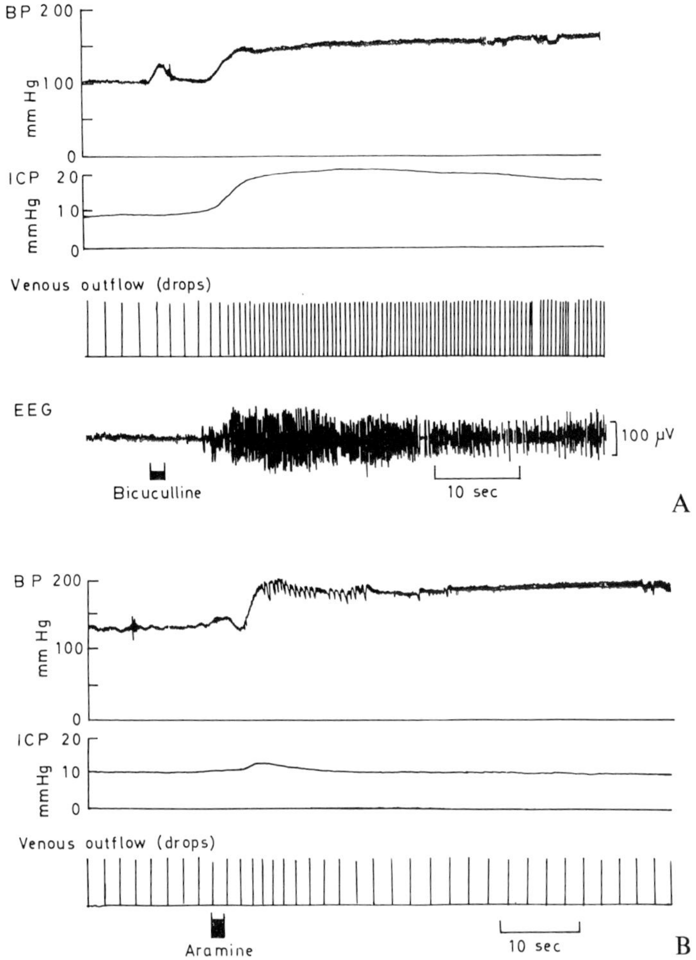

FIG. 3. A. Responses of BP, ICP and cerebral venous outflow at onset of seizure activity induced by i.v. injection of bicuculline, 1.2 mg kg^{-1} (bolus effect of the injection seen in the BP curve).
B. ICP and cerebral venous outflow during BP increase due to i.v. injection of metaraminol (Aramine, Merck, Sharp, and Dohme), 1 mg kg^{-1}.

Fig. 3A shows a typical CBF response to i.v. bicuculline (1.2 mg kg^{-1}) in an artificially ventilated, fed rat. Venous outflow (and ICP) increases *pari passu* with the appearance of the first spikes in the electroencephalogram (EEG) and reaches values four to six times normal within 15–20 s. Calculations of CVR indicate that maximal vasodilatation occurs within this period. In the

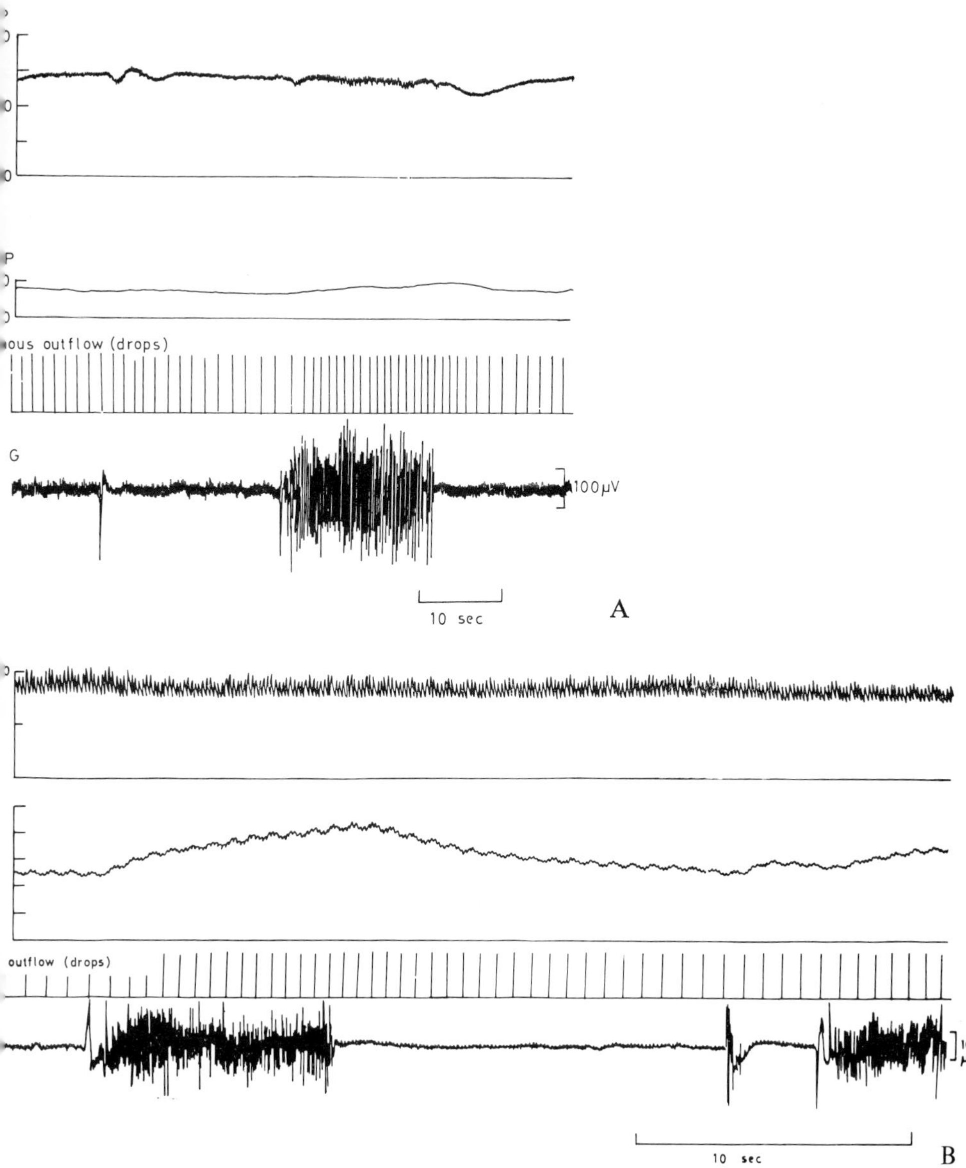

FIG. 4. BP, ICP and cerebral venous outflow during bursts-suppression pattern, after bicuculline-induced seizure activity. Record A is from an animal starved for 24 h before the experiment; hence hypoglycaemia that develops during epilepsy leads to depletion of cellular glucose and prevents increase of lactate (see Blennow *et al.* 1977). Record B is from an unstarved animal, prepared with transection of the cervical cord and occlusion of the spinal canal at the level of C-2. The ICP recording reflects the vasomotor response in the closed intracranial – C-2 space.

intact animal there is a precipitous increase in blood pressure and it may be questioned to what extent CPP influences the vasomotor response. However, as Fig. 3B shows, a similar increase in blood pressure induced by i.v. metaraminol (Aramine) produces only a small transient rise in CBF and no increase in ICP. Furthermore, a rapid decrease in CVR also occurred when the rise in blood pressure was blocked by transection of the cervical spinal cord at the level of C-2 (cf. Plum *et al.* 1968). Finally, it was found that during the burst-and-suppression EEG pattern, especially in hypoglycaemic animals (Fig. 4A) and after cord transection (Fig. 4B), each burst was accompanied by a rapid vasodilatation. These recordings show that vasodilatation followed the appearance of epileptic activity with a lag of 1 s or less.

Analyses of cerebral metabolic events during bicuculline-induced seizures (see Chapman *et al.* 1977) gave the result that (maximal) vasodilatation preceded the appearance of net tissue acidosis. Thus, although tissue lactate concentrations rose steadily during the first minute of seizure activity there was a simultaneous fall in P_{CO_2} of sufficient magnitude to induce a transient *rise* in calculated intracellular pH. Subsequent application of microelectrodes for measuring cerebral extracellular pH gave an identical result (see Astrup *et al.*, this symposium). Finally, freezing of tissue through the intact dura and analysis of total CO_2 content in superficial cortical tissue failed to indicate that acidosis developed during the first 30–60 s of seizure activity, i.e. at a time when vasodilatation was already maximal (Nilsson *et al.* 1976).

Thus, analyses of transient CBF and cerebral metabolic changes reveal a lack of coupling between CBF and tissue pH. In the steady state acidosis might well help to maintain a raised CBF. However, other results indicate that this influence may not be large. Thus, during seizures induced by homocysteine there is a more pronounced lactic acidosis than after bicuculline but CBF rises to only about 170% of control (Blennow *et al.* 1976).

The results prompted a study of changes in tissue concentrations of adenosine during induced seizures. Animals were injected with bicuculline during continuous recording of EEG and the brains were frozen through the exposed skull bone either 10 s or 20 min after injection. Since seizures started about 7 s after drug administration, freezing started after 3 s of seizure activity. However, epileptic activity must have continued for a longer period since it takes 10–15 s to freeze the tissue used for analyses. Fig. 5 shows that there was already a rise in lactate and a fall in phosphocreatine concentration in the '10 s' group. As previously reported (Chapman *et al.* 1977), seizures were accompanied by only a small decrease in energy charge. It is observed that there was no change in tissue adenosine concentration, a result compatible with the fact that the AMP concentration did not change (see below).

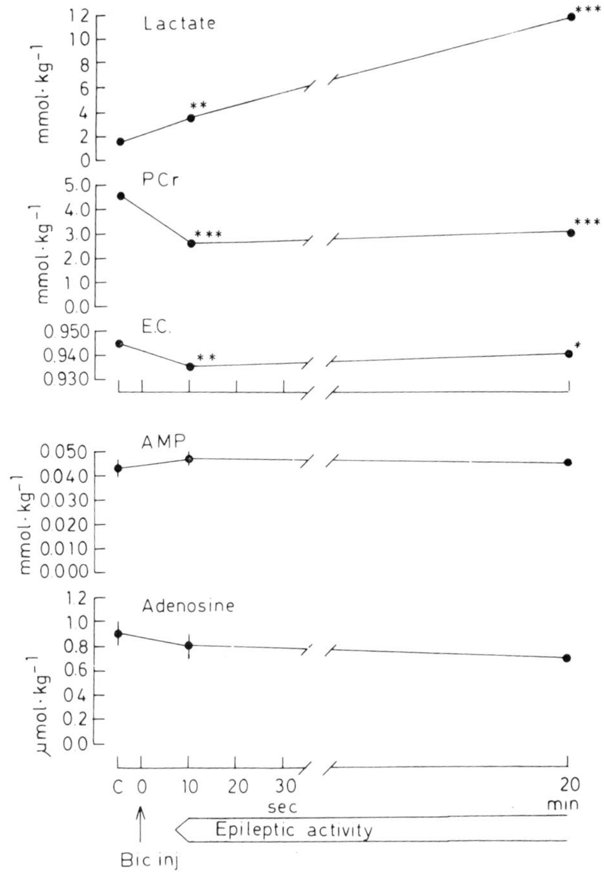

FIG. 5. Lactate, phosphocreatine (PCr) and energy charge $\left(\text{E.C.} = \dfrac{\text{ATP} + 0.5\ \text{ADP}}{\text{ATP} + \text{ADP} + \text{AMP}}\right)$ as well as AMP and adenosine concentrations in rat cerebral cortex during seizures induced by bicuculline (1.2 mg kg^{-1} i.v.). The brains were frozen with liquid nitrogen 10 s ($n = 4$) and 20 min ($n = 6$) after injection of bicuculline. C = control state ($n = 10$). Values are given as means ± S.E.M. * = $P < 0.05$; ** = $P < 0.01$; *** = $P < 0.001$.

Obviously, of possible factors responsible for the increase in CBF during seizures, adenosine is a poor candidate.

CEREBRAL BLOOD FLOW AND METABOLISM IN HYPOXIA

As stated in the introduction, there is some indirect evidence that the CBF increase in hypoxia is mediated via anaerobic production of lactic acid. It is well established that an increase in CBF occurs at Pa_{O_2} values that are associated with accumulation of lactic acid in tissue (for references, see Siesjö *et al.* 1975). Further support was provided by results showing that restriction of substrate supply by hypoglycaemia prevents the increase in CBF during hypoxia (Kogure *et al.* 1970).

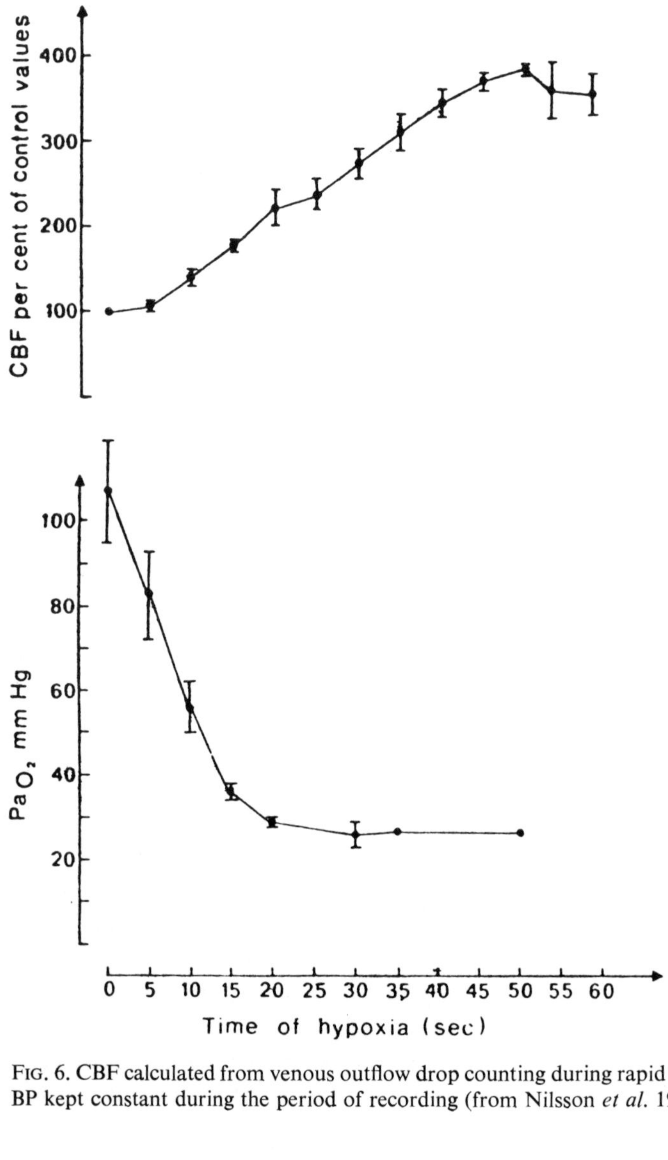

FIG. 6. CBF calculated from venous outflow drop counting during rapid induction of hypoxia. BP kept constant during the period of recording (from Nilsson *et al.* 1975).

During the last two to three years, results have been obtained that are incompatible with the pH hypothesis. Calculation of changes in CBF from $AVDo_2$ measurements showed that flow varied inversely with arterial Po_2 around normal levels, i.e. at degrees of hypoxia that seem to be unassociated with alterations in cellular concentrations of lactic acid (Borgström *et al.* 1975). Furthermore, although a precipitous rise in CBF occurred below Pao_2 values ($<$ 50 mmHg) that were also associated with a progressive lactic acidosis, a kinetic analysis showed the same type of dissociation between increase in flow and fall in pH that was observed during seizures (see above). When Pao_2 was rapidly reduced to about 25 mmHg in artificially ventilated rats the cellular concentration of lactic acid increased during the first minute but, since there was also a fall in Pco_2, calculated intracellular pH remained normal or even rose (Norberg & Siesjö 1975). Derivation of CBF from $AVDo_2$ measurements suggested that there was already a marked rise in CBF in this period (Borgström *et al.* 1975), and subsequent measurements of venous outflow showed that maximal vasodilatation occurred before a net acidosis could have developed (Nilsson *et al.* 1975) (Fig. 6). Further evidence was obtained when extracellular pH was found to remain normal or raised during the first 30–60 s of hypoxia (Astrup *et al.*, this symposium). The combined results leave little doubt that there may be a four- to fivefold rise in CBF during the initial period of hypoxia in the absence of an acid shift in pH.

In order to study whether adenosine might be a coupling factor we recently analysed cerebral cortical tissue for adenosine, adenine nucleotides and lactate in animals whose arterial Po_2 was reduced for 1–15 min (Rehncrona *et al.* 1977). Fig. 7 illustrates results obtained in animals maintained at Pao_2 values of 75, 55, 45, 35 and 25 mmHg for 15 min. For comparison, previously reported CBF values are included. These data illustrate a finding discussed above, namely that CBF increases at degrees of arterial hypoxia that are unassociated with significant changes in the concentration of lactate. Most importantly, there were no changes in concentrations of adenosine (or AMP) even if Pao_2 was reduced to levels accompanied by a four- to fivefold rise in CBF. Measurements of adenosine at 1 and 2 min of hypoxia (Pao_2 about 25 mmHg) indicated that a small rise in adenosine concentration could have been present. Thus, although not significantly different from the concentrations in controls (1.1 ± 0.1 μmol kg^{-1}), mean adenosine concentrations at 1 and 2 min were 1.3 ± 0.2 and 1.5 ± 0.1 μmol kg^{-1}, respectively. However, a further series with 2 min of hypoxia (Pao_2 19.0 ± 0.3 mmHg) showed unchanged values for tissue adenosine (and AMP) concentration. We thus conclude that adenosine does not qualify as a coupling factor mediating vasodilatation in hypoxia.

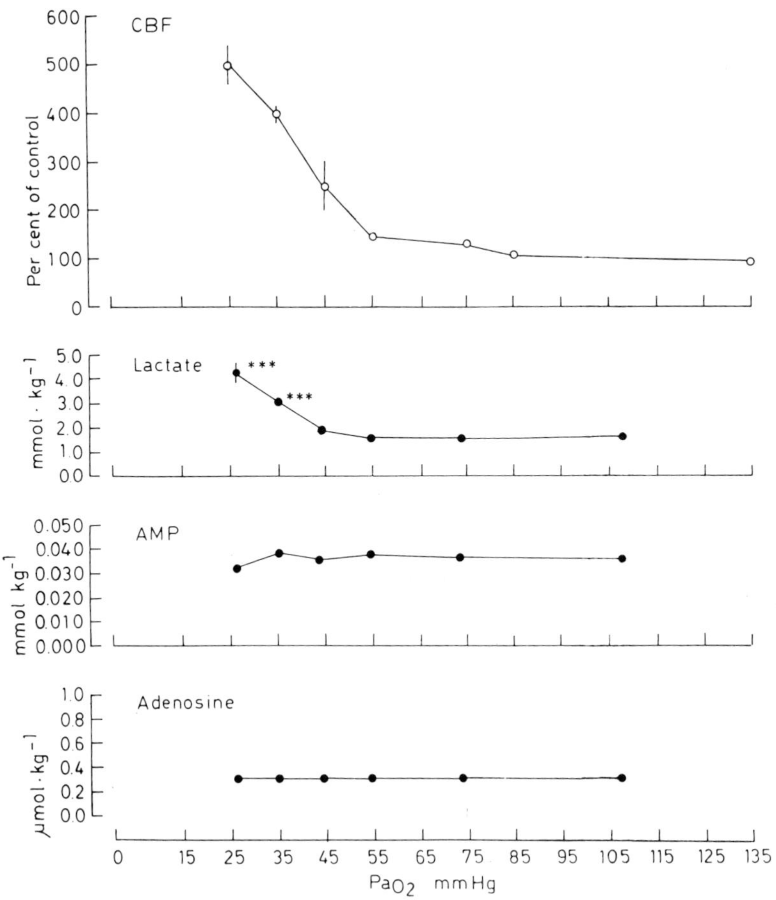

FIG. 7. Lactate, AMP and adenosine concentrations in rat cerebral cortex after 15 min of hypoxia at different arterial oxygen tensions (Pa_{O_2}). The values are means ± S.E.M. for groups of 4 animals. For comparison the percentage changes in CBF at corresponding Pa_{O_2} values after 15 min are given at the top (values taken from Borgström *et al.* 1975).

CEREBRAL BLOOD FLOW AND METABOLISM IN HYPOGLYCAEMIA

Regulation of CBF has been less extensively studied during hypoglycaemia than during seizure activity or hypoxia. However, hypoglycaemia provides an interesting example of an uncoupling of changes in CBF and in acid–base balance. Although most clinical studies have failed to reveal that severe hypoglycaemia is accompanied by consistent changes in CBF, at least one study (Della Porta *et al.* 1964) indicates that CBF may increase in hypoglycaemic coma (for further references, see Norberg & Siesjö 1976). Recently, it was found that insulin-induced hypoglycaemia in rats leads to a depletion of tissue concentrations of many metabolic acids, including lactic acid, and that acidosis does not develop at any stage of hypoglycaemia (Lewis *et al.* 1974). In spite of this, there is a significant increase in CBF (Norberg & Siesjö 1976). The absence of net acidosis in cerebral extracellular fluid has recently been confirmed (Astrup *et al.*, this symposium).

At present, there seems to be no information on tissue adenosine concentrations in hypoglycaemia. However, since vasodilatation occurs at degrees of hypoglycaemia that do not affect the tissue concentration of AMP there are no *a priori* reasons to suspect that accumulation of adenosine occurs (see below).

GENERAL COMMENTS

The results quoted clearly show that CBF increases markedly in conditions unassociated with acidosis or accumulation of adenosine. In addition to the data described above, some observations in other conditions should be briefly discussed.

It has been known for a long time that deep barbiturate anaesthesia reduces CBF to about 50% of control values at constant plasma P_{CO_2} (see Fig. 2). To our knowledge, it has not been shown that this reduction in flow is associated with an alkaline shift in cerebral extracellular pH, and data obtained on phenobarbitone-injected rats have failed to show any change in the pH of the cerebrospinal fluid (Messeter *et al.* 1972). Recently, it has been demonstrated that CBF increases after administration of amphetamine (Carlsson *et al.* 1975), and during immobilization stress (Carlsson *et al.* 1977). In neither of these conditions has it been possible to detect changes in tissue lactate concentrations, and in amphetamine-injected animals direct measurements of extracellular pH have failed to show that acidosis occurs (Astrup *et al.*, this symposium). Obviously, there are several conditions in which CBF is altered and in which appropriate changes in extracellular pH cannot be observed.

There are less extensive data on adenosine concentrations in tissue or extracellular fluid. *In vitro* experiments leave no doubt that adenosine accumulates after electrical stimulation, or in hypoxia (Pull & McIlwain 1972). However, since cerebral tissue *in vitro* lacks the compensatory increase in CBF, these conditions are accompanied by hydrolysis of ATP and by accumulation of AMP (see McIlwain & Bachelard 1971). This is of crucial importance since the activity of 5′-nucleotidase (EC 3.1.3.5), the enzyme catalysing breakdown of AMP to adenosine, is largely determined by substrate availability (Kluge *et al.* 1972). Thus, since even marked hypoxia *in vivo* does not lead to AMP accumulation it is hardly surprising that there are no signs of enhanced formation of adenosine. During bicuculline-induced seizures a moderate rise in AMP concentration has been observed (Chapman *et al.* 1977) but the present results show that this rise is not invariably present.

CONCLUSIONS

There is clear evidence from many studies, particularly those involving microapplication of solutions to pial vessels, that cerebral vessels react to changes in pH or adenosine concentrations. However, our results emphasize that there are several conditions in which such changes cannot explain the CBF responses, thus excluding H^+ ions and adenosine as general coupling factors. Obviously, we have to consider a more complex pattern of metabolic and neurogenic signals to be able to understand the mechanisms of cerebral vasomotor regulation.

ACKNOWLEDGEMENTS

This study was supported by grants from the Swedish Medical Research Council (project No. 14X-263) and from USPHS Grant No. 5 R01 NS07838-08 from the National Institutes of Health.

References

Astrup, J., Heuser, D., Lassen, N. A., Nilsson, B., Norberg, K. & Siesjö, B. K. (1978) Evidence against H and K as main factors for the control of cerebral blood flow: a microelectrode study, in this volume.

Betz, E. (1972) Cerebral blood flow: its measurement and regulation. *Physiol. Rev. 52*, 595–630

Betz, E. & Heuser, D. (1967) Cerebral cortical blood flow during changes of acid-base equilibrium of the brain. *J. Appl. Physiol. 23*, 726–733

Blennow, G., Folbergrová, J., Nilsson, B. & Siesjö, B. K. (1976) Changes in cerebral metabolism and circulation during seizures induced by DL-homocysteine. *First Eur. Soc. Neurochem. Meeting*, p. 114C, University of Bath

Blennow, G., Folbergrová, J., Nilsson, B. & Siesjö, B. K. (1977) Cerebral blood flow and oxygen utilization in rats during bicuculline-induced seizures. Effects of substrate depletion, in *Cerebral Function, Metabolism and Circulation* (Ingvar, D. H. & Lassen, N. A., eds.), pp. 12.2–12.3, Munksgaard, Copenhagen

Borgström, L., Jóhannsson, H. & Siesjö, B. K. (1975) The relationship between arterial P_{O_2} and cerebral blood flow in hypoxic hypoxia. *Acta Physiol. Scand. 93*, 423–432

Borgström, L., Chapman, A. G. & Siesjö, B. K. (1976) Glucose consumption in the cerebral cortex of rat during bicuculline-induced status epilepticus. *J. Neurochem. 27*, 971–973

CARLSSON, C., HÄGERDAL, M. & SIESJÖ, B. K. (1975) Influence of amphetamine sulphate on cerebral blood flow and metabolism. *Acta Physiol. Scand. 94*, 128–129

CARLSSON, C., HÄGERDAL, M. & SIESJÖ, B. K. (1976) The effect of hyperthermia upon oxygen consumption and upon organic phosphates, glycolytic metabolites, citric acid cycle intermediates and associated amino acids in rat cerebral cortex. *J. Neurochem. 26*, 1001–1006

CARLSSON, C., HÄGERDAL, M., KAASIK, A. E. & SIESJÖ, B. K. (1977) A catecholamine-mediated increase in cerebral oxygen uptake during immobilization stress in rats. *Brain Res. 119*, 223–231

CHAPMAN, A. G., MELDRUM, B. S. & SIESJÖ, B. K. (1977) Cerebral metabolic changes during prolonged epileptic seizures in rats. *J. Neurochem. 28*, 1025–1035

DELLA PORTA, P., MAIOLO, A. T., NEGRI, V. U. & ROSSELLA, E. (1964) Cerebral blood flow and metabolism in therapeutic insulin coma. *Metabolismo 13*, 131–140

HÄGERDAL, M., HARP, J., NILSSON, L. & SIESJÖ, B. K. (1975) The effect of induced hypothermia upon oxygen consumption in the rat brain. *J. Neurochem. 24*, 311–316

JÓHANNSSON, H. & SIESJÖ, B. K. (1975) Cerebral blood flow and oxygen consumption in the rat in hypoxia. *Acta Physiol. Scand. 93*, 269–276

KETY, S. S. & SCHMIDT, C. F. (1948) The nitrous oxide method for the quantitative determination of cerebral blood flow in man: theory, procedure and normal values. *J. Clin. Invest. 27*, 476–480

KLUGE, H., HARTMAN, W., WIECZOREK, V. & ZAHLTEN, W. (1972) Kinetic properties of cerebral 5′-nucleotidase. *J. Neurochem. 19*, 1409–1411

KOGURE, K., SCHEINBERG, P., REINMUTH, O. M., FUJISHIMA, M. & BUSTO, R. (1970) Mechanisms of cerebral vasodilatation in hypoxia. *J. Appl. Physiol. 29*, 223–229

KUSCHINSKY, W., WAHL, M., BOSSE, O. & THURAU, K. (1972) Perivascular potassium and pH as determinants of local pial arterial diameter in cats. *Circ. Res. 16*, 240–247

LASSEN, N. A. (1968) Brain extracellular pH: the main factor controlling cerebral blood flow. *Scand. J. Clin. Lab. Invest. 22*, 247–251

LEWIS, L. D., LJUNGGREN, B., NORBERG, K. & SIESJÖ, B. K. (1974) Changes in carbohydrate substrates, amino acids and ammonia in the brain during insulin-induced hypoglycemia. *J. Neurochem. 23*, 659–671

MCILWAIN, H. & BACHELARD, H. S. (1971) *Biochemistry and the Central Nervous System*, Churchill Livingstone, Edinburgh

MELDRUM, B. S. & NILSSON, B. (1976) Cerebral blood flow and metabolic rate early and late in prolonged seizures induced in rats by bicuculline. *Brain 99*, 523–542

MESSETER, K., PONTEN, U. & SIESJÖ, B. K. (1972) The influence of deep barbiturate anesthesia upon the regulation of extra- and intracellular pH in the rat brain during hypercapnia. *Acta Physiol. Scand. 85*, 174–182

NILSSON, B. & SIESJÖ, B. K. (1975) The effect of phenobarbitone anaesthesia on blood flow and oxygen consumption in the rat brain. *Acta Anaesthesiol. Scand. Suppl. 57*, 18–24

NILSSON, B. & SIESJÖ, B. K. (1976) A method for determining blood flow and oxygen consumption in the rat brain. *Acta Physiol. Scand. 96*, 72–82

NILSSON, B. & SIESJÖ, B. K. (1978) A venous outflow method for continuous measurement of the cerebral blood flow and oxygen consumption in the rat. *Circ. Res.*, submitted for publication

NILSSON, B., NORBERG, K., NORDSTRÖM, C.-H. & SIESJÖ, B. K. (1975) Influence of hypoxia and hypercapnia on CBF in rats, in *Blood Flow and Metabolism in the Brain* (Harper, M. *et al.*, eds.), pp. 9.19–9.23, Churchill Livingstone, Edinburgh

NILSSON, B., MELDRUM, B., NORBERG, K. & SIESJÖ, B. K. (1976) Correlation of changes in blood flow and acid-base changes in the brain during induced epileptic seizures, in *Ionic Actions on Vascular Smooth Muscle* (Betz, E., ed.), pp. 105–109, Springer, Berlin

NILSSON, B., ASTRUP, J., BLENNOW, G. & SIESJÖ, B. K. (1977) Cerebral function and energy metabolism at critical thresholds of oxygen availability: a study in rats during status epilepticus induced by bicuculline, in *Cerebral Function, Metabolism and Circulation* (Ingvar, D. H. & LASSEN, N. A., eds.), pp. 5.6–5.7, Munksgaard, Copenhagen

NORBERG, K. & SIESJÖ, B. K. (1974) Quantitative measurement of blood flow and oxygen consumption in the rat brain. *Acta Physiol. Scand. 91*, 154–164

NORBERG, K. & SIESJÖ, B. K. (1975) Cerebral metabolism in hypoxic hypoxia. I. Pattern of activation of glycosis: a re-evaluation. *Brain Res. 86*, 31–44

NORBERG, K. & SIESJÖ, B. K. (1976) Oxidative metabolism of the cerebral cortex of the rat in severe insulin-induced hypoglycemia. *J. Neurochem. 26*, 345–352

NORDSTRÖM, C.-H. & REHNCRONA, S. (1977) The reduction of cerebral blood flow and oxygen consumption with a combination of barbiturate anaesthesia and induced hypothermia in the rat. *Acta Anaesthesiol. Scand.*, in press

NORDSTRÖM, C.-H., REHNCRONA, S., SIESJÖ, B. K. & WESTERBERG, E. (1977) Adenosine rat cerebral cortex: its determination, normal values, and correlation to AMP and cyclic AMP during shortlasting ischemia. *Acta Physiol. Scand. 101*, 63–71

PLUM, F., POSNER, J. B. & TROY, B. (1968) Cerebral metabolic and circulatory responses to induced convulsions in animals. *Arch. Neurol. 18*, 1–13

PULL, I. & MCILWAIN, H. (1972) Metabolism of [^{14}C]adenine and derivatives by cerebral tissues, superfused and electrically stimulated. *Biochem. J. 126*, 965–973

REHNCRONA, S. NORDSTRÖM, C.-H., SIESJÖ, B. K. & WESTERBERG, E. (1977) Adenosine in rat cerebral cortex during hypoxia and bicuculline-induced seizures, in *Cerebral Function, Metabolism and Circulation* (Ingvar, D. H. & Lassen, N. A., eds.), pp. 11.12–11.13, Munksgaard, Copenhagen

RUBIO, R., BERNE, R. M., BOCKMAN, E. L. & CURNISH, R. R. (1975) Relationship between adenosine concentration and oxygen supply in rat brain. *Am. J. Physiol. 228*, 1896–1902

SIESJÖ, B. K., JÓHANNSSON, H., NORBERG, K. & SALFORD, L. G. (1975) Brain function, metabolism and blood flow in moderate and severe arterial hypoxia, in *Brain Work (Alfred Benzon Symp. 8)* (Ingvar, D. H. & Lassen, N. A., eds.), pp. 101–125, Munksgaard, Copenhagen

WAHL, M. & KUCHINSKY, W. (1976) The dilatatory action of adenosine on pial arteries of cats and its inhibition by theophylline. *Pflügers Arch. Eur. J. Physiol. 362*, 55–59

Discussion

Purves: Do you think that the significant lag Professor Siesjö sees in the reaction of CBF to changes in pH is important, Professor Lübbers?

Lübbers: It depends on the problem. In our scheme of regulation of circulation we are always trying to figure out which signals come from the arterial blood or from the nervous system and which signals come from the tissue itself. One way of discriminating between those factors is by measuring the time constants of the reaction. The time constant of tissue signals seems to be longer than that of the arterial signal.

Plum: From the description of your experiments one would have anticipated enough hysteresis in the method for the question to be almost unanswerable. How can one know the biological factors delaying flow in the vascularized areas?

Siesjö: The pH changes have been studied with three different methods. Firstly, we can calculate cellular pH values from P_{CO_2} and from changes in lactate concentration; secondly we can measure pH with extracellular electrodes; and thirdly we can derive it from measured values for total CO_2 and P_{CO_2}. All three methods give the same results. Essentially, pH remains constant or even increases in the period during which flow increases to maximal values.

Nilsson: With regard to the *time course* of the vasomotor response, the most sensitive variable in our venous outflow preparation is the continuous intracisternal pressure recording. In the experiment shown in Fig. 4B the sensitivity is increased by occlusion of the spinal canal at the level of C-2, thus changing the elastance of the intracranial pressure-volume system. It can be seen that each burst of epileptic activity and even single spikes during status epilepticus elicit vasodilatation within 1 s.

Purves: This seems to raise a possible way in which you could test your system, Dr Sokoloff. Have you done any hypoxic studies as one way of discriminating between changes in metabolism and flow?

Sokoloff: Rats breathing 7% oxygen look awfully sick but we didn't find any significant change in glucose consumption. We have not yet done any studies with lower oxygen concentrations. We didn't measure blood flow, but I presume it would have been increased.

Siesjö: In our modification of the method described by Hawkins *et al.* (1974), we measured specific activities between 2 and 4 min after injection (Borgström *et al.* 1976). During the first 2 min of hypoxia glucose uptake doubled but after 15 min of hypoxia the increase was very moderate ($P < 0.05$). That means that there is an initial increase in glycolytic rate but, subsequently, glycolytic rate may be normal or just marginally increased.

Sokoloff: That is exactly our reasoning too. We wondered how long the Pasteur effect could continue in the brain during hypoxia. If glycolysis continues without pyruvate being oxidized, lactate continues to accumulate in the tissue because transport of lactate from tissue back to the blood is limited. It is unlikely that lactate can accumulate *ad infinitum*—it has to level off, but how will it level off if it can't get out? It can do so by inhibiting glycolysis, by its effect on tissue pH or something like that. All the enzymes involved in glycolysis have pH optima, and if the pH gets too low, the enzyme activity will be reduced. Glucose consumption probably increased initially in our experiments but was not maintained, and because of the long time that our method takes, we must have missed the early Pasteur effect.

Siesjö: There is usually a very small gradient for lactate even under conditions of hypoxia. The blood level is increased so there should be very little transport of lactate from the tissue.

Purves: In hypoxia were you able to show the same correlation between the distribution of glucose uptake an dflow in different parts of the brain but with a change in slope, Dr Sokoloff?

Sokoloff: We didn't measure blood flow in our experiments, but I presume that there would still be a correlation, although not as good as in normal states.

Lübbers: If we stimulate the brain cortex with an element which contains several wires to provide measurements of P_{O_2} and flow, etc., we can see flow increase in less than 1 s after stimulation. Using photometric methods the quickest change we observed in circulation took 0.2–0.3 s.

Siesjö: We have been arguing since 1975 (Nilsson *et al.* 1975; Siesjö *et al.* 1975) that pH changes cannot be responsible for triggering the increase in flow in hypoxia and seizures. Now we hear the argument that perhaps the initial event is unrelated to pH but that the later adjustment is due to pH or, at least, is influenced by pH. Anyone who is interested in testing that hypothesis should induce epileptic seizures or hypoxia, and simultaneously hyperventilate the animal to lower the P_{CO_2}. It should then be possible to separate pH from the flow increase, perhaps even during the first 2 or 3 min.

Raichle: In all these discussions in which we are trying to relate a signal to a response we end up saying, as you did with the adenosine, that there was no change therefore that is not the signal. But isn't a feedback system made in order to bring the signal back down to its normal level, so if adenosine or anything else is normal at the time the response is maximal, isn't that precisely what the system would do? In order to see whether that was the signal one would have to block the response.

Siesjö: That is a valid point. However, one would expect to see, at least in a non-steady state, that the signal is there. Furthermore, if the system has not an indefinite gain some signal should be detectable even in the steady state.

Raichle: These are discrete measurements along the curve, aren't they?

Siesjö: Yes.

Lübbers: This argument wouldn't work with the pH.

Raichle: I am not arguing for any specific thing, but adenosine gave a very flat curve when the response was maximal, so one would say that it is a beautifully organized system. It worked perfectly.

Rosendorff: But if one followed these variants with time one would expect to see an error signal.

Raichle: It is just a problem with the discrete measurement. If the putative signal was being followed continuously, the error would possibly be seen, depending, of course, on the response time of the measuring device.

Siesjö: That was why we froze the tissue 10 s after injecting bicuculline to induce seizure, at a time when maximal vasodilatation hasn't yet appeared.

This is about 3 s after the seizure has started, and there is no increase in adenosine concentration at that time.

Purves: This should be within the time constant of the feedback system. With a continuous method one should be able to see the change.

Moskowitz: By just measuring the level of a particular molecule in brain, one is sometimes unable to detect a shift of physiologically active molecules from one compartment to the next.

Plum: You have demonstrated that H^+ cannot be held to be the messenger in all physiological circumstances, but evidence remains during seizures that there is still a messenger, and the bed is not pressure-passive. Howse *et al.* (1974) in our laboratory gave a pressor agent (phenylephrine) intravenously at the height of the hypertensive response and monitored both the systemic pressure rise and the chemical change in the brain. The degree of pressure rise depended on the point after the induction of the seizure when the phenylephrine was given. Chemical assay of the tissue indicated that tissue pH returned to control levels but did not turn alkaline during the attempt at increased hypertensive washout. Thus the vascular bed did not appear to be pressure-passive. Instead, the receptor for vascular resistance was merely activated at a much higher flow rate during the increased metabolism of the seizure. The smooth muscle retained its capacity to contract, but at a greater degree of vasodilatation.

Jöbsis: This conversation reminds me of the discussions long ago on the first donor of free energy in muscle contraction. The argument went about the same way as Dr Raichle described. What was not quite understood at that time was the speed of the reactions. It was agreed that ATP ought to break down, with ADP and AMP being formed, but none of these things could be found to occur. There were problems in sensitivity analysis and in the rate of freezing tissue. Finally it turned out that a measurement could be made if the creatine phosphokinase reaction was inhibited. Only then could ADP, AMP and adenosine catabolites be shown to accumulate. Rates of freezing of less than 100 ms were required for these events to be seen, and the amount of breakdown of various substances was equalized by the longer times of freezing, of about 300–400 ms. If the turnover is quite rapid, IMP should be accumulating. IMP itself can be catabolized further down, though it may be different in the brain than in other tissues. So what is the amount of adenosine necessary, and for how long should it be there to produce the changes that you expect?

Siesjö: I think substantial increases in extravascular adenosine concentration are needed if maximal dilatation of the vessels is to be achieved. Dr Rubio may have a comment.

Rubio: The dilatation–concentration curve for adenosine is an S-shaped curve. The concentration required to obtain a 50% maximal dilatory effect is about 10^{-6} M, or about 1 nmol/g. It is perfectly saturated at 10^{-4} M. The physiological range of adenosine is 10^{-7} to 10^{-5} M. To get maximal vasodilation one needs about 5×10^{-6} M.

Siesjö: That would mean a 5- to 10-fold increase in adenosine in order to explain maximal vasodilatation.

Rubio: It depends in whose hands.

Purves: These are actual concentrations. You are really talking about rates, aren't you?

Rubio: The only thing we can measure so far is the accumulation of adenosine.

References

BORGSTRÖM, L., NORBERG, K. & SIESJÖ, B. K. (1976) Glucose consumption in rat cerebral cortex in normoxia, hypoxia and hypercapnia. *Acta Physiol. Scand. 96*, 569–574

HAWKINS, R. A., MILLER, A. L., CREMER, J. E. & VEECH, R. L. (1974) Measurement of the rate of glucose utilization by rat brain *in vivo*. *J. Neurochem. 23*, 917–923

HOWSE, D. C., CARONNA, J. J., DUFFY, T. E. & PLUM, F. (1974) Cerebral energy metabolism, pH and blood flow during seizures in the cat. *Am. J. Physiol. 227*, 1444–1451

NILSSON, B., NORBERG, K., NORDSTRÖM, C.-H. & SIESJÖ, B. K. (1975) Influence of hypoxia and hypercapnia on CBF in rats, in *Blood Flow and Metabolism in the Brain* (Harper, N. *et al.*, eds.), pp. 9.19–9.23, Churchill Livingstone, Edinburgh

SIESJÖ, B. K., JOHANNSSON, H., NORBERG, K. & SALFORD, L. G. (1975) Brain function, metabolism and blood flow in moderate and severe arterial hypoxia, in *Brain Work* (Ingvar, D. H. & Lassen, N. A., eds.) *(Alfred Benzon Symp. 8)*, pp. 101–125, Munksgaard, Copenhagen

Central neuroendocrine regulation of brain water permeability

*MARCUS E. RAICHLE, *ROBERT L. GRUBB and JOHN O. EICHLING

Division of Radiation Sciences, The Edward Mallinckrodt Institute of Radiology, and
**Department of Neurology and Neurological Surgery, Washington University School of Medicine, St Louis, Missouri*

Abstract The brain vasculature, especially capillaries, may function in a very dynamic fashion under neuroendocrine control to regulate the internal environment of the brain. This is exemplified by new observations on the regulation of brain water permeability using the tracer $H_2{}^{15}O$ *in vivo* in adult rhesus monkeys. These studies reveal that brain water permeability, and hence brain water content and volume, are, at least in part, under the influence of the central noradrenergic system and centrally released vasopressin.

The brain vasculature permits the rapid movement of critical substrates between blood and brain, while at the same time excluding substances which might be toxic to brain cells (Davson 1976). The functional characteristics of the blood–brain barrier have generally been viewed as being fixed early in life, and only disrupted under severe stress. Accumulating evidence now suggests that this may be too restrictive a view. The barrier may function, under neural and hormonal influence, in a very dynamic fashion to regulate the internal environment of the brain. This is exemplified by the ability of the blood–brain barrier to regulate brain water permeability (Raichle *et al.* 1975).

Precise adjustment of brain water content and, hence, brain volume is of demonstrated importance to the normal functioning of the central nervous system (Fishman 1974). Because brain and blood osmolality are identical under normal circumstances, the moment-to-moment adjustment of brain water content is dependent upon the hydrostatic pressure gradient between blood and brain, which will vary with changes in posture, blood pressure and intracranial pressure, and with the permeability of the blood–brain barrier to water.

Several pieces of evidence suggest that the brain vasculature, especially capillaries, may play an important role in the regulation of brain water content through an ability to affect brain water permeability in a manner analogous to the mammalian kidney and other membranes known to regulate water permeability (e.g. toad urinary bladder) (Bindslev *et al.* 1974; Mullen *et al.* 1976; Scott & Sapirstein 1974; Strum & Danon 1974). First, the brain capillaries exhibit a number of features unique to membranes known to regulate water permeability. These include tight junctions between constituent epithelial cells (Bennett *et al.* 1959); a high mitochondrial content of constituent endothelial cells (Oldendorf *et al.* 1977); a similar complement of intracellular enzymes (Goldstein 1977), and a prompt increase in water permeability when subjected to osmotic stress (Raichle *et al.* 1977). Second, brain is not freely permeable to water, as we have previously shown (Raichle *et al.* 1976), and in fact it exhibits a permeability similar to that of membranes known to regulate water permeability (Bindslev & Wright 1976). Finally, changes in brain water permeability can be produced by stimulation of central noradrenergic neurons (Raichle *et al.* 1975) which arise from the locus coeruleus and terminate, in part, in brain capillaries (Hartman *et al.* 1972; Rennels & Nelson 1975; Swanson *et al.* 1977). This observation demonstrates the presence of at least one system in brain analogous, we believe, to the peripheral sympathetic nervous system, and which is capable of regulating brain water permeability and, thus, water content and volume. This is complemented by the recent observation from our laboratory that stimulation of peripheral sympathetic nerve fibres from the superior cervical ganglion, known to innervate small parenchymal blood vessels in brain other than capillaries (Edvinsson 1975), also produces a significant, although less pronounced, increase in brain water permeability (Grubb *et al.* 1977). It is of interest that peripheral adrenergic fibres have been noted in close association with epithelial cells lining the urinary bladder of the bullfrog (Strum & Danon 1974), a structure also specifically concerned with the regulation of water permeability; and that peripheral sympathetic stimulation affects vascular permeability in other organs (Linde 1976; Bello-Reus *et al.* 1976).

In this communication, by examining the role of centrally released vasopressin, we explore further the ability of the brain to regulate its water permeability. All membranes known to regulate water permeability are under the influence of circulating vasopressin. An increase in vasopressin concentration in blood produces a prompt and profound increase in water permeability. Recently, vasopressin and its carrier protein neurophysin II have been demonstrated in significant concentrations in cerebrospinal fluid (CSF) (Robinson & Zimmerman 1973). These studies further demonstrate that this peptide hormone and its carrier protein enter the CSF directly from brain and not from the systemic circulation. The function of this centrally released vasopressin has not been explained. It seems reasonable to suggest that the centrally released vasopressin plays an important role in the regulation of brain water permeability. On the basis of this hypothesis, we would anticipate an increase in brain water permeability in parallel with an increase in CSF vasopressin concentration. Furthermore, we would anticipate that brain water permeability would not be affected by changes in the concentration of vasopressin in blood. This is based on the observation that all vasopressin-sensitive membranes respond only on one side to the hormone (Peachey & Rasmussen 1961). Teleologically, this would make sense for the brain also in that a system designed to regulate brain water content and presumably volume should only be sensitive to the internal milieu of the brain.

METHODS

We tested the hypothesis that centrally released vasopressin is involved in the regulation of brain water permeability by administering 2 units of vasopressin (Pitressin) into the lateral ventricle in a volume of 0.1 ml and sequentially following the changes in cerebral blood flow (CBF) and the extraction of ^{15}O-labelled water. CBF and the fraction of labelled water extracted by the brain during a single capillary transit were determined by the injection of 0.2 ml of whole blood labelled with $H_2{}^{15}O$ into the right internal carotid artery of the adult rhesus monkey (*Macaca mulatta*). The details of the animal preparation, injection procedures and *in vivo* detection of the radioisotopes are described elsewhere (Raichle *et al.* 1976). The monkeys were anaesthetized with phencyclidine (2 mg/kg), paralysed with gallamine and passively ventilated on 100% oxygen. The end-tidal P_{CO_2}, arterial blood pressure and rectal temperature were continuously monitored.

The single capillary model of Renkin (1959) and Crone (1963) was used to calculate the brain PS product (capillary permeability coefficient and surface area product) for water. The relationship of CBF and the extraction fraction of labelled water (E) to the brain PS product is expressed in the equation

$$\ln(1-E) = -PS/CBF$$

Assuming a constant value for the brain capillary surface area available for water diffusion, changes in the PS product should reflect changes in brain permeability to the labelled water. Confidence in this assumption is based on the experimental observation that P·S does not change when large variations are induced in CBF by acute changes in arterial carbon tension (Raichle *et al.* 1976). *T* tests were used to test the significance of observed changes in PS product and CBF.

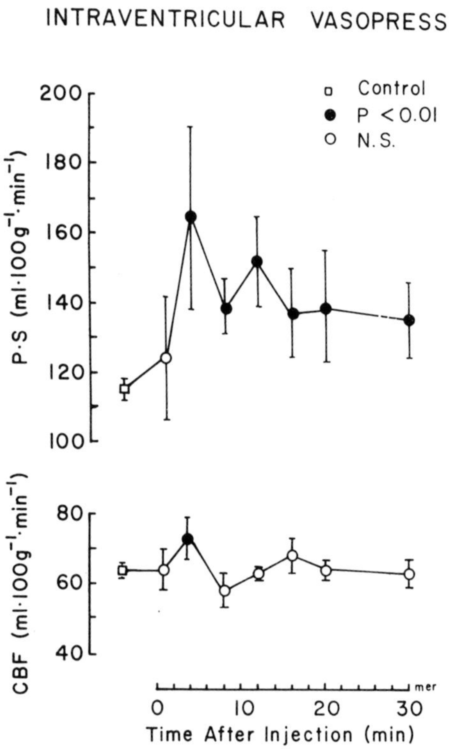

FIG. 1. The effect of intraventricular vasopressin on the brain capillary permeability coefficient and surface area product (P · S) and cerebral blood flow (CBF) in five adult rhesus monkeys. Error bars: 2 S.E.M.

RESULTS AND DISCUSSION

The effect of intraventricular vasopressin on CBF and brain water permeability in five animals is shown in Fig. 1. There was a striking increase in P · S after the intraventricular administration of vasopressin. A slight but significant increase in CBF occurred in all animals shortly after the administration of vasopressin, but did not persist. No changes were observed in any of the animals in arterial blood pressure, end-tidal carbon dioxide tension or arterial blood gases.

These results are to be contrasted with those observed after the intravenous administration of vasopressin. Doses in excess of 10 units in a single bolus failed to produce any changes in P · S.

These results provide the first demonstration of a specific function of a 'hypothalamic' peptide hormone within the central nervous system which, although similar to its action peripherally, is probably designed to meet specific needs of the brain. The fact that vasopressin has a significant effect on brain water permeability further supports the idea that regulation of brain water content is an important function of the brain vasculature mediated in part by the action of centrally released vasopressin. It is of particular interest that there is a close anatomical association between the central neuroendocrine cells of the hypothalamus, especially those concerned with the synthesis of the hormone carrier complex oxytocin–neurophysin I and vasopressin–neurophysin II, and central noradrenergic neurons (Swanson 1977; Scott *et al.* 1977), in the light of the known effect of stimulation of the latter, through the locus coeruleus, on brain water permeability (Raichle *et al.* 1975).

It would not be too surprising to find that neurons capable of releasing vasopressin and, possibly, oxytocin in brain and the central noradrenergic system are part of one coordinated neuroendocrine system in brain designed to regulate brain water content. An analogous relationship has been well described between the release of vasopressin in blood and the activity of the peripheral sympathetic nervous system (Schrier *et al.* 1977).

The existence of the proposed system in brain may explain the absence of cerebral oedema (i.e. increased brain water content) under circumstances known to increase the hydrostatic pressure gradient between blood and brain. Several investigators have made the observation that acute arterial hypertension alone (Johansson 1976) or in combination with experimentally induced seizures (Petito *et al.* 1976) produces apparent disruption of the blood–brain barrier with an extravasation of large protein molecules from blood into brain parenchyma. These dramatic demonstrations of an apparent disruption in the blood–brain barrier have been puzzling because in no instance where tissue water content has actually been measured has brain oedema been found (Johansson 1976; Petito *et al.* 1976). In order to examine the ability of our proposed system to respond to such an acute stress, we produced acute arterial hypertension in a group of anaesthetized, paralysed, passively ventilated monkeys by the administration of angiotensin II or aramine intravenously. The results of this study are shown in Fig. 2. This observation is important for several reasons. First, it demonstrates the ability of brain to appropriately adjust its water permeability in order to compensate for an increased hydrostatic gradient between blood and brain. Such an adjustment would be appropriate for the prevention of an increase in brain water content and the development of oedema. Second, this particular stress, pharmacological hypertension, is known to reduce sympathetic activity (Coote & Sato 1977) as well as reduce the release of vasopressin from brain (Schrier *et al.* 1977). It obviously remains

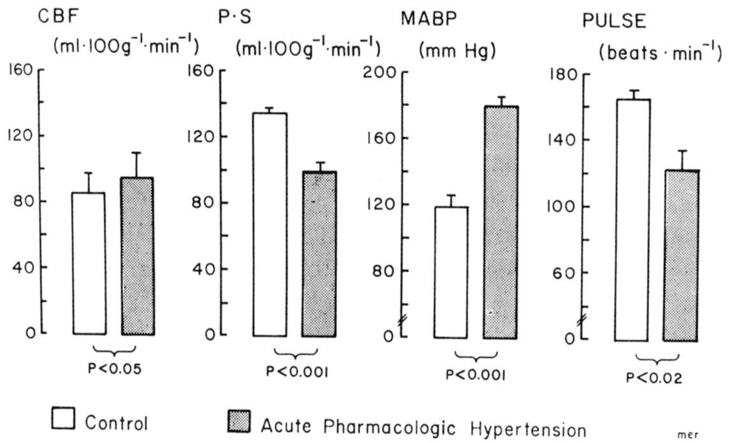

FIG. 2. The effect of acute pharmacological hypertension induced by either intravenous aramine or angiotensin II infusion on cerebral blood flow (CBF), the brain capillary permeability coefficient and surface area product (P·S), mean arterial blood pressure (MABP) and pulse rate in 11 adult rhesus monkeys. Error bars: 1 S.E.M.

to be specifically demonstrated that centrally released vasopressin and/or central noradrenergic activity is also attenuated by this manoeuvre. Finally, this observation complements the work of Cuypers *et al.* (1976), who showed that cerebral venous hypertension, even in the absence of an intact calvarium, failed to produce an increase in brain water content, despite the development of a significant hydrostatic pressure gradient between brain blood vessels and brain tissue.

Our observations, plus a significant amount of information in published work related to brain fluid and electrolyte metabolism and the brain vasculature, suggest that the latter, under the influence of a central neuroendocrine system, is probably capable of regulating brain water permeability in accordance with the brain's need to maintain a constant volume. The existence of such a system, possibly one of many within brain (Scott *et al.* 1977), is not surprising considering the need to maintain homeostasis in the closed environment of the cranial vault. Disruption of such a system would obviously have significant implications with regard to the development of brain oedema in a number of disease states.

References

BELLO-REUS, E., TREVINO, D. L. & GOTTSCHALK, C. W. (1976) Effect of renal nerve stimulation on proximal water and sodium reabsorption. *J. Clin. Invest. 57*, 1104–1107

BENNETT, H. S., LUFT, J. H. & HAMPTON, J. C. (1959) Morphological classification of vertebrate blood capillaries. *Am. J. Physiol. 196*, 381–390

BINDSLEV, N. & WRIGHT, E. M. (1976) Thermodynamic analysis of nonelectrolyte permeation across toad urinary bladder. *J. Membr. Biol. 29*, 289–312

BINDSLEV, N., TORMEY, J. MCD., PIETRAS, R. J. & WRIGHT, E. M. (1974) Electrically and osmotically induced changes in permeability and structure of toad urinary bladder. *Biochim. Biophys. Acta 332*, 286–297

COOTE, J. H. & SATO, J. (1977) Reflex regulation of sympathetic activity in the spontaneously hypertensive rat. *Circ. Res. 40*, 571–577

CRONE, C. (1963) Permeability of capillaries in various organs as determined by use of indicator diffusion method. *Acta Physiol. Scand. 58*, 292–305

CUYPERS, J., MATAKAS, F. & POTOLICCHIO, S. J. JR. (1976) Effect of central venous pressure on brain tissue pressure and brain volume. *J. Neurosurg. 45*, 89–94

DAVSON, H. (1976) The blood brain barrier. *J. Physiol. (Lond.) 255*, 1–28

EDVINSSON, L. (1975) Neurogenic mechanisms in the cerebrovascular bed. *Acta Physiol. Scand. Suppl. 427*, 1–35

FISHMAN, R. A. (1974) Cell volume, pumps, and neurologic functions: brain's adaptation to osmotic stress. *Res. Publ. Assoc. Res. Nerv. Ment. Dis. 53*, 159–172

GOLDSTEIN, G. W. (1977) Cerebral edema: role of fatty acid metabolism of brain capillaries. *N. Engl. J. Med. 296*, 632

GRUBB, R. L. JR., RAICHLE, M. E. & EICHLING, J. O. (1977) Peripheral sympathetic regulation of brain water permeability. *Acta Neurol. Scand. 56, Suppl. 64*, 490–491

HARTMAN, B. K., ZIDE, D. & UDENFRIEND, S. (1972) The use of dopamine β-hydroxylase as a marker for the central noradrenergic nervous system in rat brain. *Proc. Natl. Acad. Sci. U.S.A. 69*, 2722–2726

JOHANSSON, B. B. (1976) Water content of rat brain in acute arterial hypertension, in *Dynamics of Brain Edema* (Pappius, H. M. *et al.*, eds.), pp. 28–31, Springer, New York

LINDE, B. (1976) Studies on the vascular exchange function in canine adipose tissue. *Acta Physiol. Scand. Suppl. 433*, 1–43

MULLEN, T. L., KASHGARIAN, M., BIEMESDERFER, D., GIEBISCH, G. H. & BIBER, F. U. L. (1976) Ion transport and structure of urinary bladder epithelium of *Amphiuma*. *Am. J. Physiol. 231*, 501–508

OLDENDORF, W. H., CORNFORD, M. E. & BROWN, W. J. (1977) The large apparent work capability of the blood-brain barrier: a study of the mitochondrial content of capillary endothelial cells in brain and other tissues of the rat. *Ann. Neurol. 1*, 409–417

PEACHEY, L. D. & RASMUSSEN, H. (1961) Structure of toad urinary bladder as related to its physiology. *J. Biophys. Biochem. Cytol. 10*, 529–553

PETITO, C. K., SCHAEFER, J. A. & PLUM, F. (1976) The blood-brain barrier in experimental seizures, in *Dynamics of Brain Edema* (Pappius, H. M. *et al.*, eds.), pp. 38–42, Springer, New York

RAICHLE, M. E., HARTMAN, B. K., EICHLING, J. O. & SHARPE, L. G. (1975) Central noradrenergic regulation of cerebral blood flow and vascular permeability. *Proc. Natl. Acad. Sci. U.S.A. 72*, 3726–3730

RAICHLE, M. E., EICHLING, J. O., STRAATMANN, M. G., WELCH, M. J., LARSON, K. B. & TER-POGOSSIAN, M. M. (1976) Blood-brain barrier permeability of ^{11}C-labeled alcohols and ^{15}O-labeled water. *Am. J. Physiol. 230*, 543–552

RAICHLE, M. E., GRUBB, R. L. JR. & EICHLING, J. O. (1977) Osmotically induced changes in brain water permeability. *Fed. Proc. 36*, 470

RENKIN, E. M. (1959) Transport of potassium-42 from blood to tissue in isolated mammalian skeletal muscles. *Am. J. Physiol. 197*, 1205–1210

RENNELS, M. L. & NELSON, E. (1975) Capillary innervation in the mammalian central nervous system: an electron microscopic demonstration. *Am. J. Anat. 144*, 233–241

ROBINSON, A. G. & ZIMMERMAN, E. A. (1973) Cerebrospinal fluid and ependymal neurophysin. *J. Clin. Invest. 52*, 1260–1267

SCHRIER, R. W., BERL, T., ANDERSON, R. J. & MCDONALD, K. M. (1977) Nonosmolar control of renal water excretion, in *Disturbances of Body Fluid Osmolality* (Andreoli, T. E. *et al.*, eds.), pp. 149–178, American Physiological Society, Bethesda

SCOTT, W. N. & SAPIRSTEIN, V. S. (1974) Partition of tissue functions in epithelial localization of enzymes in 'mitochondria-rich' cells of toad urinary bladder. *Science (Wash. D.C.) 184*, 797–799

SCOTT, D. E., KROBISCH-DUDLEY, G., PAULL, W. K. & KOZLOWSKI, G. P. (1977) The ventricular system in neuroendocrine mechanisms. III: Supraependymal neural networks in the primate brain. *Cell Tiss. Res. 179*, 235–254

STRUM, J. M. & DANON, D. (1974) Fine structure of the urinary bladder of the bullfrog *(Rana catesbeiana)*. *Anat. Rec. 178*, 15–40

SWANSON, L. W. (1977) Immunohistochemical evidence for a neurophysin-containing autonomic pathway arising in the paraventricular nucleus of the hypothalamus. *Brain Res. 128*, 346–353

SWANSON, L. G., CONNELLY, M. A. & HARTMAN, B. K. (1977) Ultrastructural evidence for central monoaminergic innervation of blood vessels in the periventricular nucleus of the hypothalamus. *Brain Res. 136*, 166–173

Discussion

Sandler: You are on record as saying (Raichle *et al.* 1975) that derangements of the system you describe 'have obvious implications with regard to diseases of the brain'. There is an old report (Goltman 1935–36) of a patient with migraine who had a bony defect in his skull. Every time he had a migraine attack the membranes bulged out, returning to normal after the attack. This points to transitory brain oedema. Could your techniques, or modifications of them, be applied to the investigation of such disease states as migraine or, for that matter, depression? We have recent data (Bonham Carter *et al.* 1978) of a biochemical lesion common to migraine and depression that could be interpreted in terms of a transport deficit.

Raichle: If there is a neuroendocrine system in brain which is capable of adjusting permeabilities in response to osmotic and hydrostatic stress it is easy to believe that a disorder of this system might lead to brain swelling. Although the work I have presented is suggestive, I believe much more work is necessary to establish the role of such a system. Furthermore, vasopressin is not the only peptide hormone in the nervous system capable of affecting the vasculature. Its presence in the ventricular fluid in high concentrations suggests that its behaviour might serve as a model for a variety of systems that could behave in somewhat the same way, related not only to the vascular system but to the cells of the nervous system itself.

Purves: Professor Owman, do you agree with Dr Raichle's picture of innervated capillaries?

Owman: I do. There is now increasing evidence that capillaries receive innervation. The question is whether other parts of the circulatory system might be directly influenced by the central neurons. Structurally, these neurons do not have any close relationship to the vessels. But long-distance diffusion of the transmitters might influence the vessels either to produce a contraction or to change the permeability properties. Do you think, Dr Raichle, that in addition to the sympathetic (extrinsic) effects on cerebral arteries and arterioles there is also a central (intrinsic) effect from long-distance transmitter diffusion?

Raichle: I think there is a central effect, though it depends on what you mean by long-distance. The distances here are not much longer than those in other tissues where there is an effect. Whether the effect goes beyond the capillaries and involves other vessels or not I don't know. This has been an area of great confusion. The original description of an anatomical association between central noradrenergic fibres and blood vessels in brain suggested only that these were small vessels (Hartman *et al.* 1972). One of the puzzling things was how a nerve could come from brain substance across the perivascular space and affect a vessel. That seemed an aberrant way to affect the vessel. We now believe that the central noradrenergic system primarily affects the capillaries, while the peripheral sympathetic system affects other vessels which may also have important exchange properties.

The observations of Drs Edvinsson and Owman at this meeting of changes in brain permeability with peripheral sympathetic stimulation don't surprise me. The fact that they go in a different direction from our observations with peripheral sympathetic stimulation doesn't surprise me because we have seen this dichotomy between, for example, an increase in protein permeability or large molecule permeability at the time that the water permeability is going down. These are highly complex things.

Purves: There is a terminal on either the pericyte or the endothelial cell but all you really know is that it is not part of the extrinsic adrenergic system. What is your evidence for the origin of this type of fibre?

Raichle: There are several groups of noradrenergic neurons in the brain-stem. One of the most concentrated is in the area of the locus coeruleus, though some may be coming from other areas. The locus coeruleus is probably the only place reasonably accessible to stimulation.

Siesjö: In the regulation of tissue water content a steady state must be determined by the differences in osmotic pressure and by intracellular oncotic pressure. I presume that you are discussing transient changes?

Raichle: The brain will adjust its osmolality with time. It must however make an immediate response to the challenge, such as a change in plasma osmolality or hydrostatic pressure.

Siesjö: But at a steady state, whenever that is reached, the water content of the brain must be determined by the chemical potential of water in the brain versus that in blood. Net water transport is not determined by the water permeability but by other forces. However, these permeability changes could be important in slowing down the influx of water whenever there is a suitable gradient.

Raichle: If we put a tracer in we can see the immense flux. It is a dynamic system, not a static system. Water is moving dynamically in and out and if we put a resistance in the system this is bound to determine the equilibrium.

Lübbers: How much of the capillary water would go into the brain?

Raichle: The net flow of water into brain in the steady state is close to zero. However, this is a dynamic steady state which can only be appreciated from tracer data. These data reveal that the major portion of the water conveyed by the flow of blood enters the brain. At any given moment the amount that is diffusing into brain is equivalent to the blood flow multiplied by the fraction of blood that is water (approximately 0.85) and the fraction that is extracted by the brain (approximately 0.93 at a normal brain blood flow of 50 ml 100 g^{-1} min^{-1}). Thus we may estimate that about 40 ml water/100 g brain enters each minute. This obviously must be balanced by an equal amount which must either back-diffuse across the capillary and leave the brain via the bloodstream or enter the cerebrospinal fluid.

Rapoport: I think that the critical factor that prevents brain oedema is not a low capillary water permeability, but a very low permeability to plasma protein and salt. Water which might enter the brain because of a change in osmotic or hydrostatic pressures across the capillary wall would not be accompanied by salt if the barrier remained intact, would dilute brain interstitial osmolality, and would thereby establish a counteracting osmotic force across the capillary so as to prevent further water accumulation. The observed capillary half-time for water diffusion indicates that a new steady state would be established within about 1 min, at which time transient changes in net water flow across the capillary would disappear.

I also wonder whether you actually measure water permeability by your method, rather than loss of water from the brain tissue as a whole, which need not be limited by capillary constraints. Another method, such as determining the half-time of entry of radiolabelled or heavy water, would be needed under the same conditions before you conclude that you are changing the capillary PS value of water.

Your findings of parallel changes in rates of transfer of ethanol and water could be interpreted as changes of capillary surface area rather than of permeability. You pointed out that ethanol is more lipid-soluble than water, and should be more permeable, but it isn't only lipid solubility that determines membrane diffusion; it is lipid solubility $\times$ (mol. wt.)$^{0.5}$.

So, first it is important for you to show by another method that you are measuring a change in capillary permeability. Second, you may be changing PS according to your model. Third, I do not see how a change in water permeability can be related to brain oedema unless there is active water transport, which, as far as I know, has never been demonstrated.

Raichle: The issue of whether we are measuring brain water permeability has been discussed in detail in a number of our publications, which are listed in my references. Suffice it to say here that we are convinced that our method does measure brain water permeability and not changes in capillary surface area. However, although we are measuring changes in brain water permeability we don't contend that this is exclusively what is going on. We probably stimulate changes in a number of things. For example, when one stimulates the renal nerve this produces changes in the tubular reabsorption of both water and sodium (Bello-Reus *et al.* 1976). We believe similar things are happening in brain. Unfortunately we can't measure sodium permeability because the sodium isotope has such high energy that we can't work with it.

I would again point out that we have yet to find a discrepancy between what we know anatomically, what we measure, and what has been observed in the kidney tubule and its analogue, the toad urinary bladder. The permeabilities for water observed in these critical organs and brain are almost the same. If the permeability for water in these organs is critical to over-all body homeostasis then it does not seem unreasonable to suggest that the ability of the brain to adjust its water permeability, or sodium permeability, might not be equally critical to its internal homeostasis and functions.

Rapoport: How do you deal with the oedema problem? Oedema can be explained in terms of Starling's Law as applied to cerebral capillaries (Rapoport 1976). Steady-state net flow across the capillary wall depends on a balance or imbalance of osmotic and hydrostatic pressure differences across the wall. How can a change in permeability modify the steady-state balance of hydrostatic and osmotic forces?

Raichle: We are suggesting that there is a *variable* resistor in the blood–brain barrier system to the movement of water and possibly sodium into and out of the brain. Because we are dealing with a dynamic steady state, that resistance must enter into a consideration of brain water content and volume.

Rapoport: It doesn't come into the equation. The balance occurs when resistance transients have disappeared.

Raichle: But there is a continuing flux of water in and out. It isn't as though there is a supply that is set at equilibrium. Furthermore, the brain is producing water as part of its metabolism. As I pointed out earlier, if we put a tracer in we can see that 90% of that water moves into the brain, which means that there is a large forward flux of water into brain.

Rapoport: But the net fluxes across the capillary are critical. Volume flow across the capillary, J_v, is given as L_p ($\Delta P - \sigma\Delta\Pi$), where L_p is the capillary hydraulic conductivity that is quantitatively related to permeability, ΔP the hydrostatic pressure difference between plasma and extracellular brain fluid, $\Delta\Pi$ the osmotic pressure difference (including osmotic contributions of salts and protein), and σ a reflection coefficient which equals 1 for salts and proteins, as cerebral capillaries are largely impermeable to these solutes (Rapoport 1976). Unless capillary permeability to salts also changes when water is forced into the brain, brain extracellular osmolality will be reduced and further water accumulation will cease.

Plum: I don't find your argument totally effective, Dr Rapoport. Isn't what Dr Raichle has demonstrated straightforward and clear: water permeability changes in association with the state of stimulation which he has induced? But a lot of other things that he hasn't had the opportunity to look at may also influence the net permeability not only of water but also of other substances which might be even more crucial to either metabolism or function. That is the challenging and intriguing thing about the observation, and not whether this is a protection against brain oedema—which is, after all, only a small pathological part of what one is concerned about.

Raichle: This is a model system of the ability of the brain vasculature to modify the movement of things between blood and brain. The model may have implications well beyond water. We used water because it seemed a logical and, for us, a convenient way to demonstrate this sort of behaviour.

Siesjö: It is a beautiful model. All we are discussing here is whether changes in permeability could affect the steady-state water content of the tissue and determine whether oedema occurs.

Raichle: That is a specific issue that needs to be thought about in detail. I would just hope that this discussion will provoke you and others to think about it seriously.

Reis: What is your evidence that all of this is happening at the capillary junction and not in some cell outside the capillary?

Raichle: It is based on the tracer method and the central volume principle (see references in contribution).

Reis: Couldn't the barrier be on glia just adjacent to the capillary?

Raichle: We couldn't distinguish a small difference in volume but we know for sure that the changes occur in the vascular wall complex.

Reis: But you are relying heavily on the innervation of the capillary. You are attributing the phenomenon to the events at the capillary wall. But I am not convinced that you have proved that the water is being diffused across the capillary. Secondly, is your finding with vasopressin just a pharmacological phenomenon? A vasopressin transmitter system has not yet been demonstrated descending through the brain. At least with the locus coeruleus there is a very diffuse system. It is hard to understand how the central vasopressin system is working at the general capillary level if it doesn't distribute to many capillaries.

Raichle: The central noradrenergic system with some of its dendrites lying at or near the ventricular surface would be a nice way to sense changes in the vasopressin that might be occurring in the ventricular system and then rapidly disseminating appropriate responses to the microvasculature. Again I would point out that vasopressin, given systemically, produces absolutely no effect on the brain vasculature. This is typical of membranes regulating water permeability, in that they respond to only one side. We have focused on the capillaries because the brain capillary endothelial cells seem to be exactly like other membranes that regulate water permeability. So why go looking for another cell? I agree that our tracer technique possibly couldn't discern a difference between the glial foot process and the endothelial cell, but other people have reported that the endothelial cell is a better candidate.

Pickering: This meeting may be falling into a trap. If arterial pressure is raised acutely and the permeability of the brain vessels changes, that effect may be due to the breakdown of the blood–brain barrier and water regulation. However, something else that I mentioned earlier (p. 87) can account for that effect. The simplest example is seen in man. Patients with very high pressure may have exudates or foci of whitish cotton-wool spots in their eyes. Those exudates are due to fluid containing a lot of protein which in turn is due to focal necrosis of the arterioles caused by high arterial pressure. If the arterial pressure is reduced those exudates disappear. If arterial pressure is not reduced these affections of the small arteries and arterioles destroy the kidney, eventually killing the patient. They may also produce foci of oedema in the brain. When pharmacological agents are used which raise the pressure to the extent that you showed, we know that focal necrosis of arterioles occurs and that dye will come out of the vessels. That may be the explanation of what you have observed.

Raichle: We would expect brain water permeability to go up but in fact it goes down, which is hardly a pathological event. Rather, it suggests an attempt by the brain vasculature to adjust to increased hydrostatic forces in order to prevent swelling.

Pickering: Arteriolar necrosis is focal and so is the oedema.

Owman: I would like to draw attention again to the problem of knowing which region is really stimulated. The locus coeruleus is innervated by adrenergic neurons which have an inhibitory effect on it (Fuxe *et al.* 1974; Cederbaum & Aghajanian 1976). You may be stimulating the locus coeruleus directly, or local stimulation of these incoming adrenergic neurons may inhibit locus coeruleus output. It may therefore be a good idea to use labelled noradrenaline, for example, to show that the stimulation you apply really liberates noradrenaline from the locus coeruleus neurons rather than inhibits its release.

Raichle: These things are all possible experiments.

Purves: Isn't it possible that there is cholinergic innervation of the locus coeruleus?

Owman: Yes, from the studies by Lewis & Shute (1967). Recent evidence also indicates a serotonergic input to locus coeruleus (Pickel *et al.* 1977).

Rosendorff: I accept that there is a reasonable density of innervation around the capillaries and that these nerve terminals have as their origin the noradrenergic nerves that come from the locus coeruleus. Are these the only terminals of the locus coeruleus neurons or are there others that terminate on arteriolar smooth muscle? Are there others that terminate freely in the parenchyma, presumably in association with neurons? Ostensibly they would have nothing to do with blood vessels, at least directly. If all three kinds exist, what is the ratio of innervation of these structures? I think that the point should be made here that capillaries are probably not selectively innervated by the intracellular noradrenergic pathway (INP). Is it possible that no structures are selectively innervated by the INP at all, but that INP stimulation produces a 'field' or neuromodulator effect?

Raichle: The anatomical evidence is that some of these nerve fibres are related to the vessels and some are clearly in the parenchyma of the brain.

Rosendorff: You are saying that capillaries are just one group of a whole family of brain osmoreceptors?

Raichle: That is food for thought. The brain neuron itself is an osmometer or more precisely, an oncometer. When subjected to an osmotic stress its response is to decrease its sodium and potassium content in order to achieve a normal size. As Fishman (1974) has pointed out, if the brain must sacrifice volume or osmolality, cellular volume is relatively preserved and osmolality is altered to protect brain function. There is a beautiful parallel to this in the circulating red cells of certain species (Kregenow *et al.* 1976), where the changes in cell volume are mediated by noradrenaline. It does not seem unreasonable to suggest that regulation of brain cell volume may be influenced by centrally released noradrenaline.

Reis: In the rat the nucleus of the locus coeruleus contains only 1400 neurons on each side, yet the number of synapses in the adult brain attributed to noradrenergic fibres is close to 1% of the total. This would be an awful lot of synapses. So there is an extremely ramified system of cells which have processes from the locus coeruleus. All the noradrenergic innervation of the encephalon comes from the locus coeruleus in the rat, as does a large portion of the cerebellar innervation; some of it goes to the hypothalamus and even down into the brain-stem. One of the perplexities of this neuronal system has been that there are very few nerve cells but such a widely ramified field that it becomes rather unlikely that the locus coeruleus plays a substantial role in the normal integrative neural transmission of one cell to one cell. Many people, including myself, would like to believe that the locus coeruleus may serve as a private channel for a very important neural hormone in the brain, serving in very large measure a metabolic role, in addition to possibly integrating the action of the large fields of cells. The fact that a branch would go to a capillary and another branch to a neuron is not surprising. Secondly, the evidence is that very few of the synapses which are formed by locus coeruleus neurons are of the classic junctional type. The locus coeruleus seems to have very loose ramifications, and classic synapses are not that common. The idea is that these cells are releasing their transmitter into an area rather than close to the post-synaptic element. That would suggest that the neuronal system might release a chemically active substance affecting many neuronal elements simultaneously. Have you looked at these capillaries in the electron microscope, then made a lesion of the locus and looked at regeneration?

Raichle: We are working on isolated capillaries as well as other things. There are obviously many areas that people could explore.

Rubio: Some recent work on the heart has indicated that fatty acids of large molecular weight can move across the capillary wall, not necessarily through the endothelial cell gap, i.e. by a process of simple diffusion. This work indicates that the capillaries are capable of transporting solutes by a process of facilitated diffusion (Rose & Goresky 1975).

How did you discard the possibility of changes only in the surface(s) in the PS product? You were attributing the changes in PS only to a change in the P value.

Raichle: One way to change the available surface area is just to increase the arterial CO_2 tension and increase the flow. This causes a recruitment of capillaries and an increase in available vascular surface area, but absolutely no change in the PS as we measure it. Secondly, if an osmotic stress is produced and the water PS is changed, which is what we have done, the change in the PS is totally independent of the change in flow.

Rubio: Some recent evidence using microcirculatory techniques shows that a given change in flow is not necessarily associated with a change in capillary density (Pittman 1977).

Sokoloff: With the vasodilatation caused by CO_2, there must certainly be a change in surface area, but you don't pick up a change in PS. Doesn't that worry you?

Raichle: No. As Professor Lübbers showed (this volume) capillaries are probably not changing their surface area. Thus, in a tracer method based on *relative* flow and surface area, where we recruit a capillary and its tissue or Krogh cylinder we would not expect a change in the PS. If we used a whole-organ method we would, as others do, see a change in the PS. I would emphasize that our tracer method is related to a relative volume of tissue.

Sokoloff: It is a very large volume of tissue.

Raichle: These cylinders are unique to a given capillary. The probability of a tracer introduced from one capillary leaving by way of another is not very great.

References

Bello-Reus, E., Trevino, D. L. & Gottschalk, C. W. (1976) Effect of renal sympathetic nerve stimulation on proximal water and sodium reabsorption. *J. Clin. Invest.* *57*, 1104–1107

Bonham Carter, S., Sandler, M., Goodwin, B. L., Sepping, P. & Bridges, P. K. (1978) Decreased urinary output of tyramine and its metabolites in depression. *Br. J. Psychiatry*, in press

Cederbaum, J. M. & Aghajanian, G. K. (1976) Noradrenergic neurons of the locus coeruleus: inhibition by epinephrine and activation by the α-antagonist piperoxane. *Brain Res.* *112*, 413–419

Fishman, R. A. (1974) Cell volume, pumps, and neurologic dysfunction: brain adaptation to osmotic stress. *Res. Publ. Assoc. Res. Nerv. Ment. Dis.* *53*, 159–171

Fuxe, K., Lidbrink, P., Hökfelt, T., Bolme, P. & Goldstein, M. (1974) Effects of piperoxane on sleep and waking in the rat. Evidence for increased waking by blocking inhibitory adrenaline receptors in the locus coeruleus. *Acta Physiol. Scand.* *91*, 566–567

Goltman, A. M. (1935–6) The mechanism of migraine. *J. Allergy* *7*, 351–355

Hartman, B. K., Zide, D. & Udenfriend, S. (1972) The use of dopamine-β-hydroxylase as a marker for the central noradrenergic nervous system in rat brain. *Proc. Natl. Acad. Sci. U.S.A. 69*, 2722–2726

KREGENOW, F. M., ROBBIE, D. E. & ORVOFF, J. (1976) Effect of norepinephrine and hypertonicity on K influx and cyclic AMP in duck erythrocytes. *Am. J. Physiol. 231*, 306–312

LEWIS, P. R. & SHUTE, C. C. D. (1967) The cholinergic limbic system: projections to hippocampal formation, medial cortex, nuclei of the ascending cholinergic reticular system and the subfornical organ and supra-optic crest. *Brain 90*, 521–540

PICKEL, V. M., JOH, T. H. & REIS, D. J. (1977) A serotonergic innervation of noradrenergic neurons in nucleus locus coeruleus: demonstration by immunocytochemical localization of the transmitter specific enzymes tyrosine and tryptophan hydroxylase. *Brain Res. 131*, 197–214

PITTMAN, R. N. (1977) Influence of vasodilators on the tissue oxygen delivery in the hamster cheek pouch. *Fed. Proc. 36*, 471

RAICHLE, M. E., HARTMAN, B. K., EICHLING, J. O. & SHARPE, L. G. (1975) Central noradrenergic regulation of cerebral blood flow and vascular permeability. *Proc. Natl. Acad. Sci. U.S.A. 72*, 3726–3730

RAPOPORT, S. I. (1976) *Blood-Brain Barrier in Physiology and Medicine*, Raven Press, New York

ROSE, C. P. & GORESKY, C. A. (1975) The kinetics of transport of free fatty acids across the endothelium and their uptake by the myocyte in the dog heart. *Fed. Proc. 34*, 457

Osmotic opening of the blood–brain barrier

STANLEY I. RAPOPORT

Laboratory of Neurophysiology, National Institute of Mental Health, Bethesda, Maryland

Abstract The blood–brain barrier at cerebral blood vessels is due to a continuous lining of endothelial cells, which are connected by tight junctions that restrict intercellular diffusion. The endothelium excludes most water-soluble solutes and proteins but supports facilitated stereospecific transport of monosaccharides and large neutral and basic amino acids. The barrier in different species can be made permeable by infusing a hypertonic solution of urea or arabinose into the internal carotid artery. Endothelial cells presumably shrink and tight junctions between them widen to proteins and normally restricted solutes. Thus, intravascular protein tracers such as Evans' blue–albumin, ^{125}I-labelled albumin, horseradish peroxidase (EC 1.11.1.7) and α-mannosidase (EC 3.2.1.24) are allowed into the brain, and uptake of [^{3}H]norepinephrine (noradrenaline) is increased more than twofold above a normal rate of accumulation by brain. Osmotic barrier opening to amines has been used to demonstrate their effect on cerebral blood flow from within the brain parenchyma. Osmotic barrier opening is reversible, may be graded with respect to molecular size and is not followed by evidence of brain damage or of brain oedema (when measured two days after hypertonic infusion). Transient cerebral changes probably accompany osmotic opening, however, as glucose uptake and cerebral metabolism of glucose are increased after hypertonic infusion.

ULTRASTRUCTURE AND TRANSPORT AT CEREBRAL VESSELS

The blood–brain barrier at the cerebral vasculature is due to a continuous lining of endothelial cells that are connected by tight junctions. The junctions restrict intercellular diffusion and make the barrier as a whole have the permeability and transport properties of the endothelial cells and their membranes (Crone 1965; Reese & Karnovsky 1967). Lipid-soluble solutes and CO_2 and O_2 pass rapidly across the barrier, whereas water-soluble solutes including ions and proteins do not. Protein transfer is low also because vesicular transport is slight or absent at the vascular endothelium.

The endothelium, together with the choroid plexus and arachnoid membrane, acts as a regulatory system that determines the composition of the brain and cerebrospinal fluid with respect to that of blood (reviewed by Rapoport 1976*a*). In addition to restricting exchange of proteins, ions and water-soluble non-electrolytes, the endothelium can transport, by facilitated, stereospecific saturable mechanisms, substances that are involved in brain metabolism. Furthermore, enzymes within the vascular endothelium can trap aromatic amino acids such as L-dopa.

At cerebral capillaries, monosaccharides with a pyranose ring in the C_1-chair form are transported by a saturable stereospecific mechanism that is comparable to that found in red cells. D-Glucose, D-galactose, D-mannose, 2-deoxy-D-glucose and 3-*O*-methyl-D-glucose compete for the common carrier system. As competitors of glucose are rarely found in the blood, the main function of the system is to deliver sufficient glucose to the brain to support cerebral metabolism. In man, signs of hypoglycaemia appear when blood glucose falls to below 19 mg/100 ml or, in the occasional case of galactosaemia, when large quantities of blood galactose inhibit glucose entry into brain (Kety *et al.* 1948; Neame 1970; Rapoport 1976*a*).

Large neutral and large basic amino acids that are essential for brain metabolism are also transported at cerebral capillaries by an L-system and a basic amino acid system, respectively (Oldendorf 1971; Rapoport 1976*a*). Competition among amino acids in the same transport class determines relative rates of passage from blood to brain and, therefore, subsequent cerebral metabolism. For example, the blood concentration of tryptophan, as compared to that of competing neutral amino acids, affects tryptophan uptake as well as serotonin synthesis by the brain (Fernstrom & Wurtman 1972).

Lactic and pyruvic acids normally leave the brain by a facilitated mechanism that is specific for short-chain monocarboxylic acids. As the monocarboxylic acid carrier saturates at low substrate concentrations, these acids may accumulate in brain if production is excessive, and thereby affect cerebral blood flow (Oldendorf 1972).

As far as is known, the above transported substrates move from a high to a low concentration across the cerebrovascular endothelium, independently of energy requirements or of ionic gradients.

OSMOTIC OPENING OF THE BLOOD–BRAIN BARRIER

The cerebrovascular endothelium can be made permeable to normally excluded proteins and solutes by infusing a hypertonic solution of a poorly lipid-soluble solute into the internal carotid artery. In this paper, I shall

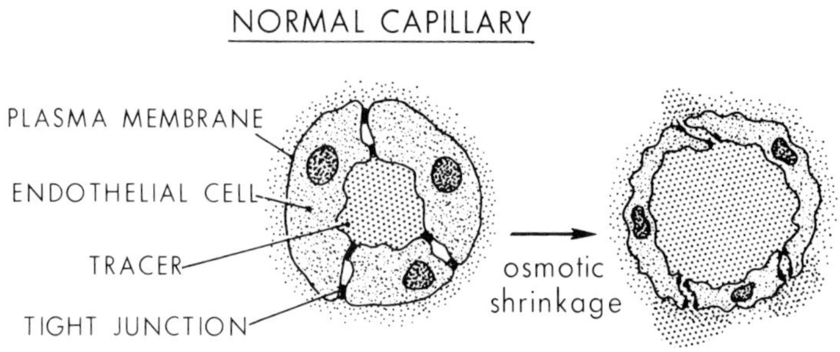

FIG. 1. Model for normal barrier and for barrier opening by widening of interendothelial tight junctions. When endothelial cells shrink in a hypertonic environment, their membranes stress tight junctions and make them permeable to intravascular tracer.

present physiological and ultrastructural evidence that indicates that the permeability increment is caused by osmotic shrinkage of endothelial cells and widening of tight junctions. I shall also show that the method can be used to study central effects of various substances on cerebral blood flow (CBF) and cerebral function.

Tight junctions between cells are networks of fibrillar strands that limit intercellular diffusion. In epithelial tissues, osmotic or hydrostatic pressure stresses can alter structure and permeability of these junctions by physically deforming them (Ussing 1971; reviewed by Rapoport 1976*a*). A model which can account for osmotic opening of the blood–brain barrier, based partially on these observations, is illustrated in Fig. 1. Its premise is that tight junctions between cerebrovascular endothelia are also distorted and made permeable when endothelial cells shrink in hypertonic solutions.

The model is consistent with the following evidence: (*a*) osmotic thresholds (minimal osmolal concentrations), both for opening of the blood–brain barrier and for shrinkage of single cells, increase with increasing solute lipid solubility, (*b*) osmotic barrier opening is reversible, (*c*) osmotic opening produces observable transfer of intravascular protein (exogenous horseradish peroxidase [EC 1.11.1.7]) between cerebrovascular endothelial cells and not through them, (*d*) osmotic opening may be graded with respect to the size of penetrating molecule. Reversible graded barrier opening that follows the rules of osmotic cell shrinkage would not be expected if endothelial cells were irreversibly damaged, or if vesicular transport were stimulated so as to increase barrier permeability.

TEST OF MODEL FOR OSMOTIC BARRIER OPENING

Overton (1895) and Collander (1937) showed that single plant or animal cells shrank reversibly when placed in a hypertonic solution of a lipid-insoluble solute. Shrinkage by equiosmolal solutions of non-electrolytes which were slightly lipid-soluble declined when lipid solubility increased. The results indicated that cell membranes were ideally semi-permeable to lipid-insoluble solutes, allowing water but not the solutes to pass, and partially semi-permeable to somewhat lipid-soluble solutes. It seemed reasonable to suppose that cerebrovascular endothelial cells also would shrink in hypertonic solutions as a function of solute lipid solubility, and that tight junctions between the cells might widen as illustrated in Fig. 1.

To test this hypothesis, hypertonic solutions of solutes with different lipid solubilities were applied to the arachnoid surface of the rabbit or cat brain for 10 min and were then removed (Rapoport 1970; Rapoport *et al.* 1972). Barrier opening was studied by evaluating the pH response at the arachnoid surface to an intravenous injection of $NaHCO_3$ (a measure of barrier integrity to ions), or by determining the minimal osmolal concentration (threshold osmolality) that produced extravasation of blood-borne Evans' blue–albumin from pial vessels. In the latter experiments, reversibility of opening was determined by injecting Evans' blue intravenously 30 min after, rather than before, a threshold osmolality had opened the barrier at the arachnoid surface.

The results are summarized in Table 1, where test substances are ranked according to their octanol/water partition coefficient, a measure of lipid solubility. Osmolal thresholds at the barrier site (presumably at the vascular endothelium) were estimated by taking into account differences in diffusion at the pia-arachnoid membranes.

The data in the table support the interpretation that hypertonic solutions open the barrier by shrinking endothelial cells, as illustrated in Fig. 1. Electrolytes, and non-electrolytes less lipid-soluble than propionamide, opened the barrier reversibly. More lipid-soluble solutes acted irreversibly, probably by destroying endothelial cell membranes. The table also shows that osmolal thresholds of the reversibly acting solutions increased with increasing lipid solubility, as expected from the inverse relation between lipid solubility and shrinkage of single cells by hypertonic solutions (Overton 1895; Collander 1937).

The topical observations in Table 1 were extended to vessels within the brain by perfusing hypertonic solutions into the internal carotid artery of different species (Thompson 1970; Rapoport *et al.* 1972; Studer *et al.* 1974; Rapoport 1976*a*). Patterns of reversible and irreversible opening held at intracerebral vessels just as they did at the pial vasculature. Intracarotid

TABLE 1

Effect of topically applied concentrated solutions on blood-brain barrier in the rabbit.

Substance	*Octanol/water partition*	*Reversibility of opening*	*Threshold osmolality at barrier*[a]
LiCl	—	Yes	0.87
Na_2SO_4	—	Yes	0.82
NaCl	—	Yes	1.0
Sucrose	0.0002	Yes	1.1
Glucose	0.0005	Yes	1.0
Urea	0.0016	Yes	1.7
Glycerol	0.003	Yes	2.1
Lactamide	0.005	Yes	—
Ethylene glycol	0.012	No	—
Methyl urea	0.016	Yes	2.2
Formamide	0.02	Yes	2.9
Propylene glycol	0.039	No	—
Acetamide	0.055	Yes	3.5
Propionamide	0.16	Yes	3.2
Cyanamide	0.16	No	—
Methanol	0.20	No	—
Ethanol	0.48	No	—
Methyl carbamate	0.50	No	—
Ethyl carbamate	0.71	No	—

[a]Thresholds relative to NaCl threshold = 1.
A solution was applied to a cortical region for 10 min, then removed. Intravascular Evans' blue–albumin was used as a barrier tracer. The osmolal threshold for barrier opening was calculated from the surface osmolality by taking into account diffusion through the pia-arachnoid. Reversibility of opening indicates that the barrier closed 30 min after arachnoidal application of a threshold concentration of a particular solute. Solutes are ranked according to their octanol/water partition coefficients. Data are from Rapoport *et al.* (1972).

infusion of hypertonic solutions of lactamide or urea opened the barrier reversibly on the hemisphere homolateral to infusion, whereas hypertonic solutions of propylene glycol or ethanol acted irreversibly.

ULTRASTRUCTURAL STUDIES, REVERSIBILITY AND GRADED OPENING

Electron microscope studies confirmed that hypertonic solutions, whether infused into the carotid artery or applied to the brain surface, increased cerebrovascular permeability by opening interendothelial tight junctions. Carotid infusion of 2M to 3M-urea or of Hypaque 50 (a hypertonic contrast

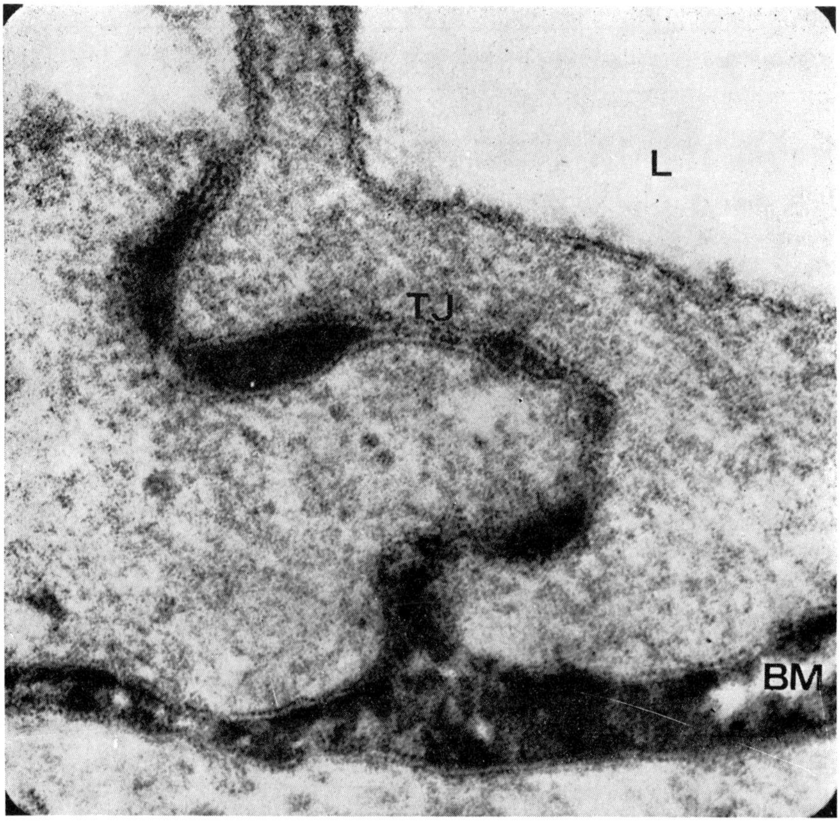

FIG. 2. Opening of tight junctions between cerebrovascular endothelial cells to peroxidase tracer, after intracarotid infusion of 3 M-urea in the rabbit. Peroxidase was administered intravenously before infusion, and the animal was killed 90 s after infusion. The tracer was washed from the capillary lumen (L) during fixation. Reaction product is present along the interface between endothelial cells, in the gaps between tight junctions (TJ) and in the basement membrane (BM) (× 88 000). (From Brightman *et al.* 1973.)

medium employed in cerebral angiography) allowed intravascular horseradish peroxidase into the rabbit brain via interendothelial tight junctions (Fig. 2) (Brightman *et al.* 1973; Sterrett *et al.* 1976). Reaction product did not flood vascular endothelial cells and pinocytosis was not stimulated.

Although tight junctions can be made permeable to protein without apparent separation of apposing cell membranes (Fig. 2), in some cases membranes do separate fully following hypertonic treatment. Separation by a distance of 0.1 μm, without cell damage, has been noted in rats after carotid infusion of an arabinose solution of 1.4–1.6 mol/kg (M. Sato, M. W. Brightman &

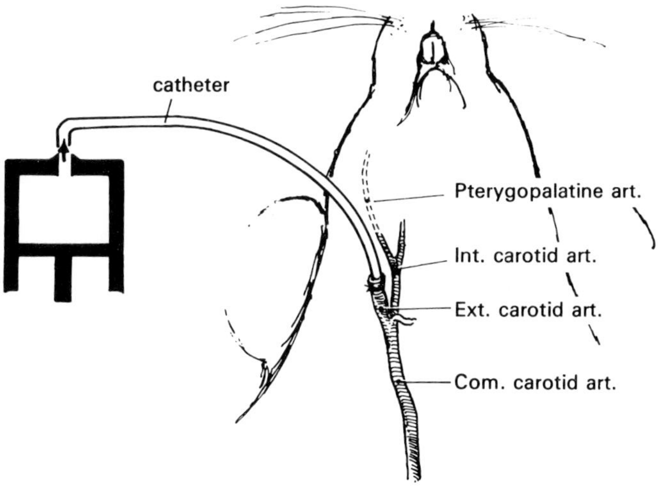

FIG. 3. Brain perfusion via a catheterized external carotid artery in the rat. Adapted from Greene (1963).

S. I. Rapoport, unpublished observations). In addition, hypertonic arabinose infusion appears to increase the number of endothelial pinocytotic vesicles that contain reaction product of horseradish peroxidase. Transendothelial vesicular transport is not stimulated, however, because the vesicles are found in brains that have been infused *in situ* with concentrated glutaraldehyde before the intravascular administration of horseradish peroxidase. Glutaraldehyde fixation stops vesicular transport (Westergaard & Brightman 1973). It is possible that the vesicles contribute to channels that are 'frozen' *in situ* by glutaraldehyde fixation (cf. Sterrett *et al.* 1976; Simionescu *et al.* 1975).

Different extents of tight junctional widening could account for the observed gradation of opening with respect to the size of test molecule (Rapoport 1970; Thompson 1970; Studer *et al.* 1974). For example, carotid infusion of a sucrose solution, 1.2 mol/kg, in the rat opens the barrier to ^{22}Na but not to the larger ^{125}I-labelled albumin molecule, whereas a 4.2 mol/kg sucrose solution opens the barrier to both tracers (Table 2). A 1.6 to 1.8 mol/kg solution of arabinose, infused into a catheterized external carotid artery of the rat (Fig. 3), allows enzymes such as human placental α-mannosidase (EC 3.2.1.24) and yeast invertase (β-fructofuranosidase, EC 3.2.1.26) into the brain (Barranger *et al.* 1977). These molecules have molecular weights of the order of 200 000 daltons and remain intracerebrally for at least 24 h after barrier opening.

TABLE 2

Brain spaces of tracers injected intravenously in rats after infusion of different solutions into internal carotid artery.

Infusate	^{125}*I-labelled albumin space* $\times$ *10*^{2}		^{22}*Na space* $\times$ *10*^{2}	
	30 min[a]	*4 h*	*30 min*	*4 h*
Control	1.73	1.73	10.8	10.8
Isotonic saline	1.61	1.75	11.0	11.5
Sucrose, 4.2 mol/kg	2.15[b]	1.66	19.7[b]	11.6
Sucrose, 1.2 mol/kg	1.72	1.81	17.0[b]	11.2

[a]Time after infusion; [b]Significantly different from control ($P < 0.05$)
The brain space is the ratio of brain concentration to blood concentration. Data are from Studer *et al.* (1974).

TABLE 3

Barrier opening to [^{14}C]fructose in dog by infusion of hypertonic solutions into vertebral artery

Time after infusion	*3*M-*urea infusion (6)*[a]	*0.9*M-*NaCl infusion (5)*[a]
	% Change in capillary permeability	
5 min	$+ 437 \pm 9$[b]	$+ 1013 \pm 272$[b]
90 min	$+ 145 \pm 53$[b]	$+ 583 \pm 94$[b]

[a]No. of animals; [b]Mean $\pm$ S.E.M. differs from zero ($P < 0.05$)
Permeability was measured by indicator dilution technique. Data are from Pollay (1975*b*).

As summarized in Table 1 and noted after urea infusion into the carotid artery of the rabbit (Rapoport *et al.* 1972), the barrier to intravascular Evans' blue–albumin may remain open for less than 30 min after osmotic treatment. Studies with [^{14}C]fructose, ^{22}Na or ^{125}I-labelled albumin as barrier tracers suggest, on the other hand, that the barrier can remain patent for 90 min to 4 h after hypertonic infusion (Tables 2 and 3) (Pollay 1975*b*; Studer *et al.* 1974).

Reversible barrier opening without neurological sequelae or obvious brain damage or oedema can be produced in rhesus monkeys and baboons that are infused, via a catheterized lingual artery, with 3 mol/kg urea or 2.5 mol/kg lactamide solution, and in rats infused with 1.8 mol/kg arabinose solution (Fig. 3). Measurable, long-term brain damage associated with the osmotic

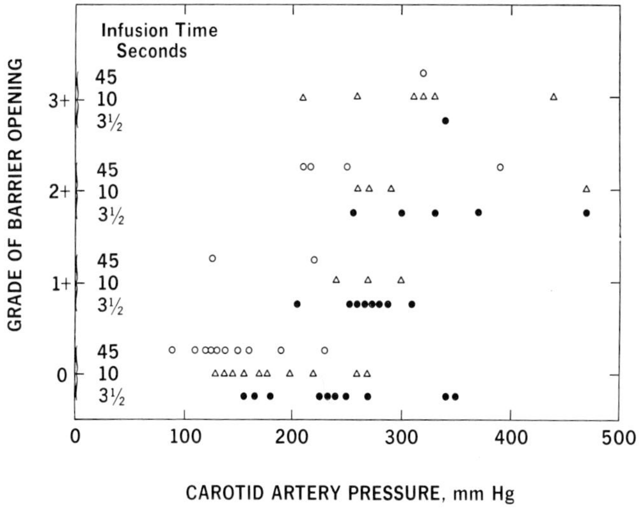

FIG. 4. Relation of barrier opening to carotid artery pressure during infusion for 3.5, 10 or 45 s in rat. Isotonic saline was infused at different rates into the common carotid artery when the external carotid was ligated and carotid pressure was calculated after subtracting the pressure drop due to the catheter system. Barrier opening to intravascular Evans' blue–albumin was graded from 0 (no brain staining) to 3+ (deep blue staining). Each symbol represents 1 animal. (From Rapoport 1976*b*.)

procedure is prevented if the cerebral circulation is not permanently compromised, if cerebral oxygenation is maintained to counteract effects of possible apnoea or bradycardia due to hypertonic infusion, if filtered solutions of purified solutes are used for infusion, and if carotid hypertension is prevented (Rapoport & Thompson 1973; Rapoport 1976*a*, *b*; Rapoport *et al.* 1977; MacKenzie *et al.* 1976; Pickard *et al.* 1977; Chiueh *et al.* 1978). Rapid infusion rates can result, for example, in hypertensive barrier opening and brain oedema through carotid artery pressure being raised during infusion to levels beyond 170 mmHg (Fig. 4).

Additional studies are needed to determine the optimal agents and their concentrations for maximal osmotic opening without associated brain damage, as solutions of the same osmolality may differ with respect to toxicity. For example, X-ray contrast media that are used in cerebral angiography can open the barrier at a common 1.2 osmolal threshold and nevertheless have different clinical neurotoxicities. The latter correlate with solute lipid solubility (Rapoport *et al.* 1974; Rapoport & Levitan 1974; Sterrett *et al.* 1976).

QUANTITATIVE MEASURES OF BARRIER OPENING BY HYPERTONIC SOLUTIONS

Transported substrates

The osmotic method allows normally excluded solutes into the brain but may also increase brain uptake of solutes that enter by facilitated transport. The method is proportionally more effective with respect to excluded agents, however. For example, carotid infusion of 3 M-urea in the rabbit increases brain uptake of glycine, which is not transported, but not of the transported amino acid, phenylalanine (Pollay 1975*a*).

TABLE 4

Cerebrovascular permeability to [^{14}C]glucose and cerebral blood flow in dog, after vertebral artery infusion of hypertonic urea or NaCl solution.

Solution	*Time after infusion (min)*	*% Change CBF*	*% Change permeability*
Urea, 3 M	5	15.3 ± 2.9[a]	39.7 ± 5.9[a]
Urea, 3 M	90	− 0.4 ± 3.8	18.0 ± 7.2
NaCl, 0.9 M	5	− 18.6 ± 5.3[a]	− 12.6 ± 3.2[a]
NaCl, 0.9 M	90	− 23.9 ± 6.9[a]	− 17.6 ± 8.4

[a]Mean ± S.E.M. ($n = 5$) differs from 0 ($P = 0.05$)
Permeability was calculated by the indicator dilution technique. Data are from Pollay (1975*b*)

TABLE 5

Brain uptake index (BUI) of [^{14}C]2-deoxy-D-glucose in rabbit after carotid artery infusion of various solutions

Solution	*Molarity*	*Brain uptake index*		*% Inhibition*
		No inhibition	*Self-inhibition*[a]	
Ringer	0.16	48.8 ± 0.8[b]	14.4 ± 1.8	71
Urea	2–3	72.9 ± 2.3	20.0 ± 2.0	74
Urea, 20 min	2–3	48.1 ± 4.2		
Acetamide	5.0	68.7 ± 1.0	18.7 ± 2.3	73
NaCl	0.5	67.2 ± 3.3	11.5 ± 0.8	83

[a]BUI tested with injection of 50mM-2-deoxy-D-glucose; [b]Mean ± S.E.M.
Except as noted, BUI values were determined immediately after infusion. Data are from Spatz *et al.* (1976).

Infusion of 3 M-urea solution into the dog vertebral artery increases cerebrovascular permeability to [^{14}C]glucose, as determined by the indicator dilution technique (Table 4) (Pollay 1975*b*). Increased permeability is accompanied by an increased CBF, but changes in both CBF and permeability disappear within 90 min. Hypertonic NaCl solution affects neither CBF nor [^{14}C]glucose permeability, however, although permeability to normally excluded [^{14}C]-fructose is augmented (Tables 3 and 4).

In rabbits, infusion of hypertonic solutions of non-electrolytes or of NaCl reversibly increases the brain uptake index (BUI) of [^{14}C]2-deoxy-D-glucose (Table 5) and [^{14}C]3-*O*-methyl-D-glucose (Spatz *et al.* 1976). The elevated BUI values of these tracers are inhibitable by non-tracer material to the same extent as are BUI values in control, unperfused brain regions.

As 3-*O*-methyl-D-glucose is not phosphorylated within brain (Narahara & Özand 1963), an increase in its BUI after hypertonic treatment suggests that monosaccharide transport is stimulated independently of changes in cerebral metabolism. One possibility is that capillary surface area increases when CBF is elevated. It should be remembered, however, that permeability coefficients as determined by the BUI or indicator dilution techniques are not entirely certain because of assumptions concerning CBF and the reference tracer (Crone 1965; Rapoport 1976*a*).

Osmotic barrier opening may be accompanied by transient, localized increases in cerebral glucose consumption (Pappius *et al.*, 1978). Carotid infusion of 1.4 M-mannitol solution in the conscious rat, by the method of Fig. 3, results in local increments in uptake of intravenously injected [^{14}C]2-deoxy-D-glucose, as measured by autoradiography (Sokoloff *et al.* 1977). These local 'hot spots' of phosphorylated tracer reflect increased glucose metabolism, caused possibly by entry of K into brain from blood (cf. Katzman & Pappius 1973).

OSMOTIC BARRIER OPENING FOR THE STUDY OF CBF

In the baboon, carotid infusion of hypertonic urea solution is followed by changes in overall brain CBF that disappear within 30 min, whereas barrier opening may last up to 4 h (Tables 2 and 3) (MacKenzie *et al.* 1976; Pickard *et al.* 1977). The osmotic method can therefore be employed to study central effects of normally excluded agents on CBF, 30 min to 2 h after barrier opening. As illustrated in Table 6, when either norepinephrine (noradrenaline), serotonin or prostaglandin-E_2 is injected into the carotid artery 30 min after hypertonic treatment, changes in CBF are more significant than in the absence of barrier opening. The findings suggest that these agents, when admitted

TABLE 6

Response of cerebral blood flow in baboons to intracarotid infusion of drugs before and after barrier opening by 2M-urea solution (data from Pickard *et al.* 1977).

Condition	*PGE₂* 10^{-7} *g/(kg min)*	*Serotonin* 10^{-7} *g/(kg min)*	*Norepinephrine* 5×10^{-8} *g/(kg min)*
	% Change in cerebral flow		
Pre-urea	— 19 ± 4	— 6 ± 4	+ 2 ± 4
Post-urea	— 39 ± 9[a]	— 30 + 4[a]	+ 49 ± 13[a]

[a]Mean ± S.E.M. significantly different from pre-urea change ($P < 0.05$).

TABLE 7

Entry of ^{3}H into rat brain during continuous intravenous infusion of [^{3}H]norepinephrine, after barrier opening by 1.8 mol/kg arabinose solution.

			Unperfused hemisphere		*Perfused hemisphere*		
No. of animals	*Time after opening min*	*Blood concentration counts/(min ml)*	*Concentration counts/(min g)*	*Space %*	*Concentration counts/(min g)*	*Space %*	*Perfused/Unperfused*
4	10	43 200[a] ± 2 830	5 300 ± 470	12.3	11 500 ± 1 660	26.7	2.2
3	60	87 300 ± 9 600	38 000 ± 8 800	43.5	66 000 ± 19 000	75.7	1.7

[a]Mean ± S.E.M.
Space is brain concentration/blood concentration. Data are from Chiueh *et al.* (1978).

to the brain parenchyma, can modify CBF, possibly by affecting smooth muscles controlling arteriolar resistance or by altering brain metabolism and influencing CBF indirectly. These conclusions should be tempered, however, as local changes in cerebral metabolism or CBF, which follow osmotic barrier opening, may not be reflected in measurements of these parameters over an entire cerebral hemisphere (Pappius *et al.* 1978).

Osmotic barrier opening in fact increases brain uptake of amines (or their metabolites) two- to threefold, as measured by the BUI technique (J. E. Hardebo, personal communication) and more directly by studying compartmental blood-to-brain transfer (Chiueh *et al.* 1978). In the latter experiments (Tables 7 and 8), ^{125}I-labelled albumin was injected and [^{3}H]norepinephrine was infused intra-

TABLE 8

Entry of ^{125}I-labelled albumin into rat brain after intravenous injection, after barrier opening by arabinose solution, 1.8 mol/kg.

No. of animals	*Time after opening*	*Blood concentration*	*Unperfused hemisphere*		*Perfused hemisphere*		*Perfused/ Unperfused*
			Concentration	*Space*	*Concentration*	*Space*	
	min	*counts/ (min ml)*	*counts/ (min g)*	%	*counts/ (min g)*	%	
4	10	311 300 ± 30 460	6 900 ± 190	2.2	13 850 ± 930	4.4	2.0
3	60	294 500 ± 9 400	9160 ± 310	3.1	20 300 ± 5 000	6.9	2.2

*Mean ± S.E.M.
Space is brain concentration/blood concentration. Data are from Chiueh *et al.* (1978).

venously (at a rate of 2.5 μCi/min) immediately after barrier opening by an arabinose solution, 1.8 mol/kg, in rats by the method of Fig. 3. Ten min or 60 min later, brain spaces of both tracers in the perfused hemisphere were twofold greater than corresponding spaces in the unperfused hemisphere. In regions such as the caudate nucleus, uptake was increased three to five times.

The ^{3}H space in control unperfused brain regions was 12.3% after 10 min of intravenous infusion of [^{3}H]norepinephrine and 43% after 60 min infusion, whereas albumin spaces were 2 to 3%. Control brain continually accumulated [^{3}H]norepinephrine or its metabolites, possibly at vascular endothelial cells or at nerve endings. Due to a blood–brain barrier, brain uptake of ^{3}H is less than uptake in other tissues (Whitby *et al.* 1961), but nevertheless is measurable and significant in the adult rat.

References

BARRANGER, J. A., PENTCHEV, P. G., RAPOPORT, S. I. & BRADY, R. O. (1977) Augmentation of brain lysosomal enzyme activity following enzyme infusion with concomitant alteration of the blood-brain barrier. *Ann. Neurol. 1*, 496

BRIGHTMAN, M. W., HORI, M., RAPOPORT, S. I., REESE, T. S. & WESTERGAARD, E. (1973) Osmotic opening of tight junctions in cerebral endothelium. *J. Comp. Neurol. 152*, 317–326

CHIUEH, C. C., SUN, S. L., KOPIN, I. J., FREDERICKS, W. R. & RAPOPORT, S. I. (1978) Entry of ^{3}H-norepinephrine, ^{125}I-albumin and Evans blue from blood into brain following unilateral osmotic opening of the blood-brain barrier. *Brain Res.*, in press

COLLANDER, R. (1937) The permeability of plant protoplasts to nonelectrolytes. *Faraday Soc. Trans. 33*, 985–990

CRONE, C. (1965) The permeability of brain capillaries to nonelectrolytes. *Acta Physiol. Scand. 64*, 407–417

FERNSTROM, J. D. & WURTMAN, R. J. (1972) Brain serotonin content: physiological regulation by plasma neutral amino acids. *Science (Wash. D.C.) 178*, 414–416

GREENE, E. C. (1963) *Anatomy of the Rat*, Hafner, New York

KATZMAN, R. & PAPPIUS, H. M. (1973) *Brain Electrolytes and Fluid Metabolism*, Williams & Wilkins, Baltimore

KETY, S. S., POLIS, B. D., NADLER, C. S. & SCHMIDT, C. F. (1948) The blood flow and oxygen consumption of the human brain in diabetic acidosis and coma. *J. Clin. Invest. 27*, 500–510

MACKENZIE, E. T., MCCULLOCH, J., O'KEANE, M., PICKARD, J. D. & HARPER, A. M. (1976) Cerebral circulation and norepinephrine: relevance of the blood-brain barrier. *Am. J. Physiol. 231*, 483–488

NARAHARA, H. T. & ÖZAND, P. (1963) Studies of tissue permeability. IX. The effect of insulin on the penetration of 3-methyl-glucose-H^3 in frog muscle. *J. Biol. Chem. 238*, 40–49

NEAME, K. D. (1970) Transport of monosaccharides, amines and certain other metabolites, in *Handbook of Neurochemistry*, vol. 4 (Lajtha, A., ed.), pp. 329–359, Plenum Press, New York

OLDENDORF, W. H. (1971) Brain uptake of radiolabeled amino acids, amines and hexoses after arterial injection. *Am. J. Physiol. 221*, 1629–1639

OLDENDORF, W. H. (1972) Blood-brain barrier permeability to lactate. *Eur. Neurol. 6*, 49–55

OVERTON, E. (1895) Über die osmotischen Eigenschaften der lebenden Pflanzen und Tierzelle. *Vierteljahresschr. Naturforsch. Ges. Zür. 40*, 159–201

PAPPIUS, H. M., SAVAKI, H., FIESCHI, C., RAPOPORT, S.I. & SOKOLOFF, L. (1978) Cerebral glucose utilization after opening of blood-brain barrier. *9th Annu. Meet. Am. Soc. Neurochem.*, in press

PICKARD, J. D., DURITY, F., WELSH, F. A., LANGFITT, T. W., HARPER, A. M. & MACKENZIE, E. T. (1977) Osmotic opening of the blood-brain barrier: value in pharmacological studies on the cerebral circulation. *Brain Res. 122*, 170–176

POLLAY, M. (1975*a*) Evaluation of altered blood-brain barrier permeability to amino acids. *Res. Commun. Chem. Pathol. Pharmacol. 10*, 763–766

POLLAY, M. (1975*b*) Effect of hypertonic solutions on the blood-brain barrier. *Neurology 25*, 852–856

RAPOPORT, S. I. (1970) Effect of concentrated solutions on blood-brain barrier. *Am. J. Physiol. 219*, 270–274

RAPOPORT, S. I. (1976*a*) *Blood–Brain Barrier in Physiology and Medicine*, Raven Press, New York

RAPOPORT, S. I. (1976*b*) Opening of the blood–brain barrier by acute hypertension. *Exp. Neurol. 52*, 467–479

RAPOPORT, S. I. & LEVITAN, H. (1974) Neurotoxicity of X-ray contrast media. Relation to lipid solubility and blood–brain barrier permeability. *Am. J. Roentgenol. Radium Ther. Nucl. Med. 122*, 186–193

RAPOPORT, S. I. & THOMPSON, H. K. (1973) Osmotic opening of the blood-brain barrier in the monkey without associated neurological deficits. *Science (Wash. D.C.) 180*, 971

RAPOPORT, S. I., HORI, M. & KLATZO, I. (1972) Testing of a hypothesis for osmotic opening of the blood–brain barrier. *Am. J. Physiol. 223*, 323–331

RAPOPORT, S. I., THOMPSON, H. K. & BIDINGER, J. M. (1974) Equi-osmolal opening of the blood–brain barrier in the rabbit by different contrast agents. *Acta Radiol. Diagn. 15*, 21–32

RAPOPORT, S. I., MATTHEWS, K., THOMPSON, H. K. & PETTIGREW, K. D. (1977) Osmotic opening of the blood–brain barrier in the rhesus monkey without measurable brain edema. *Brain Res., 136*, 23–29

REESE, T. S. & KARNOVSKY, M. J. (1967) Fine structural localization of a blood–brain barrier to exogenous peroxidase. *J. Cell Biol. 34*, 207–217

SIMIONESCU, N., SIMIONESCU, M. & PALADE, G. E. (1975) Permeability of muscle capillaries to small heme-peptides. Evidence for the existence of patent transendothelial channels. *J. Cell Biol. 64*, 586–607

SOKOLOFF, L., REIVICH, M., KENNEDY, C., DES ROSSIERS, M. H., PATLAK, C. S., PETTIGREW, K. D., SAKURADA, O. & SHINOHARA, M. (1977) The [^{14}C]deoxyglucose method for the measurement of local cerebral glucose utilization: theory, procedure, and normal values in the conscious and anesthetized albino rat. *J. Neurochem.*, *28*, 897–916

SPATZ, M., RAP, Z. M., RAPOPORT, S. I. & KLATZO, I. (1976) Effects of hypertonic solutions and of mercuric chloride on the uptake of [^{14}C] glucose analogues by rabbit brain. *Neuropathol. Appl. Neurobiol. 2*, 53–61

STERRETT, P. R., BRADLEY, I. M., KITTEN, G. T., JANSSEN, H. F. & HOLLOWAY, L. S. (1976) Cerebrovasculature permeability changes following experimental angiography. A light- and electronmicroscopic study. *J. Neurol. Sci. 30*, 385–403

STUDER, R. K., WELCH, D. M. & SIEGEL, B. A. (1974) Transient alteration of the blood–brain barrier: effect of hypertonic solutions administered via carotid artery injection. *Exp. Neurol. 44*, 266–273

THOMPSON, A. M. (1970) Hyperosmotic effects of brain uptake of nonelectrolytes, in *Capillary Permeability* (Crone, C. & Lassen, N. A., eds.) *(Alfred Benzon Symp. 2)*, pp. 459–467, Munksgaard, Copenhagen

USSING, H. H. (1971) Introductory remarks. *Philos. Trans. R. Soc. Lond. B. Biol. Sci. 262*, 85–90

WESTERGAARD, E. & BRIGHTMAN, M. W. (1973) Transport of proteins across normal cerebral arterioles. *J. Comp. Neurol. 152*, 17–44

WHITBY, L. G., AXELROD, J. & WEIL-MALHERBE, H. (1961) The fate of ^{3}H-norepinephrine in animals. *J. Pharmacol. Exp. Ther. 132*, 193–201

Discussion

Reis: Clinically, hypertonic agents are used to reduce cerebral oedema. Is the right drug being used for the wrong reason? Are some of these agents opening up the barrier and allowing other materials to get into the brain to do their work, rather than themselves removing fluid from oedematous cells?

Rapoport: I don't think so. In the treatment of clinical oedema, plasma osmolality usually is not raised above 0.34 osmol (Buckell & Walsh 1964), and this steady-state level is insufficient to open the blood-brain barrier. If plasma osmolality is maintained for some time above 0.38 osmol, however, the barrier is opened when cerebral microhaemorrhages are produced (Luttrell *et al.* 1959). When we osmotically open the barrier, on the other hand, we infuse a solution whose osmolality is 1.2 osmol or higher into the carotid artery, and we do not produce gross brain damage because the infusion time is only 20 to 30 s. Contrast media used in cerebral angiography also have osmolalities above 1.2 osmol (Rapoport *et al.* 1974).

Sandler: If chicks up to the fourth or fifth week of life are injected with certain putative monoamine neurotransmitters, these will get across to the brain without any adjuvant when administered parenterally. Are there ultra-structural differences in the chick which enable solutes which otherwise would not get across the blood-brain barrier to cross it? This model has been used extensively, in particular by Marley (Marley & Stephenson 1972) who studied the direct central effects of these compounds after peripheral dosage.

Rapoport: These amines might diffuse into the brain of the newly hatched chick via the choroid plexus, as tight junctions between choroidal epithelia are incomplete immediately after hatching (Doolin & Birge 1969). Although cerebrovascular tight junctions are complete at the time of hatching (Delorme *et al.* 1970), amines could enter the brain across capillaries if the tight junctions were somewhat permeable, or if enzymic trapping mechanisms were deficient, as they appear to be in cerebral capillaries of the immature rat (Loizou 1970).

Raichle: There are several methodological difficulties in the methods you refer to for the measurement of permeability. Most importantly one can't measure flow. The information obtained, the extraction fraction or the brain uptake index, is not only a function of permeability but also of flow, yet in no instance do these methods measure flow. Secondly, they use water as a freely permeable reference standard, but water is not freely permeable, as discussed in and after my paper. If you impose a change in your experimental conditions you have to know what the standard is doing and what, if anything, has happened to the blood flow. The techniques are very simple in design but there are obviously many pitfalls in interpretation.

Rapoport: The BUI and indicator dilution techniques provide important information about relative rates of capillary transport under well-established normal conditions with constant blood flow. If blood flow is altered, these methods cannot be used to calculate permeability unless the alteration is measured. It would be important to be able to measure permeability independently of flow.

Raichle: A fair amount of evidence contradicts what you have shown for the tight junctions. What is your response to the people who say that they cannot see the changes in the tight junctions?

Rapoport: First, the work has been confirmed in part by Sterrett *et al.* (1976), using hypertonic angiographic contrast media. Second, contrary results with respect to hypertonic solutions have not been published, although we do find (M. Sato, M. W. Brightman & S. I. Rapoport, unpublished observation) that transendothelial channels may also form in response to hypertonic arabinose infusion in the rat. Non-junctional mechanisms certainly can contribute to increased cerebrovascular permeability under a number of conditions. Is there disagreement also about the hypertonic findings?

Plum: Dr Rapoport, do you think that the blood–brain barrier changes reported in hypertension by Hansson *et al.* (1975) and during seizures by Petito *et al.* (1977) reflect a singular, species-specific change? Or do you believe that hypertension and osmotic changes differently open the barrier? What Petito *et al.* demonstrated was that at the peak of the hypertension response, when CBF was at a maximum, pinocytosis greatly increased across the endothelial wall. The changes appeared to be in capillaries and venules. They were proportional to the number of venules and the route of the vesicles appeared to be from the luminal to the abluminal side. A careful search failed to disclose opening of the endothelial tight junctions. Gross anatomical studies using Evans' blue in these animals with seizures gave the impression that the maximal barrier break was central in the distribution of the drainage into the great cerebral vein. Such a distribution implies a mechanical impediment to flow, an inference supported by the finding that venous endothelium was affected more than arteriolar.

Ultrastructurally, reaction product was located in the intercellular space on the abluminal side of the capillary, in the basement membrane and in the pericyte, but not intracellularly within neurons or astrocytes. Pinocytotic staining declined rapidly after the last seizure with its associated hypertensive response.

Rapoport: We found in the rabbit that tight junctions opened in response to infusion of hypertonic urea mainly at the capillaries, and that larger vessels were affected but less frequently. We could not be certain if these larger vessels were arterioles or venules.

A sufficient number of investigators have reported increased pinocytotic activity at cerebrovascular endothelia, in response to altered physiological conditions, to convince me that vesicular transport can be an important cause of increased permeability. However, it is necessary to demonstrate that what one sees with the electron microscope is vesicular transport (uptake and discharge of tracer by vesicles) rather than pinocytotic uptake alone. We tested for vesicular transport in rats infused with hypertonic arabinose solution by fixing the brain with dilute osmium fixative for 1 hour after infusion, at which time peroxidase was injected intravascularly. As prefixation stops transport (Westergaard & Brightman 1973), the pinocytotic vesicles that we saw could not have contributed to transendothelial transport.

Plum: The curious thing is that all vesicular activity apparently is going outwards.

Purves: Dr Rapoport saw a channel. Do you see that, Dr Plum?

Plum: We looked for channels in all our sections in about 40 rats. We found a single apparently opened intercellular junction not unlike what Dr Rapoport showed.

Rapoport: Critical experiments have yet to be done to determine, in specific instances of increased cerebrovascular permeability, the quantitative contributions of vesicular transport, tight junctional opening or trans-endothelial channel formation.

Siesjö: Your studies with noradrenaline uptake indicate that you already have a substantial uptake without opening the barrier, and you can double the uptake by opening the barrier. But many published findings indicate that some physiological effects of noradrenaline represent threshold phenomena. For example, noradrenaline does not increase flow if it is infused without opening the barrier but an effect is seen after the barrier is opened. How can those two things be put together?

Rapoport: Uptake of ^3H or its metabolites by normal cerebral regions of animals infused intravenously with [^3H]noradrenaline (Table 7 in my paper) could be due to uptake by vascular endothelium or by nerve endings in contact with blood. It is my understanding from Professor Owman's comments that monoamine oxidase can trap noradrenaline at endothelia. After osmotic barrier opening, we know that intercellular channels are transiently established to allow noradrenaline into the brain parenchyma, from where it could exert specific effects on cerebral blood flow.

Lübbers: It is dangerous to talk about the permeability of a capillary. We know, at least from other capillaries, that permeabilities at the arterial and venous ends of the capillary are quite different. The exchange process may change very much so it is always very difficult to know what is being measured, especially if flow is uneven.

Rapoport: It is dangerous to talk about permeability, but necessary to do so if we want to quantify and compare our results. Furthermore, as capillary surface area in grey matter may be as high as 240 cm^2/g tissue, I would guess that capillary exchange processes would dominate exchange processes at venules and arterioles because the surface area of these vessels must be much less than capillary surface area.

Lübbers: The differences between the methods may be responsible for different results. Even under steady-state conditions quite different balances for the tissue may be observed. You said that one can forget about the resistance with steady-state values but this can only be true if there is the same resistance on both sides of the capillary or for the different parts of the capillary.

Rapoport: I agree. When one measures permeability in complex organs one is getting an overall average for a component.

References

BUCKELL, M. & WALSH, L. (1964) Effect of glycerol by mouth on raised intracranial pressure in man. *Lancet 2,* 1151–1152

DELORME, P., GAYET, J. & GRIGNON, G. (1970) Ultrastructural study on transcapillary exchanges in the developing telencephalon of the chicken. *Brain Res. 22*, 269–283

DOOLIN, P. F. & BIRGE, W. J. (1969) Ultrastructural differentiation of the junctional complex of the avian choroidal epithelium. *J. Comp. Neurol. 136*, 253–268

HANSSON, H. A., JOHANNSON, B. & BLOMSTRAND, C. (1975) Ultrastructural studies on cerebrovascular permeability in acute hypertension. *Acta Neuropathol. 32*, 187–198

LOIZOU, L. A. (1970) Uptake of monamines into central neurons and the blood–brain barrier in the infant rat. *Br. J. Pharmacol. 40*, 800–813

LUTTRELL, C. N., FINBERG, L. & DRAWDY, L. P. (1959) Hemorrhagic encephalopathy induced by hypernatremia. II. Experimental observations on hyperosmolarity in cats. *Arch. Neurol. 1*, 153–160

MARLEY, E. & STEPHENSON, J. D. (1972) Central actions of catecholamines, in *Handb. Exp. Pharmacol.*, vol. 33: *Catecholamines* (Blaschko, H. & Muscholl, E., eds.), pp. 463–537, Springer, Berlin

PETITO, C. K., SCHAEFER, J. A. & PLUM, F. (1977) Ultrastructural characteristics of the brain and blood–brain barrier in experimental seizures. *Brain Res. 127*, 251–267

RAPOPORT, S. I., THOMPSON, H. K. & BIDINGER, J. M. (1974) Equiosmolal opening of the blood–brain barrier in the rabbit by different contrast agents. *Acta Radiol. Diagn. 15*, 21–32

STERRETT, P. R., BRADLEY, I. M., KITTEN, G. T., JANSSEN, H. F. & HOLLOWAY, L. S. (1976) Cerebrovascular permeability changes following experimental angiography. A light- and electronmicroscopic study. *J. Neurol. Sci. 30*, 385–403

WESTERGAARD, E. & BRIGHTMAN, M. W. (1973) Transport of proteins across normal cerebral arterioles. *J. Comp. Neurol. 152*, 17–44

Control of cerebral vascular smooth muscle during general anaesthesia

D. GORDON McDOWALL, YOSHIAKI OKUDA*, DIETER HEUSER and N. P. KEANEY†

Department of Anaesthesia, University of Leeds and Institute of Physiology, University of Tübingen

Abstract The effects of some general anaesthetics, for example thiopentone, Althesin (alphaxalone + alphadolone) and ketamine, on cerebral vascular smooth muscle are those which would be expected from their metabolic actions. With other anaesthetics, mainly those administered by inhalation, and especially the volatile agents, cerebral blood flow increases in excess of the metabolic activity, which is usually depressed to varying degrees. During general anaesthesia with any of these agents, responses to changes in arterial P_{CO_2} or blood pressure are maintained. Furthermore, when seizure activity occurs during enflurane administration, there is a flow response to the associated metabolic stimulation.

The time course of the flow response to the metabolically depressant drug Althesin has been measured in baboons and shown to be very rapid. With this drug cerebrovascular resistance begins to increase within 2 s of its arrival in the brain. This rapid flow change occurs also after sympathetic denervation. Extracellular fluid pH of the cortex does not alter until after the initiation of the vascular smooth muscle response.

The simple concept of the effects of general anaesthesia on the brain is that a progressive depression of brain function occurs which is accompanied by reductions in metabolism and flow proportional to the depth of anaesthesia. This view appears to have validity, particularly for barbiturate anaesthesia, and also for anaesthesia with Althesin (alphaxalone + alphadolone) (Pierce *et al.* 1962; Pickerodt *et al.* 1972). The effects of certain other anaesthetic drugs, however, are different. The best-known exception is ketamine, which produces a seizure type of EEG activity, together with increases in cerebral oxygen uptake and in cerebral blood flow (CBF) (Takeshita *et al.* 1972). These changes occur while the patient is in a clinical state normally termed 'general anaesthesia',

*Present address: Department of Anesthesiology, Yamaguchi University School of Medicine, 1144 Kogushi, Ube-shi, Yamaguchi-ken 755, Japan

†Present address: Department of Pharmacology, University of Manchester, Stopford Building, Oxford Road, Manchester M13 9PT.

though rapid eye movements and twitching movements of the limbs may be seen.

Ketamine, though the most obvious, is not the only anaesthetic drug to produce EEG activation. The volatile anaesthetic enflurane, although it usually causes EEG depression with reduction of metabolism and flow, can also lead to seizure-like EEG activity with increased metabolism and flow (Michenfelder & Cucchiara 1974). This change tends to be triggered by high concentrations of enflurane, hypocapnia and auditory stimulation. Even a drug like Althesin, whose obvious effect is EEG depression, can be shown with the use of depth electrodes to produce increased activity in certain deep grey matter nuclei, for example in the hippocampus of the cat (Kayama 1974). The barbiturates indeed produce an initial increase in frequency and amplitude of the EEG which originates in the mesencephalic reticular formation (Rosner & Clark 1973).

The conclusion, then, must be that the state of general anaesthesia, though often associated with electrical and metabolic depression of the brain, need not necessarily be so. The clinical state of general anaesthesia can exist in the presence of an activated EEG with increased cerebral metabolism and flow. It has been suggested that this apparent anomaly results from very abnormal temporal patterns of neuronal spike discharges (i.e. grouped rather than single discharges) (Creutzfeldt 1975), and from changes in the pattern of inhibitory and excitatory input to the cortical neurons. However, ketamine has been shown also to increase oxygen consumption in isolated brain slices, which would suggest that the drug has a direct cortical effect that is not dependent on secondary changes in afferent input (Martin *et al.* 1972).

One point which is clear, largely as a result of the work of Siesjö and his colleagues (Nilsson & Siesjö 1970, 1974; MacMillan & Siesjö 1973), is that during general anaesthesia with clinically appropriate dosage of anaesthetics, metabolic energy stores such as ATP and creatine phosphate are high, so that if metabolism is depressed the reduction is secondary to a reduction in functional activity and not vice versa. Michenfelder (1974) came to the same conclusion on the basis of his experiments with thiopentone, in which he gave massive doses of the drug and measured cerebral oxygen uptake. He found that there was a progressive fall in oxygen uptake as EEG activity declined, but once the EEG had become isoelectric further doses of thiopentone had no further effect on oxidative metabolism. He concluded from this that oxygen uptake is reduced by thiopentone only so long as functional depression is increasing. Of course, what causes functional depression with general anaesthetics is another question, to which many answers have been suggested —some physical, e.g. changes in cell membrane permeability; some physicochemical, e.g. changes in the free to bound intracellular calcium; and some neuropharmacological, e.g. changes in neurotransmitters.

All the above comments refer to dose ranges of anaesthetic drugs which produce clinical anaesthesia. At higher dose levels biochemical changes do occur, e.g. uncoupling of oxidative phosphorylation in mitochondrial suspensions with halothane (H. Smith 1973) and accumulation of lactate in brain tissue in intact animals (Michenfelder & Theye 1975). These changes, however, are clearly not necessary for the production of general anaesthesia.

In their effects on cerebral perfusion, the general anaesthetics can be divided into those that have an appropriate action, when flow and metabolism move in the same direction, and those that have an inappropriate action, when flow and metabolism move in opposite directions. In the appropriate group are thiopentone and Althesin which reduce both flow and metabolism, and ketamine which increases both flow and metabolism. In the inappropriate group belong the volatile anaesthetic agents ether, chloroform, trichloroethylene, halothane, methoxyflurane, enflurane and isoflurane, which all depress metabolism while increasing flow (McDowall 1975; Lassen & Christensen 1976). The inhalational agents nitrous oxide and cyclopropane also depress oxygen uptake and increase CBF (Alexander *et al.* 1970; Smith *et al.* 1970; Michenfelder & Theye 1972; Wollman *et al.* 1965; Sakabe *et al.* 1976; McDowall & Harper 1965). Whether anaesthetic drugs produce appropriate or inappropriate changes in cerebral perfusion, the cerebral circulation still responds to changes in arterial P_{CO_2} (see Table 1) and continues to show autoregulation to changes in blood pressure. As regards thiopentone, it has been said that the response to Pa_{CO_2} change is diminished (Pierce *et al.* 1962) but this is difficult to evaluate since the normocapnic flow value is much reduced by thiopentone. With Althesin, which also reduces normocapnic CBF, the percentage change in flow with change in P_{CO_2} (CBF at a P_{CO_2} of 40 mmHg being 100%) yields a value very similar to that in conscious man (Sari *et al.* 1976). Halothane has been said to increase the sensitivity to change in P_{CO_2} (McHenry *et al.* 1965) and isoflurane and enflurane have been shown to have similar actions to halothane (Michenfelder & Cucchiara 1974; Cucchiara *et al.* 1974). Under light general anaesthesia, autoregulation to change in blood pressure is preserved, though it may be impaired with deep anaesthesia (Smith *et al.* 1970; Keaney *et al.* 1973). There are two particularly interesting drugs among the inhalational agents: enflurane and cyclopropane. Enflurane under normal conditions of general anaesthesia behaves as do the other volatile agents, depressing oxidative metabolism while increasing cerebral perfusion. However, it is possible to produce a seizure-like EEG pattern with this agent, and when this occurs there is a sudden increase in CBF and

TABLE 1

Responsiveness of CBF to changes in arterial P_{CO_2} in conscious man compared with responsiveness in anaesthetized man and animals

Species	*Conscious/ anaesthetic techniques*		*%ΔCBF/ mmHg* ΔP_{CO_2}[a]	*CBF methodology*	*Reference*
Monkey	Pentobarbitone		2.2	Interior jugular venous thermistor flowmeter	Reivich 1964
Baboon	Halothane (F_I 0.7%/N_2O)	Mean flow	3.9	^{133}Xe clearance	Okuda *et al.* 1976
Dog	Enflurane (F_I 2.2%)		3.5	Direct venous outflow	Michenfelder & Cucchiara 1974
Dog	Methoxyflurane (F_I 0.25%)		3.2	Direct venous outflow	Michenfelder & Theye 1973
Dog	Isoflurane (F_I 1.4%)		2.3	Direct venous outflow	Cucchiara *et al.* 1974
Dog	Thiopentone/ N_2O(F_I 80%)	Fg	2.8	^{85}Kr clearance	Harper & Glass 1965
Dog	Pentobarbitone	Fg	5.7	^{85}Kr clearance	Häggendal & Johansson 1965
Dog	Pentobarbitone		1.6	^{131}I-labelled antipyrine (with venous sampling from superior sagittal sinus)	Colton & Frankel 1972
Dog	Althesin		2.7	Direct venous outflow	Sari *et al.* 1976
Man	Awake		1.6	N_2O Kety-Schmidt	Patterson *et al.* 1955
Man	Awake		3.0	N_2O Kety-Schmidt	Wasserman & Patterson 1961
Man	Awake		2.2	^{85}Kr Kety-Schmidt	McHenry *et al.* 1965
Man	Halothane (F_I 1.2%)		2.9	^{85}Kr Kety-Schmidt	Wollman *et al.* 1964
Man	Halothane (F_I 1.2%)		2.8	^{85}Kr Kety-Schmidt	Alexander *et al.* 1964
Man	Halothane (F_I 1.2%)		2.6	^{85}Kr Kety-Schmidt	McHenry *et al.* 1965
Man	Cyclopropane (F_I 21%)		2.8	^{85}Kr Kety-Schmidt	Alexander *et al.* 1968
Man	Thiopentone		1.7	N_2O Kety-Schmidt	Pierce *et al.* 1962
Man	Thiopentone/N_2O		2.2	^{85}Kr Kety-Schmidt	Wollman *et al.* 1965
Man	Droperidol/ fentanyl/N_2O	Fg Fw	2.9 2.0	^{123}Xe clearance	Wilkinson & Browne 1970

F_I: initial flow; Fg: flow in grey matter; Fw: flow in white matter.

[a] CO_2 responsiveness is expressed as % change from the normocapnic value per mmHg Pa_{CO_2} change, to allow comparison between drugs which produce different normocapnic values for CBF.

in cerebral metabolic rate ($CMRO_2$) (Michenfelder & Cucchiara 1974). It would seem therefore that, at least with this agent, not only is responsiveness to $Paco_2$ preserved, but so also is the responsiveness to whatever mechanism normally matches perfusion to oxidative metabolism. The other drug with special features is cyclopropane, which produces a varying pattern of cerebral metabolic effects at different inspired concentrations (Alexander *et al.* 1970), which seems to relate to varying degrees of metabolic stimulation by raised concentrations of blood catecholamine (Michenfelder & Theye 1972).

Most of the work referred to above has been based either on flow methods, which measure large areas of brain, or flow methods which are regional, but with only one region measured. Ketamine, however, has been studied with multiple regional detectors by Hougaard *et al.* (1974). These workers found marked inter-regional differences in cortical flow with this drug, while confirming previous work of an increase in mean CBF. They suggested that these regional differences in perfusion reflect regional variations in cortical activation and oxidative metabolism, a feature of the clinical use of this drug being that patients suffer from hallucinations on occasions.

The control of cerebrovascular smooth muscle during general anaesthesia would therefore appear to vary with the anaesthetic drug used. Drugs of the appropriate group may exert their vascular effects by the usual mechanisms which match flow to metabolic requirement. However, the volatile agents which increase flow while depressing oxidative metabolism must have some additional action on vascular smooth muscle. Nonetheless flow responses to Pco_2, blood pressure and cerebral activation are preserved. The observed increase in sensitivity to $Paco_2$ during halothane anaesthesia might be held to explain the vasodilatation which occurs with halothane at normocapnia, as illustrated in Fig. 1. However, this merely pushes the question one step backwards, for what is it that alters the sensitivity to Pco_2?

It is certain that the cerebral vasodilatation seen with these drugs is not due to tissue acidosis, for lactate levels are low and brain tissue Pco_2 falls with the new balance between perfusion and metabolism. A. Smith (1973) has attempted to relate the flow changes with the volatile agents to cerebral venous oxygen content, arguing that since the cerebral venous oxygen content was similar with three different volatile anaesthetics, at the same depth of anaesthesia, the venous oxygen might be a control factor for vascular resistance. However, it seems more likely that cerebral venous oxygen merely reflects the action of some other flow/metabolic link. Discussion of the vasodilatation associated with this inappropriate group of drugs cannot profitably be carried much further, although it is easy to hypothesize at length. Certainly the *in vitro* action of these agents on cerebrovascular smooth muscle is one of

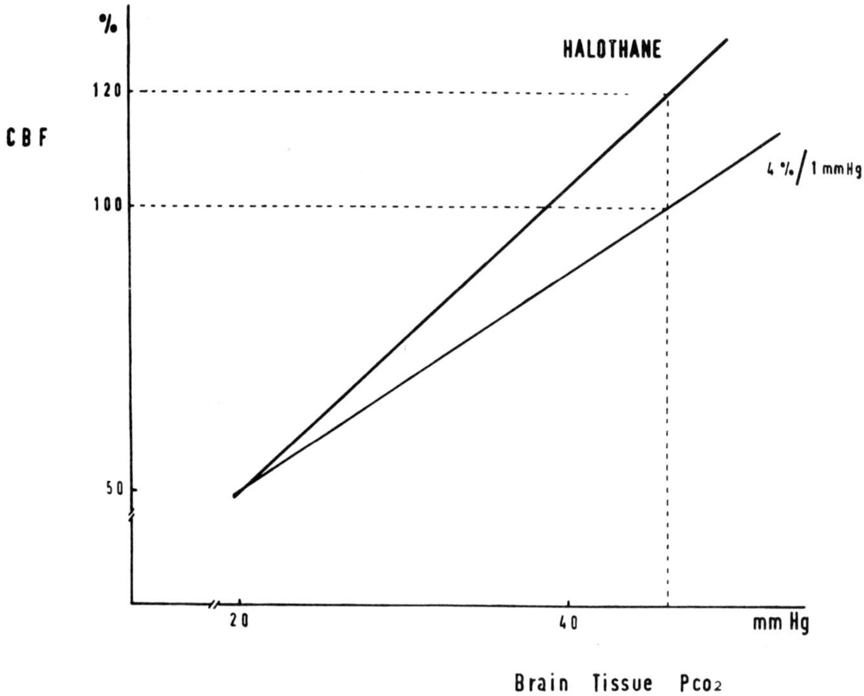

FIG. 1. Diagram showing how an increased sensitivity of CBF to Pa_{CO_2} change, induced by halothane, might account for the cerebral vasodilatation that occurs with this drug at normocapnia.

dilatation, and therefore the background vascular tone may be altered by such factors as changes in cyclic AMP concentrations.

Some authorities have laid much emphasis on small differences in the balance struck between flow and metabolism with individual agents. In some studies such detailed comparisons are not valid, since the flow measurement techniques employed give values for flow in different territories from those which provide the metabolic data. Furthermore, not all differences between cerebral metabolism and perfusion should necessarily be related to events occurring within the brain. The example of the influence of the blood catecholamine level on responses to cyclopropane should be borne in mind. Furthermore, statements that cerebral metabolic depression and depth of anaesthesia are not related have limited fundamental relevance, since the patterns of excitation and inhibition within the brain vary at different concentrations of an anaesthetic drug. Cerebral metabolism, as usually measured, is based on mean values for approximately one cerebral hemisphere.

This mean metabolic rate includes a range of different metabolic activities in different structures. Following the introduction of the deoxyglucose method for quantitative determination of local cerebral utilization of glucose (Sokoloff 1975), reports of the effects of anaesthetics on local metabolic activity in specific brain structures are beginning to appear (Shapiro *et al.* 1975).

In Leeds we have been particularly interested in the intravenous anaesthetic drug Althesin, which is a mixture of two steroid hypnotics, alphadolone and alphaxalone, which are rendered soluble in water by a polyoxyethylated castor oil. This particular drug is of interest because it produces marked EEG changes with a corresponding major reduction in cerebral oxygen uptake with only a modest fall in blood pressure (Pickerodt *et al.* 1972). It seemed therefore to be a useful tool for studying the mechanism of the flow–metabolism link in the appropriate group of anaesthetics (Keaney *et al.* 1975). Experiments were performed in lightly anaesthetized baboons during normocapnic controlled ventilation. Internal carotid blood flow was measured by electromagnetic flowmeter and CBF by xenon clearance after intracarotid injection. Althesin (50 μl/kg) was injected as a bolus into a central vein and was mixed with $^{99}Tc^{m}$ so that its arrival in the brain could be detected with a scintillation detector. Blood pressure, internal carotid blood flow and EEG were continuously recorded and subsequently carotid vascular resistance was calculated.

Althesin produced marked EEG slowing after every i.v. injection, in most instances producing periods of burst suppression. The first slowing of the EEG frequency occurred 9.1 $\pm$ 0.4 s after Althesin injection, while the arrival of the drug was timed in the brain at 7.6 $\pm$ 0.3 s. The first significant change in carotid blood flow and carotid vascular resistance occurred between 9 and 10 s after injection, i.e. approximately 2 s after the drug arrived in the brain, and virtually at the same time as the EEG changes. In some animals Althesin injections were given after cervical sympathectomy or during α-adrenergic blockade produced with phenoxybenzamine. There was no change in the time relationship of the cerebrovascular response to Althesin (Keaney *et al.* 1978).

The rapidity of the vascular response, i.e. within 2 s of arrival of the drug in the brain, made it difficult to believe that the vascular change was due to a metabolic signal secondary to the observed depression in cerebral oxidative metabolism. From earlier studies (Pickerodt *et al.* 1972) the quantitative change in oxidative metabolism produced by this dose of Althesin was known, and with this information the maximum fall in mean cortical tissue P_{CO_2} was calculated for the 2 s time lag between drug arrival and cerebrovascular resistance change. This turned out to be a change in mean cortical tissue P_{CO_2} of less than 0.3 mmHg (Keaney *et al.* 1978).

In some of the baboons the effects of intracarotid Althesin were also tested, and no immediate change in the EEG was seen, so that it appeared to be necessary for the drug to reach the brain-stem to produce the marked EEG depression seen after i.v. injection. At the same time there was little immediate change in internal carotid blood flow after intracarotid injection. In some animals in which the intracarotid dose of Althesin was large, there was a later small EEG change and flow reduction, due presumably to the drug reaching the brain-stem on recirculation.

In a further series of experiments, extracellular fluid pH of the cortex was measured, using a micro-pH electrode inserted approximately 1 mm into the cortical mantle (McDowall *et al.* 1978). In these experiments internal carotid blood flow was again measured. It was found that the carotid vascular resistance increased at the same time as in the earlier experiments after Althesin injection, and at a time when there was no change in extracellular fluid pH. Approximately 30 s later an alkaline shift in extracellular fluid pH was seen but this clearly followed, and did not precede, the changes in flow and vascular resistance.

The conclusions from these experiments would appear to be that the reduction in cerebral perfusion which is associated with Althesin-induced cerebral metabolic depression is not initiated by a change in cortical extracellular fluid pH or P_{CO_2} and that it is not mediated through the sympathetic innervation of the cerebral vessels. The results would be consistent with a neurogenic mechanism, such as that described by Ponté & Purves (1974). This initial neurogenic signal, if such it be, appears to be followed by a metabolic signal consisting of an alkaline shift in extracellular fluid pH which appears approximately 30 s after the initiation of the response.

ACKNOWLEDGEMENT

The studies on the timing and mechanism of the response to Althesin were supported by the Medical Research Council.

References

Alexander, S. C., Wollman, H., Cohen, P. J., Chase, P. E. & Behar, M. (1964) Cerebrovascular response to Pa_{CO_2} during halothane anesthesia in man. *J. Appl. Physiol. 19*, 561–565

Alexander, S. C., James, F. M., Colton, E. T., Gleaton, H. R. & Wollman, H. (1968) Effects of cyclopropane on cerebral blood flow and carbohydrate metabolism in man. *Anesthesiology 29*, 170

Alexander, S. C., Colton, E. T., Smith, A. L. & Wollman, H. (1970) The effects of cyclopropane on cerebral and systemic carbohydrate metabolism. *Anesthesiology 32*, 236–245

COLTON, J. S. & FRANKEL, H. M. (1972) Cerebrovascular response to CO_2 during hyperthermia. *Am. J. Physiol. 223*, 1041–1043

CREUTZFELDT, O. D. (1975) Neurophysiological correlates of different functional states of the brain, in *Brain Work* (Ingvar, D. H. & Lassen, N. A., eds.) *(Alfred Benzon Symp. 8)*, pp. 21–26, Munksgaard, Copenhagen

CUCCHIARA, R. F., THEYE, R. A. & MICHENFELDER, J. D. (1974) The effects of isoflurane on canine cerebral metabolism and blood flow. *Anesthesiology 40*, 571–574

HÄGGENDAL, E. & JOHANSSON, B. (1965) Effects of arterial carbon dioxide tension and oxygen saturation on cerebral blood flow autoregulation in dogs. *Acta Physiol. Scand. Suppl. 258*, 27–53

HARPER, A. M. & GLASS, H. I. (1965) Effects of alterations in the arterial CO_2 tension on the blood flow through the cerebral cortex at normal and low arterial blood pressure. *J. Neurol. Neurosurg. Psychiatry 28*, 449–452

HOUGAARD, K., HANSEN, A. & BRODERSEN, P. (1974) The effect of ketamine on regional cerebral blood flow in man. *Anesthesiology 41*, 562–567

KAYAMA, Y. (1974) Comparison of the effects of Althesin and barbiturates on the neocortex and hippocampus of cats. *Br. J. Anaesth. 46*, 912–917

KEANEY, N. P., PICKERODT, V. W. A., MCDOWALL, D. G., CORONEOS, N. J., TURNER, J. M. & SHAH, Z. P. (1973) Cerebral circulatory and metabolic effects of hypotension produced by deep halothane anaesthesia. *J. Neurol. Neurosurg. Psychiatry 36*, 899–905

KEANEY, N. P., MCDOWALL, D. G., PICKERODT, V. W. A., TURNER, J. M., LANE, J. R., OKUDA, Y., DESHMUKH, V. D. & CORONEOS, N. J. (1975) The time course of the cerebral circulatory response to metabolic depression, in *Cerebral Circulation and Metabolism* (Langfitt, T. W. *et al.*, eds.), pp. 375–377, Springer, Berlin

KEANEY, N. P., MCDOWALL, D. G., PICKERODT, V. W. A., TURNER, J. M., LANE, J. R., OKUDA, Y., DESHMUKH, V. D. & CORONEOS, N. J. (1978) Time course of the cerebral circulatory response to metabolic depression. *Am. J. Physiol.*, in press

LASSEN, N. A. & CHRISTENSEN, M. S. (1976) Physiology of cerebral blood flow. *Br. J. Anaesth. 48*, 719–734

MCDOWALL, D. G. (1975) The influences of anaesthetic drugs and techniques on intracranial pressure, in *A Basis and Practice of Neuroanaesthesia* (Gordon, E., ed.), pp. 135–169, Excerpta Medica, Amsterdam

MCDOWALL, D. G. & HARPER, A. M. (1965) Blood flow and oxygen uptake of the cerebral cortex of the dog during anaesthesia with different volatile agents. *Acta Neurol. Scand. Suppl. 14*, 146

MCDOWALL, D. G., HEUSER, D., OKUDA, Y., JONES, G. M. & WADON, A. (1978) Relationships between blood flow and extracellular fluid pH of the brain during cerebral metabolic depression induced by Althesin, in preparation

MCHENRY, L. C., SLOCUM, H. C., BIVENS, H. E., MAYES, H. A. & HAYES, G. (1965) Hyperventilation in awake and anesthetised man. *Arch. Neurol. 12*, 270

MACMILLAN, V. & SIESJÖ, B. K. (1973) The effect of phenobarbitone anaesthesia upon some organic phosphates glycolytic metabolites and citric acid cycle associated intermediates of the rat brain. *J. Neurochem. 20*, 1669

MARTIN, A. V., ALONSO, J. M. A. & CASADO, J. C. (1972) Effect of ketamine hydrochloride on oxygen and glucose uptake by brain tissue *in vitro*. *Experientia (Basel) 28*, 1070–1071

MICHENFELDER, J. D. (1974) The interdependency of cerebral function and metabolic effects following maximum doses of thiopental in the dog. *Anesthesiology 41*, 231–236

MICHENFELDER, J. D. & CUCCHIARA, R. F. (1974) Canine cerebral oxygen consumption during enflurane anesthesia, and its modification during induced seizures. *Anesthesiology 40*, 575–580

MICHENFELDER, J. D. & THEYE, R. A. (1972) Effects of cyclopropane on canine cerebral blood flow and metabolism. *Anesthesiology 37*, 32–39

MICHENFELDER, J. D. & THEYE, R. A. (1973) Effects of methoxyflurane on canine cerebral metabolism and blood flow. *Anesthesiology 38*, 123–127

MICHENFELDER, J. D. & THEYE, R. A. (1975) *In vivo* toxic effects of halothane on canine cerebral metabolic pathways. *Am. J. Physiol. 229*, 1050

NILSSON, L. & SIESJÖ, B. K. (1970) The effects of anaesthetics upon labile phosphates and upon extra- and intracellular lactate, pyruvate and bicarbonate concentrations in the rat brain. *Acta Physiol. Scand. 80*, 235

NILSSON, L. & SIESJÖ, B. K. (1974) Influence of anaesthetics on the balance between production and utilisation of energy in the brain. *J. Neurochem. 23*, 29

OKUDA, Y., MCDOWALL, D. G., ALI, M. M. & LANE, J. R. (1976) Changes in CO_2 responsiveness and in autoregulation of the cerebral circulation during and after halothane-induced hypotension. *J. Neurol. Neurosurg. Psychiatry 39*, 221–230

PATTERSON, J. L. JR., HEYMAN, A., BATTEY, L. L. & FERGUSON, R. W. (1955) Threshold of response of the cerebral vessels of man to increase in blood carbon dioxide. *J. Clin. Invest. 34*, 1857–1863

PICKERODT, V. W. A., MCDOWALL, D. G., CORONEOS, N. J. & KEANEY, N. P. (1972) Effect of Althesin on cerebral metabolism and intracranial pressure in the anaesthetized baboon. *Br. J. Anaesth. 44*, 751–757

PIERCE, E. C., LAMBERTSEN, C. J., DEUTSCH, S., CHASE, P. E., LINDE, H. W., DRIPPS, R. D. & PRICE, H. L. (1962) Cerebral circulation and metabolism during thiopental anaesthesia and hyperventilation in man. *J. Clin. Invest. 41*, 1664

PONTÉ, J. & PURVES, M. J. (1974) The role of the carotid body chemo-receptors and the carotid sinus baro-receptors in the control of the cerebral blood vessels. *J. Physiol. (Lond.) 237*, 315

REIVICH, M. (1964) Arterial P_{CO_2} and cerebral haemodynamics. *Am. J. Physiol. 206*, 25

ROSNER, B. S. & CLARK, D. L. (1973) Neurophysiologic effects of general anesthesia. *Anesthesiology 39*, 59–81

SAKABE, T., KURAMOTO, T., KUMAGAE, S. & TAKESHITA, H. (1976) Cerebral response to the addition of nitrous oxide to halothane in man. *Br. J. Anaesth. 48*, 957–962

SARI, A., MAEKAWA, T., TOHJO, M., OKUDA, Y. & TAKESHITA, H. (1976) Effects of althesin on cerebral blood flow and oxygen consumption in man. *Br. J. Anaesth. 48*, 545–550

SHAPIRO, H. M., GREENBERG, J. H., REIVICH, M., SHIPKO, E., VAN HORN, K. & SOKOLOFF, L. (1975) Local cerebral glucose utilisation during anaesthesia, in *Blood Flow and Metabolism in the Brain* (Harper, M. *et al.*, eds.), p. 9.42, Churchill Livingstone, Edinburgh

SMITH, A. L. (1973) Dependence of cerebral venous oxygen tension on anesthetic depth. *Anesthesiology 39*, 291–298

SMITH, A. L., NEIGH, J. L., HOFFMAN, J. C. & WOLLMAN, H. (1970) Effects of general anesthesia on autoregulation of cerebral blood flow in man. *J. Appl. Physiol. 29*, 665–669

SMITH, H. (1973) Effect of halothane upon rabbit brain mitochondria. *Biochem. Pharmacol. 22*, 773

SOKOLOFF, L. (1975) The ^{14}C deoxyglucose method for the quantitative determination of local cerebral glucose utilisation, in *Blood Flow and Metabolism in the Brain* (Harper, M. *et al.*, eds.), p. 15.3, Churchill Livingstone, Edinburgh

TAKESHITA, H., OKUDA, Y. & SARI, A. (1972) The effects of ketamine on cerebral circulation and metabolism in man. *Anesthesiology 36*, 69–75

WASSERMAN, A. J. & PATTERSON, J. L. JR. (1961) The cerebral vascular response to reduction in arterial CO_2 tension. *J. Clin. Invest. 40*, 1297–1303

WILKINSON, I. M. S. & BROWNE, D. R. G. (1970) The influence of anaesthesia and arterial hypocapnia on regional blood flow in the normal human cerebral hemisphere. *Br. J. Anaesth. 42*, 472–482

WOLLMAN, H., ALEXANDER, S. C., COHEN, P. J., CHASE, P. E., MELMAN, E. & BEHAR, M. G. (1964) Cerebral circulation of man during halothane anesthesia. *Anesthesiology 25*, 180–184

WOLLMAN, H., ALEXANDER, S. C., COHEN, P. J., SMITH, T. C., CHASE, P. E. & VAN DER MOLEN, R. A. (1965) Cerebral circulation during general anesthesia and hyperventilation in man. *Anesthesiology 26*, 329–334

Discussion

Astrup: You didn't measure the potassium ion concentration with Althesin. In activation potassium seems a good candidate for the initiation of flow changes. It may also be a candidate in deactivation. There is some indication that extracellular potassium goes down when electrical activity ceases. The decrease is small—from 3 to 2.5 mmol l^{-1}, but it may be significant.

McDowall: Will it go down quickly enough?

Astrup: It goes down immediately.

Sandler: Although it is a truism, it is still necessary to say that drugs may have many different actions. Ketamine (Dundee & Wyant 1974), for example, has a profound effect on catecholamine economy and it does other things too, such as produce post-anaesthetic hallucinations.

McDowall: Most of the effects fit in with the concept that ketamine is mainly a stimulant drug. The hallucinations which occur correspond with the increases in regional cerebral perfusion in the visual association areas (as shown by Hougaard *et al.* 1974). There seems therefore to be a correlation between the regional flow changes and the visual hallucinations with this drug.

Heistad: I am not sure that the percentage increase in blood flow is the proper way to evaluate CO_2 responses. If flow increased from 40 to 80 ml min^{-1} during hypercapnia without anaesthesia, and from 20 to 40 during hypercapnia with anaesthesia, you would conclude that CO_2 responsiveness was the same. That is not necessarily valid. Secondly, you concluded that autoregulation is impaired by anaesthesia. However, we use chloralose and urethane anaesthesia and have found no change in flow with arterial pressure between 60 and 140 mmHg. Thirdly, flowmeters on the carotid artery in the baboon may measure some extracranial flow. How does Althesin affect extracranial resistance?

McDowall: Maybe the conclusion about the P_{CO_2} response under anaesthesia isn't valid, but it is very difficult to compare the responsiveness of the cerebrovascular bed to Pa_{CO_2} change under different forms of anaesthesia, because the normocapnic values for CBF differ so greatly. A comparison of percentage changes in relation to normocapnic flow is perhaps more relevant than changes in absolute values; for example, how do you compare a change of 1 ml 100 g^{-1} min^{-1} in CBF with Pa_{CO_2} alteration during halothane anaesthesia, when the normocapnic flow may be 60 ml 100 g^{-1} min^{-1} with the same absolute change during thiopentone anaesthesia when the normocapnic value may be 30 ml 100 g^{-1} min^{-1}?

Heistad: I don't think one way is necessarily more valid than the other.

McDowall: The different agents consistently produce similar changes in CBF with P_{CO_2} alteration when these changes are converted to percentages.

Plum: It would be interesting to make the calculations. Some of your changes are about 1% or 1.5%. When Martin Reivich (1964) plotted the full length of the CO_2–CBF response in the monkey, he noted a fairly linear response between about 20 mmHg on the low side and 60 mmHg on the high side. Between those limits he got a figure for ΔP_{CO_2} to ΔCBF equal to 1.11 ml 100 g^{-1} min^{-1} for each 1 mmHg change, not a percentage of the initiating point in terms of perturbing the system. Approximately similar values were found in published reports from human studies.

McDowall: But if you start from a totally different level and do a P_{CO_2} response, you get a similar linear relationship from any two points within that. The whole curve has shifted.

Purves: Hence the danger of pooling results. There is a fairly wide spectrum for any given animal and the similarity that you showed could be obscuring quite marked differences.

McDowall: I agree. The only valid comparison is in the same animal with the same technique. The purpose of showing that review of the literature was to demonstrate that, with all techniques of anaesthesia, there is continuing marked P_{CO_2} responsiveness.

Regarding the question of the flowmeter on the carotid artery in baboons, we confirmed in all the studies that the changes in carotid blood flow were also seen in xenon clearance measurements after Althesin administration. There may, however, still be a small non-cerebral flow contribution in our flowmeter measurements. Even if this is so, it cannot affect the interpretation of the Althesin studies, since this drug has a slight direct dilatory action on non-cerebral vascular smooth muscle.

Rosendorff: I am never quite sure why so many studies on the effects of anaesthetic agents on cerebral blood flow (though I do not include this study) ignore many of the elementary rules of good pharmacology. In addition to the question of the appropriate choice of animal and technique, the access of the drug to vascular receptors, the kinetics of its interaction with receptors, and its inactivation, storage and elimination, there is also the serious problem of the effects of different doses. Many compounds have dose-dependent effects which are different, sometimes quite opposite, with low doses to what they are at high doses. Most of the anaesthetic agents you discussed, as I understand it, have only been studied at one or perhaps two doses, usually at the dose that produces 'light' anaesthesia. Has anybody looked systematically at the dose-response relationships for commonly used anaesthetic agents?

Secondly, I think a tacit assumption is made that any change in cerebral blood flow with anaesthetic drugs must necessarily be secondary to changes in cerebral metabolism. This is not necessarily so. We know that barbiturates cause a dose-dependent non-competitive inhibition of contractions induced by a variety of vasoactive substances in a variety of vessels *in vitro*. In other words, barbiturates may have a direct effect on vascular smooth muscle as well as presumably acting on blood flow through organs via a change in metabolism.

There is also the complex question of receptor occupancy and activation. What receptors are we looking at? Are they neurons or vascular smooth muscle cells? Is it possible to look at one in isolation from the other? If so, how? These questions may be impossible to answer, but I think they are essential to the issue.

McDowall: The first question is fairly easy to answer. Many of these drugs have been looked at with different dose levels, so we do know the relationship to dosage. With some, the relationship is what one would expect—a progressive effect on oxidative metabolism with a parallel effect on flow, for example with thiopentone. With other drugs, however, the vascular and metabolic effects diverge. In some cases this changing flow/metabolism relationship is due to general systemic effects of high drug dosage, such as hypotension. With cyclopropane at certain dose levels there is considerable adrenergic activation, which accounts for the varying vascular and metabolic responses to different dose levels of cyclopropane (Michenfelder & Theye 1972).

I agree entirely that it is very difficult to deal with drugs that act at so many sites. That is why it was important, when we studied Althesin, to look at the direct action of the drug on the cerebrovascular smooth muscle. This was done by Dr Heuser, who applied the drug directly to the outer surface of pial vessels and saw a slight dilatory effect. From this we can confidently conclude that the increased cerebrovascular resistance seen after intravenous administration was not due to a direct action on vascular smooth muscle.

Purves: The quality of evidence from this type of experiment depends very much on the speed of response from the electrode. You assured us that when this was tested *in vitro* the electrode responded rapidly. However, what is its response like in the brain? And in this connection I am not certain of the characteristics of the electrode. Was this one of Dr Heuser's early electrodes with a tip size of about 80 μm?

Heuser: Yes, the tip diameter was about 80 μm. During dynamic calibration in a flow-through system the time constants of the electrodes were: $\tau = 0.36$ s, $2\ \tau = 0.63$ s and $3\ \tau = 0.84$ s. So we could demonstrate that the response time of the electrode *in vitro* actually was quick enough.

Purves: Yes, but what happens when the electrode is actually in the brain? For example, when the animal inhales CO_2, will the electrode give you some idea of the circulation time from lung to brain?

Heuser: In earlier experiments (Astrup *et al.* 1976) we tested the response time of the implanted pH electrode in the rat brain during CO_2 inhalation. We found first deviations from the baseline pH value 2–3 s after the onset of CO_2 inhalation.

McDowall: We also gave intravenous bicarbonate and saw an acid shift, due to evolved CO_2, virtually synchronously with the arrival of the bicarbonate in the cerebral vessels.

Rapoport: What temperature coefficients did you get?

Heuser: The normal range was 0.3–0.5 mV/1 °C.

McDowall: One error that we discovered was that because of the large and rapid change in CBF, there was a marked change in intracranial blood volume. As a result, 'brain volume' decreased and the area of contact of the electrode with brain tissue changed after Althesin injection. As a result, in the initial experiments we saw a large change in pH, with the electrode positioned on the pial surface. As soon as we positioned the electrode in brain tissue and not on the surface, we observed the smaller changes in pH reported here.

Siesjö: Some inhalation anaesthetics (e.g. halothane) reduce the oxygen uptake of the brain but give only a small decrease, or none at all, in cerebral blood flow. There is one drug, diazepam, which even in anaesthetic concentrations will fail to lower oxygen uptake in the brain but will still reduce blood flow (Carlsson *et al.* 1976*a*).

McDowall: In a lot of studies there is a considerable problem with these comparisons between flow and metabolism, because flow is measured by regional clearance techniques, while metabolic changes are calculated on arteriovenous differences which, when the venous blood is obtained from the internal jugular bulb, relate to whole hemispheric changes.

I would like to make a general point about anaesthesia for animal experimental work on cerebral circulation and metabolism. There seems to be a belief that the lighter the level of anaesthesia, the more reliable the experimental results. I think this is only partly true, though of course I agree that unnecessarily deep anaesthesia may blunt cerebrovascular responsiveness. Inadequate anaesthesia results in a fluctuating state of cerebral arousal, with unsteady conditions of flow and metabolism. A large number of papers at the recent Copenhagen meeting (Ingvar & Lassen 1977) were based on nitrous oxide anaesthesia in cats and rats. N_2O does not provide adequate anaesthesia in these species, and in many such studies there is therefore a varying degree of activation. It is quite wrong to believe that because full anaesthesia hasn't been produced the experimental conditions will be more stable than with a stable though light degree of anaesthesia, monitored either with some form of EEG analysis or by gas chromatography to ensure constant blood concentrations.

Siesjö: Nitrous oxide in a concentration of 70% may provide insufficient anaesthesia but it gives a very constant metabolic rate. In our control animals studied over a period of five years there has been no variation whatsoever. However, if one doesn't want to reduce the metabolic rate, it is dangerous to use various drugs in combination. For example, in order to obtain a more satisfactory level of anaesthesia, we added a small dose of diazepam. The combination reduced the oxygen uptake in the brain to the same level as is observed with barbiturate anaesthesia, probably because there is drug interaction (Carlsson *et al.* 1976*a*).

McDowall: That makes my point. You are studying a highly activated brain, not a normal situation. If you produce anaesthesia by adding diazepam to the N_2O, then you see a large decrease in oxygen uptake, which was previously at stimulated levels.

Siesjö: But is it really activation? In Dr Sokoloff's studies of glucose uptake in the conscious animal the figures are slightly higher than the ones we obtain with 70% N_2O.

Sokoloff: We studied animals under 70% nitrous oxide, 30% oxygen, and immobilized with gallamine, and compared them with our normal, conscious, partially restrained rats. In the N_2O-treated animals cerebral glucose utilization was 20% lower than in the conscious restrained animals. We have recently studied three conscious, free-moving rats and obtained the same values for cerebral glucose utilization as in the conscious, restrained animals.

Siesjö: We got about 10% lower values for CMR_{O_2} with 70% N_2O than when 70% N_2 was given to adrenalectomized animals (or those given propranolol) but the difference was not statistically significant (Carlsson *et al.* 1976*b*).

McDowall: A good technique of anaesthesia is to give nitrous oxide with a very low level of some supplement that is maintained for a long time. With nitrous oxide and low concentrations of halothane we get very steady CMR_{O_2} values for hours. Provided one is monitoring either the blood or the EEG one can maintain satisfactory conditions for many hours. Fitch *et al.* (1976) achieve the same result with intramuscular phencyclidine given half-hourly to supplement N_2O/O_2 anaesthesia.

Astrup: There was a drop in blood pressure when Althesin was injected. This induces a collapse of the arterioles in the brain and an increase in cerebrovascular resistance simply as a passive haemodynamic effect. This is the same argument as Dr Plum mentioned earlier: in the state of activation increased perfusion pressure is a very significant factor for the initiation of hyperaemia. Maybe you have the reverse condition here. How much of the effect is haemodynamic and how much is a metabolic control mechanism?

McDowall: In fact the fall in blood pressure was only about 10 mmHg, well within the autoregulation range.

Purves: What do you think is causing what you call an appropriate response?

McDowall: Most of the volatile inhalational agents probably have a direct smooth muscle relaxing effect, as has been demonstrated *in vitro*. This effect accounts for the inappropriate relationship between flow and metabolism seen under anaesthesia with these agents. What is interesting is that this direct action does not appear to block the other control mechanisms on the vessel, such as CO_2 response, autoregulation or response to change in metabolic activity. There is really a resetting of the vascular tone, but with the vascular muscle remaining sensitive to the usual influences.

Purves: It has been shown that the most pronounced effect of halothane as well as the barbiturates is to depress excitatory postsynaptic potentials in cortical cells (Richards 1972) and these drugs appear to be acting primarily on some function of the synapse, possibly reducing the output of the transmitter. I suppose that it is possible that these drugs could be acting in a similar way on the smooth muscle neuromuscular junction. Thus there is some evidence which would provide an explanation for the generalized depression of both metabolism and blood flow by barbiturates and volatile anaesthesia. How do you relate this to the rather different responses such as changes in metabolism and so on?

McDowall: We find a fairly general pattern of depression of cerebral metabolism, except with ketamine. Blood flow changes are different because I think some of these drugs have a direct action on smooth muscle. Ketamine and a similar agent, phencyclidine, produce a lot of activity but the pattern of activity between inhibitory and excitatory synapses is so abnormal that it is misprocessed centrally. The input to the neuron has such an abnormal pattern, both in terms of the frequency of the spikes and of the balance between inhibitory and excitatory circuits, that the brain is unable to process the data and therefore the patient is unaware of his surroundings.

Purves: With barbiturates is there a change in distribution of glucose uptake in the different parts of the brain, Dr Sokoloff?

Sokoloff: There is a generalized decrease in glucose consumption throughout the brain, but the effects are much greater in grey matter than in white matter. Among the various grey structures the effects are not markedly different. With barbiturates, of course, there can be an increased blood flow despite the decreased metabolic rate because of respiratory depression and increased arterial P_{CO_2}.

Purves: But I thought that you showed that the metabolism in different parts of the brain responded differently to barbiturates?

Sokoloff: There was a tendency for structures with normally higher metabolic rates to be more greatly affected. For example, the components of the sensory pathways, such as the auditory and visual systems, were more affected than other structures.

References

ASTRUP, J., HEUSER, D., LASSEN, N. A., NILSSON, B., NORBERG, K. & SIESJÖ, B. K. (1976) Evidence against H^+ and K^+ as the main factors in adjusting cerebral blood flow to metabolism. A microelectrode study, in *Ionic Actions on Vascular Smooth Muscle* (Betz, E. ed.), pp. 110–115, Springer, Berlin

CARLSSON, C., HÄGERDAL, M., KAASIK, A. E. & SIESJÖ, B. K. (1976*a*) The effects of diazepam on cerebral blood flow and oxygen consumption in rats and its synergistic interaction with nitrous oxide. *Anesthesiology 45*, 319–325

CARLSSON, C., HÄGERDAL, M. & SIESJÖ, B. K. (1976*b*) The effect of nitrous oxide on oxygen consumption and blood flow in the cerebral cortex of the rat. *Acta Anaesthesiol. Scand. 20*, 91–95

DUNDEE, J. W. & WYANT, G. M. (1974) *Intravenous Anaesthesia*, pp. 219–247, Churchill Livingstone, Edinburgh

FITCH, W., FERGUSON, G. G., SENGUPTA, B., GARIBI, J. & HARPER, A. M. (1976) Autoregulation of cerebral blood flow during controlled hypotension in baboons. *J. Neurol. Neurosurg. Psychiatry 39*, 1014–1022

HOUGAARD, K., HANSEN, A. & BRODERSEN, P. (1974) The effect of ketamine on regional cerebral blood flow in man. *Anesthesiology 41*, 562–567

INGVAR, D. H. & LASSEN, N. A. (eds.) (1977) *Cerebral Function, Metabolism and Circulation*, Munksgaard, Copenhagen

MICHENFELDER, J. D. & THEYE, R. A. (1972) Effects of cyclopropane on canine cerebral blood flow and metabolism. *Anesthesiology 37*, 32–39

REIVICH, M. (1964) Arterial P_{CO_2} and cerebral hemodynamics. *Am. J. Physiol. 206*, 25–35

RICHARDS, C. D. (1972) The depression of evoked cortical EPSPs by halothane. *J. Physiol. (Lond.) 222*, 152P

Histochemical and pharmacological approach to the investigation of neurotransmitters, with particular regard to the cerebrovascular bed

CHRISTER OWMAN and LARS EDVINSSON

Department of Histology, University of Lund, Sweden

Abstract The distribution of aminergic neurotransmitters can be followed with great precision by using histochemical techniques according to which the various amines are transformed to intensely fluorescent products, which can be seen in nerves by fluorescence microscopy. Additional information can be achieved by immunohistochemical localization, in nerves, of the specific enzymes involved in the biosynthesis of the transmitters. There is strong evidence that certain immunohistochemically demonstrable polypeptides may also act as neurotransmitters in the brain.

Aminergic and peptidergic nerves are distributed in complex pathways in the brain, and they also form dense networks enclosing vessels in the cerebrovascular bed. Some of these nerve systems are extrinsic, originating in ganglia outside the brain; others are entirely intracerebral. The detailed organization of the nerve terminals in relation to the brain vessels can be followed by electron microscopy: different types of nerves can be distinguished by the appearance of the synaptic vesicles, with or without administration of 'false adrenergic transmitters'.

Pharmacological studies *in vitro* and *in vivo* have suggested that the calibre of brain vessels and associated changes in local cerebral blood flow can be influenced by the various nerve systems, either by an effect directly on the vascular smooth muscle or via remote actions on the vessel wall through long-distance diffusion of the transmitter or through some kind of a mediator. The action of circulating amines is modified by interference with the blood–brain barrier, whose capacity also appears to be influenced by nervous mechanisms.

There has been a major breakthrough in neurobiological research during the last decade. This is to a considerable extent due to the rapid development of fundamentally new techniques allowing detailed investigations on the distribution and function of monoaminergic neurotransmitters—both in the central nervous system and in autonomic nerves—by histochemical, chemical, electron microscopic and cytopharmacological approaches. By these techniques the neurotransmitter itself, or specific enzymes involved in its metabolism can be demonstrated with a unique degree of precision and specificity in all portions of the neuron: in the cell body and the preterminal part of the axon as well as in the axon terminal. The ultrastructure of the neuroeffector relationship in the synaptic area can be analysed by techniques which differentiate between the various types of monoaminergic nerve endings involved in the transmission mechanism. The release of the transmitter during nerve activation can be followed by histochemical as well as by chemical methods both *in vivo* and *in vitro*, and the actions produced can be studied by a variety of physiological and pharmacological models. In the present description the main emphasis will be placed on neurohistochemical and cytopharmacological approaches related to the transmitters dopamine, noradrenaline, adrenaline, 5-hydroxytryptamine (serotonin), acetylcholine, and the possible involvement also of peptidergic neurotransmission.

GENERAL FEATURES OF THE NEUROEFFECTOR RELATIONSHIP

Intraneuronal distribution of the transmitter

The transmitter substance is present throughout the neuron, where its concentration varies in a characteristic manner in different portions. It is stored in submicroscopic structures known as 'granules' or 'vesicles'. Most information on the intraneuronal distribution of the transmitter has been gained from studies on noradrenaline in postganglionic sympathetic nerves (Dahlström 1966). The concentration of noradrenaline in the nerve cell body is of the order of 10–100 μg/g wet weight. In all probability the amine storage granules are synthesized in this part of the neuron, and their turnover has been calculated as 1–5 h. The amine-containing granules are transported from the cell body in the axon by an axoplasmic flow mechanism, at an average effective rate of 5–10 mm/h. The concentration of the amine in this 'preterminal' part of the axon, which often forms bundles or small fascicles, is of the same order of magnitude as in the soma.

When the effector region is reached, each preterminal axon splits up into fine fibres, which further divide to form a network of nerve terminals. These axon terminals are characterized by swellings ('varicosities') occurring at regular intervals along the fibres; this is in contrast to the smooth appearance of the preterminal part of the axon. The varicosities are partly or entirely devoid of the Schwann cell sheath ('neurilemma'), and form the synaptic contacts with the effector cells (Elfvin 1963). Accordingly, the varicosities contain the largest number of synaptic vesicles—about 500–1500 per varicosity—and the highest concentration of the transmitter substance—about 1000–3000 $\mu g/g$ wet weight, corresponding to a total content of approximately 5×10^{-3} μg noradrenaline in each varicosity. The noradrenaline concentration in each synaptic vesicle has been estimated as about 2.4 M (assuming that all of it is present in the interior cavity of the vesicle).

Organization of the innervation apparatus

The anatomy and distribution of the different systems of monoaminergic neurons in the central nervous system have been the subject of several excellent reviews (Fuxe 1965; Fuxe *et al.* 1968; Ungerstedt 1971; Lindvall & Björklund 1974*b*), a very recent one particularly focusing on the organization of the catecholamine neuron systems (Björklund & Lindvall 1977).

The synaptic complex in the autonomic ganglia has many similarities with the neuronal links in the brain and spinal cord. Varicosed nerve terminals enclose the soma of the postganglionic neuron in a basket-like fashion, sometimes extending for some distance on the surface of the proximal part of its axon. Experimental evidence has been presented by Libet (1970) and by Libet & Tosaka (1970) to suggest that a catecholamine, probably dopamine, is a synaptic transmitter for the slow inhibitory postsynaptic potential (S-IPSP) in mammalian sympathetic ganglion cells. The hypothetical pathway for the mediation for S-IPSP involves the synaptic termination of cholinergic preganglionic fibres on a dopaminergic interneuron, the preganglionic release of acetylcholine that acts at a muscarinic type of postsynaptic receptor of the interneuron, the subsequent release of dopamine by the interneuron at its presynaptic terminations on the ganglion cells, and the action of dopamine on specific postsynaptic receptors of the ganglion cell (Eccles & Libet 1961; Libet 1970). In order to establish the role of dopamine as a synaptic transmitter it would be desirable to obtain evidence concerning its actual presynaptic release in response to suitable stimulation of the preganglionic nerve. Experiments on isolated superior cervical sympathetic ganglia of rabbits (Libet & Owman 1974) demonstrated that dopamine in the ganglion is localized in the population of small intensely fluorescent cells (SIF cells). The histochemical results strongly indicated that the network of beaded catecholamine-containing fibres surrounding the ganglion cells represent terminating fibres originating from these dopamine-containing cells, which in all probability constitute a dopamine interneuron: preganglionic impulses, by a cholinergic synaptic action, can induce a histochemically demonstrable release of dopamine from these cells, and the ability of the ganglion to respond with a S-IPSP to orthodromic input may be viewed as being dependent on the supply of functionally releasable dopamine in these interneurons.

The organization of the peripheral autonomic neuroeffector system was well formulated by Hillarp in his classical thesis in 1946, and the description is still valid today: 'The peripheral innervation apparatus consists of the nervous ground plexus, composed of a terminal Schwann plasmodium within which terminal axon ramifications are running. Each effector cell is in direct contact with some part of this ground plexus. Within the plexus each axon has a certain extension and innervates in its course a certain number of cells, which react as a functional unit, the neuro-effector unit. One or more such units are supplied by one and the same neuron. A neuro-effector unit is not innervated by one neuron only; several neurons, the terminal axon ramifications of which run within the same strands of the ground plexus, converge towards it. By this presence of overlap in the innervation structure proper, the response of the autonomic effector system to indirect stimulation can be modified by temporal and by spatial summation effects'. The autonomic ground-plexus may have an essentially two-dimensional or three-dimensional organization (Gabella 1976). The vas deferens is a good example of a well-developed, three-dimensional neuromuscular system in which each smooth muscle cell in the whole thickness of the muscle layer is supplied by a number of varicosities belonging to several nerve terminals. In a blood vessel, on the other hand, the autonomic nerve terminals supply only the outermost smooth muscle layer by an essentially two-dimensional plexus located at the adventitia–media border. There are but a few exceptions to this rule: in, for example, the portal vein (Johansson *et al.* 1970) and alar veins of bats (Edvinsson *et al.* 1974*a*) the terminals form a three-dimensional network, which thus extends also into the deeper parts of the smooth musculature comprising the media layer.

The synapse

The term 'synapse' in a broad sense is used to describe a close relationship between two neurons or in a neuroeffector unit, irrespective of the presence of specializations within, or in the region of, the opposing cell membranes. In the mammalian nervous system the synapses are chemical, although the occurrence of electrotonic transmission cannot be excluded within the central nervous system.

Structural criteria for a synapse in the central neuropil are usually better defined than for peripheral junctions. Thus, besides the presence of a synaptic cleft not wider than 20 nm, accumulations of synaptic vesicles near the opposing membranes as well as membrane specializations are usually minimum requirements. The definition of a peripheral neuroeffector unit—i.e. the organization of a true functioning innervation of a given effector cell—is more liberal (Bennett 1972): in a vascular neuromuscular complex, for example, a distance of up to 100 nm is usually considered as a 'close contact' between an axon varicosity—partly or entirely denuded of its Schwann cell sheath—and the membrane of a smooth muscle cell (although membrane-to-membrane distances as small as 20 nm are sometimes found), membrane specializations are usually not present (though the axon varicosity may often lie in a shallow trough of the innervated smooth muscle cell), and there is usually no accumulation of synaptic vesicles near the abutting membrane of the nerve ending.

Thus, whether an arteriole, for example, can be said to have true autonomic *innervation* depends not just on the presence of nerves or transmitter in the tissue but also on the existence of a *close relationship* between axon endings (varicosities) and the membrane of smooth muscle cells. And the *degree* of innervation is not simply reflected by the general density of the perivascular nerve plexus (or the concentration of transmitter in the tissue), but also by the *number* of varicosed nerve endings *per volume* of innervated smooth musculature.

Since only a few of the cells in a bundle of smooth musculature are directly innervated by the autonomic nerves it can be anticipated that the individual smooth muscle cells are electrically (and also mechanically) coupled (Bennett 1972). This coupling is usually provided by flask-shaped protrusions from one muscle cell membrane into an adjacent muscle cell. Also plaque-like junctions along the muscle cells may be present. Gap junctions have been identified between the apposing membranes in these contact areas, thus offering the morphological substrate for low electrical resistance pathways and the electrical coupling between adjacent smooth muscle cells.

Release of the transmitter

Three different types of synaptic vesicles are usually observed in the axon varicosities of autonomic nerves supplying a smooth muscle tissue: small vesicles (30 to 60 nm diameter) which may or may not contain a granular core (15 to 25 nm diameter), and large vesicles (60 to 150 nm diameter) which always contain a granular core (40 to 70 nm diameter). Two classes of axon varicosities in smooth muscle can be identified in terms of the types of vesicles which they include: in one class of varicosity, belonging to adrenergic axons, there are both small granular and agranular vesicles, whereas in the other class of varicosity there are no small granular vesicles; these are non-adrenergic axons, often identified as cholinergic. Large granular vesicles may be present in either class of varicosity.

The axon varicosity constitutes the site of release of the transmitter substance after nerve stimulation. The enzyme dopamine-β-hydroxylase (dopamine β-monooxygenase, EC 1.14.17.1) and the protein chromogranin A, which both are found only in synaptic vesicles, are liberated together with noradrenaline from the nerve terminals, thus supporting the view that the neurotransmitter is released by a process of exocytosis. Attempts have been made to estimate the quantity of transmitter released from the varicosities during nerve activation (Bennett 1972). At a close contact the noradrenaline concentration in the extracellular space is in the order of 10^{-6}–10^{-5} g/ml. The reduced concentration of transmitter due to diffusion into the extracellular spaces between the muscle cells after the release appears to be compensated for by an increase in the receptive area over which the transmitter acts: the ratio of receptive area beneath a close contact varicosity to that of the total cell surface area is of the order of 1000. However, since the smooth muscle cells in a bundle are joined by the above-mentioned low-resistance pathways between adjacent cells to form an electrical syncytium, the effect of a low uniform concentration of transmitter throughout the bundle may have a greater effect than exposure at a few points of high concentration in the muscle. This is because electrical current escapes into neighbouring cells if there are only a few points of high concentration, whereas with a low uniform concentration current does not escape into neighbouring cells as all the cells are at the same potential. In these circumstances the relative effect of a uniform concentration throughout the muscle compared with that at a point in the muscle is simply the ratio of cell membrane resistance to the input resistance of the syncytium, which is of the order of 100. Thus, the effect of a uniform concentration of transmitter throughout the muscle bundle on the potential change in a single cell would be about 100 times more powerful than that of the same concentration applied directly to the cell. An increase in the area over which the transmitter acts may therefore enhance the potential generated in the muscle, both because the number of receptors excited increases and because the leakage of current between the cells in the smooth muscle syncytium decreases (Bennett 1972).

During sustained stimulation of the sympathetic nerves, the action of noradrenaline is terminated primarily through a re-uptake of the transmitter into the nerve terminals. It has been calculated (Langer 1970) that about 70% of the noradrenaline released during a physiological impulse frequency has this fate. Some 20% is taken up by the muscle and is metabolized mainly by catechol-*O*-methyltransferase (EC 2.1.1.6) in the region of the receptors, while the remainder (about 10%) diffuses away from the muscle. How the action of postganglionic cholinergic nerve stimulation terminates and what the fate of acetylcholine is after its release are less well understood. The immediate termination may occur by diffusion from the region of the receptors into the extracellular space; during maintained impulse firing both the diffusion from the muscle and the activity of cholinesterase play an important role.

NEUROHISTOLOGICAL TECHNIQUES FOR THE STUDY OF AMINERGIC AND PEPTIDERGIC NERVE SYSTEMS

Methodological advances in the field of neurohistology have formed the basis for a particularly rapid development in current research on neurotransmission mechanisms. The formaldehyde method of Falck and Hillarp (see Björklund *et al.* 1972) allowed, for the first time, a direct demonstration of the transmitter substance itself in neurons. The method is sensitive enough to demonstrate changes in the levels of neurotransmitter, as indicated by an altered fluorescence intensity, induced by physiological activity at the synaptic region (Owman & Falck 1975). A further dramatic increase in the sensitivity, sufficient for catecholamines in nerves to be seen, could be achieved by introducing glyoxylic acid as the reagent (Lindvall & Björklund 1974*a*). In combination with certain heavy metal salts, the histofluorescence technique has recently been further developed to give an enhanced fluorescence yield not only for the catecholamines but also for 5-hydroxytryptamine (Lorén *et al.* 1976, 1977). Since the fluorophores of the catecholamines have very similar fluorescence characteristics and can be distinguished safely only with cytospectrofluorometric techniques in combination with certain histotechnical procedures, highly sensitive methods have been introduced for the immunohistochemical demonstration of the specific enzymes involved in the synthesis of various catecholamines, e.g. dopamine-β-hydroxylase (Hökfelt *et al.* 1975*a*). Immunohistochemical methods have also been applied to the demonstration of a new class of neurons in which various types of polypeptides seem to serve as transmitters (e.g. Hökfelt *et al.* 1975*b*; Larsson *et al.* 1976). Recent modifications also allow for these molecules to be immunohistochemically localized in the electron microscope. Such techniques may also prove to be of considerable importance for the specific localization of cholinergic nerves (Rossier *et al.* 1975), though the cholinesterase technique is still the most widely used way of demonstrating this system of fibres.

Fluorescence reactions for amines

The basis for the detection of biogenic β-phenylethylamines and β-(3-indolyl)-

ethylamines in the Falck–Hillarp formaldehyde technique is their transformation into intensely fluorescent isoquinoline and β-carboline molecules, respectively (Björklund *et al.* 1972, 1975). This is achieved through combined cyclization–dehydrogenation reactions under nearly dry conditions. The latter requirement is fulfilled by using freeze-dried tissue specimens or whole mounts of tissue membranes thin enough to dry efficiently in a desiccator. Dry formaldehyde is generated by sublimation of paraformaldehyde at high temperatures. The chemical mechanisms underlying the fluorophore formation have been extensively studied and are now well understood.

The first step in the reaction between the monoamines and formaldehyde is a Pictet–Spengler cyclization resulting in tetrahydroisoquinoline and tetrahydro-β-carboline molecules, which either do not fluoresce or fluoresce only very weakly. The fluorophore formation occurs in a second step, where the tetrahydro derivatives are dehydrogenated to 3,4-dihydro compounds. According to the Pictet–Spengler cyclization, formaldehyde reacts only with molecules having a free amino group. This means that only primary or secondary β-phenylethylamines and β-(3-indolyl)ethylamines can be expected to fluoresce, whereas tertiary amines or amides will not condense with formaldehyde. Under the mild histochemical conditions of the standard Falck–Hillarp method, a cyclization will occur only with compounds having high electron density at the ring carbon atom where the closure takes place. Among the phenylethylamines 3,4-dehydroxylated compounds (such as dopamine, noradrenaline and dopa) as well as 3-hydroxylated compounds (such as metatyramine and metaraminol) give the highest fluorescence yields. The 3-methoxylated compounds (e.g. normetanephrine) give only very low fluorescence yield in the standard reaction. The secondary phenylethylamine, adrenaline, requires more intense reaction conditions (higher reaction temperature and/or longer reaction time) than the corresponding primary amine, noradrenaline. This is probably because the reaction with adrenaline has a higher energy requirement in the dehydrogenation step. In general, primary indolylethylamines have a low to moderate fluorescence yield in the standard histochemical formaldehyde reaction. The *N*-acetylated compounds (such as melatonin) have been found to give no or only very weak visible fluorescence after formaldehyde treatment: these compounds are amides and cannot be expected to enter the fluorophore-forming Pictet–Spengler reaction.

In the search for reagents other than formaldehyde that would increase the sensitivity and/or specificity of the reaction with the biogenic monoamines, the introduction of glyoxylic acid has been the most successful advancement (Lindvall & Björklund 1974*a*). This reagent has a very high over-all sensitivity for catecholamines and indolamines: when glyoxylic acid-perfused tissue is used, the reaction has been estimated to be about 10 times more sensitive for dopamine than the standard Falck–Hillarp technique. From this it follows that about 10^{-7} picomoles of dopamine would be readily detected in a varicosity with the glyoxylic acid method. Its high sensitivity allows for a demonstration of the entire course of the nerves, including cell body, preterminal and terminal parts of the axon, thus facilitating the neuroanatomical mapping of catecholamine systems in the brain that has contributed to the detection of, for example, hitherto unknown systems of dopaminergic neurons (Lindvall & Björklund 1974*b*). The fluorophore formation from primary and secondary phenylethylamines and indolylethylamines in the glyoxylic acid method has been shown to proceed in the same two principal reaction steps as in the formaldehyde method (Björklund *et al.* 1975), starting with an acid-catalysed Pictet–Spengler condensation giving very weakly fluorescent compounds that can be transformed into strongly fluorescent molecules via autooxidative decarboxylation or an intramolecularly acid-catalysed reaction with glyoxylic acid. Glyoxylic acid treatment also induces fluorescence from *N*-acetylated indolylethylamines, such as melatonin. These compounds are amides and cannot undergo a Pictet–Spengler cyclization (as mentioned above, they do not yield fluorescence with formaldehyde), which means that the fluorophore formation from the *N*-acetylated amines in the glyoxylic acid method must be due to a different type of reaction, which has so far not been clarified.

A very useful technical modification of the glyoxylic acid technique has recently been presented by de la Torre & Surgeon (1976). The method utilizes cryostat sections, and the complete processing time from fresh tissue to microscopic examination takes only 15–20 min. The outcome of the reaction for neuronal amines is excellent under optimal conditions, the only disadvantage being that the technique is slightly unpredictable and less easy to standardize than the more elaborate original procedures (Lindvall & Björklund 1974*a*). In a further recent modification by Lorén *et al.* (1976, 1977), the formaldehyde and glyoxylic acid techniques have been applied together in order to combine the advantage of freeze–dried and paraffin-embedded material with a sensitivity and precision comparable to those of the glyoxylic acid method, which is usually carried out on Vibratome-sectioned material. Perfusing the animals with a solution containing formaldehyde and glyoxylic acid in the presence of a very high magnesium content (40 g $MgSO_4$/150 ml solution) at acid pH gives a very high sensitivity and precision for the demonstration of both catecholamine and serotonin neuron systems in the brain. The mechanism of the action of the magnesium ions is not clear: it is possible that it 'locks in' the catecholamines within the nerve cell and also prevents their spontaneous release through well-known cellular mechanisms. The low pH seems to act as an external catalyst in the Pictet–Spengler cyclization step.

Histamine can also be demonstrated by fluorescence histochemistry through a reaction with *o*-phthaldialdehyde (Björklund *et al.* 1972). This reaction has proved to be very efficient for the precise localization of this diamine in mast cells and in certain endocrine cell systems, but the histotechnical problems involved in the demonstration of histamine in the nervous system have not yet been solved: the requirement for small amounts of water during the reaction tends to make the amine and/or its fluorophore diffuse away from its cellular sites, which makes a precise demonstration difficult, particularly in tissues such as the brain, where cellular water is firmly bound and hard to extract to an optimal level by the freeze–drying procedures applied.

The fluorophores formed from the various amines in the histochemical reactions have characteristic spectral properties. This offers a very exact means for differentiation between various compounds both in tissues and in model systems consisting of, for example, authentic amines included in dried protein droplets or in silica gel thin-layers. The excitation and emission spectra are best analysed in a microspectrofluorometer (Björklund *et al.* 1975), which can also be used for quantitative analysis of intracellular fluorophores.

The excitation spectrum expresses the efficiency by which the exciting light of different wavelengths induces fluorescence. This spectrum is obtained by varying the wavelength of the excited light, while the intensity of the emitted light is measured at a fixed wavelength. The excitation spectrum of a fluorescent substance is practically identical with its absorption spectrum, and is for this reason particularly helpful for identification purposes. The emission spectrum gives the spectral distribution of the emitted light and can be considered independent of the wavelength of the exciting (activating) light. It is recorded at a fixed wavelength of excitation (preferably close to the wavelength of maximal excitation), and the relative distribution of the emitted light in the visual part of the spectrum is registered.

The usefulness of the microspectrofluorometric characterization of the fluorescence characteristics is illustrated by the differentiation between the noradrenaline and dopamine fluorophores (Björklund *et al.* 1972, 1975). These are indistinguishable under the standard conditions of the formaldehyde and glyoxylic acid techniques, since the fluorophores at neutral pH are both in their quinoidal form. Upon acidification with HCl vapour, the dopamine fluorophore will be converted into the tautomeric non-quinoidal form, which exhibits an excitation maximum at 370 nm. The noradrenaline fluorophore, on the other hand, will only transiently occur in its non-quinoidal form, and is rapidly converted on prolonged treatment with HCl to the fully aromatic isoquinoline, having an excitation maximum at about 320 nm. A consequence of this shift in excitation maximum during the stepwise acidification is that the noradrenaline fluorescence, as seen in the microscope, disappears whereas the dopamine fluorescence is only slightly reduced (cf. Libet & Owman 1974).

In the quantitative analysis of the fluorophores the intensity of the intracellular fluorescence is compared to that of a standard, which may consist of a known concentration of authentic amine dissolved in gelatin which, after hardening, is treated and sectioned along with the tissue preparation (Lichtensteiger 1969). An arbitrary measure of the amine content before and after interference with its concentration in the tissue can be obtained by comparing the two tissues, which have been treated and sectioned simultaneously in the same paraffin block (Libet & Owman 1974). The quantitative estimations have to rely on a high degree of standardization of the histochemical reaction, and on the fact that there is a linear relationship between the concentration of amine and fluorescence intensity only up to a certain maximum level, after which a quenching effect is obtained (Jonsson 1971).

Immunohistochemical techniques

Immunohistochemical approaches have for several reasons been increasingly applied in the study of monoamine neuron systems. The formaldehyde technique of Falck and Hillarp, and recent highly sensitive modifications, have contributed extensively to our knowledge of the distribution of monoamine neuron systems, not only in the brain but also in peripheral tissue. However, differentiation between the various catecholamines (dopamine, noradrenaline and adrenaline) has not always been unequivocal, due to the above-mentioned similarity in excitation and emission spectra (and hence the same fluorescence colour), and therefore they have to be distinguished on the basis of other characteristics that can be elucidated only by special histochemical procedures. Moreover, the fluorescence yield of the fluorophore from 5-hydroxytryptamine is comparatively low and sensitive to the fading effect of the light source, which has restricted our knowledge about serotonergic neuron systems in the brain. An important advance in terms of increased precision and a better differentiation between the various types of monoamine neurons was obtained by immunohistochemical demonstration of the enzymes involved in the biosynthesis of the different catecholamines and 5-hydroxytryptamine (Hökfelt *et al.* 1975*a*). The principles for the histochemical demonstration of substances on the basis of immunological reactions had been worked out many years ago by Coons *et al.* (1942). The successful application of this approach to neurotransmitter research was to a great extent based on the fact that certain enzymes present in the catecholamine neurons are also found in the glandular cells of the adrenal medulla, which thus constitutes a rich source for the purification of tyrosine hydroxylase (tyrosine 3-monooxygenase, EC 1.14.16.2), dopa decarboxylase (aromatic-L-amino-acid decarboxylase, EC 4.1.1.28), dopamine-β-hydroxylase, and phenylethanolamine *N*-methyl transferase.

According to the direct immunohistochemical method (Goldman 1968), which provides the simplest reaction, a few drops of appropriately diluted fluorescein-labelled antibody are applied to tissue sections containing the cellular antigen, and after incubation the drops of conjugate are shaken off and the unbound antibody is washed away. In the indirect (antiglobulin) method (Goldman 1968), the substance actually rendered fluorescent is not the antigen under consideration, but rather an intermediate material, whose distribution corresponds precisely to that of the antigen being studied. The technique takes advantage of the fact that the antibody molecules, in addition to reacting with antigens, are themselves capable of serving as antigen which can be demonstrated by fluorescent antibodies. A pronounced increase in sensitivity over the direct method is obtained because the molecular combining ratio of antibody to antigen is always greater than 1, and may be as much as 10 or more, as the intermediate layer of unlabelled antibody multiplies the number of sites to which fluorescent markers can be attached.

Most immunohistochemical studies on the distribution and organization of monoaminergic neuron systems and various types of peptidergic nerves in the brain and peripheral tissue, as well as in cerebral vessels, have utilized fluorescence techniques. However, there is an increasing demand for immunohistochemical staining methods that can be used at the level of light microscopy without requiring fluorescence equipment, and also for use in electron microscopy. The most successfully applied techniques are (Sternberger 1974): (1) The immunoferritin method according to which ferritin is covalently bound with immunoglobulin by a double-armed reagent where one arm conjugates with ferritin and the other with immunoglobulin. Conjugation is carried out in two stages, and toluene 2,4-diisocyanate is used as the conjugating reagent. (2) The unlabelled antibody enzyme method utilizing the peroxidase (EC 1.11.1.7)–antiperoxidase complex (PAP). The enzyme, horseradish peroxidase, is attached to the tissue antigen via specific antibody without the use of a covalent labelling reaction. The site of reaction is shown by staining the peroxidase with 3,3′-diaminobenzidine tetrahydrochloride–hydrogen peroxide and osmium tetroxide for light or electron microscope demonstration.

Electron microscope techniques

The differentiation of the various types of monoamine neurons can to a certain extent be carried out by electron microscopy using indirect methods, such as selective denervation (cf. Iwayama 1970), which is most conveniently performed for studies on the peripheral nervous system. The nerves can also be identified on the basis of the selective uptake of radioactive amines or amine precursors, which can be demonstrated at the cellular level by autoradiography (Hökfelt & Ljungdahl 1972; Chan-Palay 1976). A problem, though, is that the site of accumulation of the exogenous transmitters or precursors is not necessarily identical with the storage site for the endogenous transmitter.

It is generally agreed that, at least in the adrenergic nerves, the transmitter substance is stored in the synaptic vesicles of about 50 nm diameter and present in large numbers in the varicosities of the axon terminal. It is often claimed that the presence of a dense core in these vesicles is a determining feature of the adrenergic type of the terminal. However, dense-cored synaptic vesicles do not regularly occur in adrenergic neurons from tissues fixed in glutaraldehyde and osmium, which under these conditions makes differentiation from cholinergic neurons difficult. The problem was overcome by the fixation of tissues in potassium permanganate, which was introduced by Richardson (1966) for the demonstration of noradrenaline at the ultrastructural level. This type of fixation results in the appearance of a well-defined electron-dense core in the synaptic vesicles of all adrenergic neurons, thus facilitating their differentiation from the non-adrenergic type of axon terminals which in the periphery are characterized by empty (electron-lucent) synaptic vesicles. The conditions for the reaction between the monoamines and potassium permanganate for application to the ultrastructural differentiation of various monoaminergic neurons have been studied in detail (Hökfelt & Ljungdahl 1972): not only noradrenaline but also the other biogenic monoamines—dopamine, adrenaline, and 5-hydroxytryptamine—react with potassium permanganate, to the same extent as noradrenaline; 5-hydroxytryptamine seems to cause the strongest and adrenaline the weakest reaction. The basic requirement for the technique thus seems to be that potassium permanganate and the monoamine react with each other to produce a precipitate and that both reagents are present in sufficiently high concentration at the storage sites to produce a reaction intense enough for practical purposes.

The adrenergic nerves can also be demonstrated with high precision in the electron microscope after the administration of the false adrenergic transmitter, 5-hydroxydopamine, followed by fixation in glutaraldehyde and osmium, or in potassium permanganate (Tranzer & Thoenen 1967). 5-Hydroxydopamine is selectively taken up into the adrenergic nerves and produces the appearance of a highly electron-dense core in the synaptic vesicles, whereas those of non-adrenergic nerves consequently remain empty. A corresponding approach is to treat the animals with the transmitter analogues, 6-hydroxydopamine (or 6-hydroxydopa) and dihydroxytryptamines (Fuxe *et al.* 1974), which produce a selective and efficient degeneration of the catecholaminergic and serotonergic nerves, respectively, with the appearance of characteristic degenerative phenomena that can easily be demonstrated by electron microscopy.

Histochemistry of the cholinergic system

Unfortunately, so far no direct technique is available for the histochemical demonstration of cholinergic nerves in a way analogous to that available for the demonstration of the catecholamine and serotonin neuron systems. This is partly due to the fact that the acetyl and choline moieties of the transmitter are such simple and widely distributed molecules in all cells that a discriminating histochemical technique is difficult to develop. Cholinergic nerves in both the central nervous system and the periphery are therefore traditionally localized by an indirect approach, namely cholinesterase histochemistry (Koelle 1963), according to which it is assumed that the enzyme (acetyl-cholinesterase, EC 3.1.1.7) is a good marker for nerves storing acetylcholine.

The reaction is usually done with freshly frozen or cryostat sections, but excellent results are also obtained with sections cut on a Vibratome or with whole-mounts of thin membranes, such as blood vessels which have been cut open, or choroid plexuses. The preparations are incubated in a medium containing acetylthiocholine, copper sulphate and glycine, and adjusted to a pH of 6.4 with phosphate buffer. The solution is saturated with copper thiocholine so that as soon as thiocholine is liberated enzymically precipitation will occur. The sections are then rinsed in a saline solution and immersed in yellow ammonium sulphide solution to convert the precipitated copper to copper sulphide. Presumptive sites of enzymic activity are seen as dark-brown deposits. As a technical control in the original method, sections are pre-incubated in diisopropylfluorophosphate in saline solution to inactivate the cholinesterases.

An absolute prerequisite for the reliability of the technique for the demonstration of cholinergic nerves is that pseudocholinesterase (cholinesterase EC 3.1.1.8) must be efficiently inhibited by an irreversible inhibitor. The conditions for this type of specific control have been reported by Holmstedt (1957*a*, *b*). It should be remembered that most of the detailed inhibition experiments have been performed on feline tissues and that the conditions are not necessarily directly applicable to tissues from other species. Rats, for example, in addition to the specific acetylcholinesterase and butyryl-cholinesterase, also have a propionylcholinesterase. The way this last enzyme is inhibited is intermediate between that of acetylcholinesterase and butyrylcholinesterase. This means that special care has to be taken before a positive reaction, even in combination with classical inhibitors, can be said to be due to acetylcholinesterase, thus reflecting the presence of cholinergic nerves. It should also be noted that when there is prolonged incubation with substrate (using sections preincubated for inhibition of pseudocholinesterase), a non-specific precipitation may occur which does not necessarily represent acetylcholinesterase. With the use of proper incubation times (usually below 4 h) a reaction is obtained with cholinergic nerves in the central nervous system and the cholinergic motor nerves from the autonomic and spinal systems in the periphery, whereas sensory fibres appear to contain too little of the enzyme to be clearly seen under these conditions (Ehinger 1966).

Since acetylcholinesterase is not exclusively present in tissues that store acetylcholine, attempts have been made to develop histochemical staining methods for more specific enzymes. The technique for choline acetyltransferase (EC 2.3.1.6) represents such an approach (Kása 1975). The usefulness for histochemical purposes has, however, been limited for technical reasons. Attempts are now being made to apply immunohistochemical techniques (Rossier *et al.* 1975) for a more sensitive and specific localization of cholinergic nerves.

INNERVATION OF THE CEREBROVASCULAR BED

The cerebrovascular bed has been widely held to be unique in that it lacks a perivascular innervation, the cerebral blood flow therefore being regulated entirely via so-called metabolic and chemical factors. There seem to be several reasons for this misconception. For example, available histological staining methods were not sensitive and specific enough for the relation of nerve fibres to vessels to be unequivocally demonstrated in the central nervous system; further, some of the early electron microscope studies (Pease & Molinari 1960; Samarasinghe 1965) indicated that neither extracerebral nor intracerebral arteries and arterioles received nerves or, if axon terminals could be demonstrated, they did not penetrate into the smooth muscular media from the adventitia. Negative information from electron microscope studies is, of course, of little relevance since the information at this high level of resolution obviously has to be based on an analysis of extremely small regions; moreover, it is now well established that the presence of nerves at only the surface of the vascular media in fact represents the characteristic organization of a vascular innervation apparatus. Naturally, there have been a number of physiological observations indicating that the brain circulation may be influenced by neurogenic mechanisms, but with the very meagre structural basis for such mechanisms there has been a tendency to interpret positive results as artifacts of the experimental situation caused by variables beyond the control of the investigator.

Perivascular adrenergic nerves of extracerebral origin

Conclusive proof for the existence of a well-developed sympathetic nerve supply to the cerebral vascular bed was presented 10 years ago by Nielsen & Owman (1967), using the Falck–Hillarp histofluorescence technique. The results have since been confirmed, primarily on the basis of this method, in a number of laboratory animals (for references, see Owman *et al.* 1974; Edvinsson 1975) and in humans (Edvinsson *et al.* 1976).

The arteries and arterioles of the brain are enclosed by a plexus of adrenergic nerves which is superimposed on the media, covered by the adventitia. Also cerebral veins receive an adrenergic innervation, though less well-developed than that on the arterial side. There is a rich supply of fluorescent nerves in relation to all major vessels at the base of the brain, those belonging to the carotid system being more densely innervated than those of the vertebral system. Many of the nerves in the network enclosing the vertebral and basilar arteries have a smooth appearance and a lower fluorescence intensity, characteristic of the preterminal part of the axon, whereas most other vessels are supplied with intensely fluorescent terminals with a typical varicosed appearance. Bundles of preterminal fibres are also found in the connective tissue supporting the vertebral and basilar arteries.

Denervation experiments in combination with histochemical demonstration of the adrenergic nerves and chemical determination of the noradrenaline concentration in the vessels have shown that all these adrenergic nerves originate in the superior cervical sympathetic ganglia (Nielsen & Owman 1967; Iwayama *et al.* 1970; Edvinsson *et al.* 1972*a*). It should be noted that in some animals the ganglia are located closely outside the base of the skull, and aberrant clusters of adrenergic ganglion cells may also be present in the postganglionic nerve trunk above the ganglion: this means that complete sympathetic denervation by excision of the superior cervical ganglia may be technically difficult and has to be confirmed by fluorescence histochemistry of the vascular area to be tested after the sympathectomy. There is reason to believe that the transition between the vascular innervation originating in the superior cervical ganglia and that arising from lower sympathetic ganglia of the neck is located at the level of foramen magnum: in the cat, for example, a complete intracranial vascular denervation is achieved after superior cervical ganglionectomy, whereas in the rabbit a small number of nerves, obviously belonging to lower ganglia, may remain in the caudal part of the basilar artery and in the intracranial portions of the vertebral arteries. Here, the sympathetic type of cerebrovascular nerves will be defined as adrenergic nerves disappearing after superior cervical ganglionectomy.

The perivascular plexus of sympathetic nerves can be followed on the convexities of the brain, where arterioles as small as 15–20 μm in diameter are accompanied by adrenergic nerve fibres. The nerves then follow the small arteries and arterioles as they penetrate almost at a right angle into the brain parenchyma, and the entire intracerebral system of arterioles—i.e. vessels extending beyond the termination of the perivascular space—is innervated, to an extent that varies characteristically in different regions. This has been studied in detail in material from baboons (Edvinsson & Owman 1977*c*): some 70–90% of the arterioles receive sympathetic adrenergic nerves in regions such as the thalamus, hypothalamus, parietal cortex, and medial geniculate body whereas the innervation is much less developed in the olfactory bulb, medulla oblongata, occipital cortex, and cerebellum where only 10–30% of the arterioles are accompanied by adrenergic nerves. There is reason to believe that this heterogeneity in perivascular sympathetic innervation of the brain is directly correlated with the efficiency by which sympathetic nerve stimulation and sympathomimetic amines are able to produce an alteration in cerebral perfusion (Sercombe *et al.* 1975).

One of the specialized vascular regions in the brain, the choroid plexus has been shown by fluorescence histochemical and electron microscope methods to receive a prominent adrenergic innervation (Edvinsson *et al.* 1974*b*, 1975*b*). The nerves supply both the choroid arterioles and the secretory epithelium, and there is experimental evidence to suggest that they have an inhibitory effect on the bulk production of cerebrospinal fluid, probably by an action on both effector systems (Lindvall *et al.* 1977*b*).

Electron microscope studies (Nelson & Rennels 1970; Iwayama *et al.* 1970; Nielsen *et al.* 1971*a*; Cervós-Navarro & Matakas 1974) have shown that small bundles of non-myelinated autonomic nerves, lacking varicosities and synaptic vesicles but rich in microtubuli, run in the periadventitial tissue outside the vessel together with myelinated fibres. The nerves are all enclosed in a sheath of Schwann cells. Closer to the vessel, the autonomic nerve bundles consist of both preterminal axons and terminals, the latter characterized by their varicosed appearance. In preparations (only pial arteries were studied) fixed with potassium permanganate, or after treatment of the animals with 5- or 6-hydroxydopamine (Iwayama *et al.* 1970; Nielsen *et al.* 1971*a*), about half of the total number of varicosities are seen to contain a great number of 50 nm synaptic vesicles with an electron-dense core characteristic of the adrenergic nerve terminal. These terminals, which all disappear after bilateral cervical sympathetic ganglionectomy, come in close contact with the outer smooth muscle layer of the vascular media, lose their Schwann cell sheath partially or completely, and approach to within 80 to 100 nm of the smooth muscle cells. These terminals are often located in furrows between two adjacent muscle cells or in a shallow trough on the surface of a cell. This may give the false impression that the nerves penetrate into the outer third of the vascular muscle layer. The cleft between the nerve terminals and the smooth muscle cells is always filled with a moderately electron-dense material, probably comprising the fused basement membranes from the nerve and the muscle cell. No membrane specialization is seen in the part of the varicosity facing the muscle. The picture thus agrees well with a true vasomotor innervation of both extracerebral and intracerebral small arteries and arterioles.

It has been shown by various techniques that sufficient noradrenaline can be liberated from the perivascular nerve plexus to produce a prominent vasomotor reaction of the vessel. Thus, administration of the indirectly acting sympathomimetic agent, tyramine, to an isolated artery suspended in an organ bath will produce a contraction that can be abolished by denervation of the vessel (Nielsen *et al.* 1971*b*); electrical field stimulation of the artery similarly induces a contraction that can be inhibited by tetrodotoxin or guanethidine (Bevan & Bevan 1973; Edvinsson *et al.* 1976). Furthermore, the release of neurotransmitter during the transmural stimulation has been measured directly by estimating the 'overflow' of tritiated noradrenaline (Edvinsson *et al.* 1977).

The re-uptake of liberated transmitter into the nerve terminals constitutes the principal mechanism for termination of the action of the adrenergic nerves, and it therefore represents an important parameter in functional studies on the adrenergic neuroeffector apparatus. This uptake mechanism has recently been characterized in detail by incubation of feline pial vessels from various regions in the presence of [^{3}H]noradrenaline (Edvinsson & Owman 1977*b*). The uptake (which was almost abolished by vascular sympathectomy) was found to be less efficient in preparations from the basilar and vertebral arteries than in those from other vascular regions at the base of the brain, probably because the majority of axons in the former preparations are of the preterminal rather than the terminal type (although the noradrenaline *concentration* in the vascular tissue is of the same order of magnitude as that in vessels from other regions supplied with a similarly dense network of terminal fibres). The neuronal uptake into the pial vessel preparations showed the characteristics of an active process: it was saturable, as demonstrated by the linear relationship in the Lineweaver–Burk plot, and it concentrated noradrenaline against a considerable gradient. Furthermore, the uptake process was found to be temperature-dependent, being inactivated at 0 °C, and it required the presence of Na^+–K^+-activated ATPase (EC 3.6.1.3) as evidenced by the blockade with ouabain. The mean value for the apparent K_m of noradrenaline was approximately 5×10^{-7} M, and the mean maximum rates of uptake (E_{max}) were about 4.5×10^{-7} M/(kg min); in the basilar and vertebral arteries the amount of uptake was too low for calculation of its kinetics.

The neuronal uptake of the noradrenaline transmitter has to be taken into account in the quantitative pharmacological characterization of amine receptors in the vascular smooth muscle *in vitro*, because it will tend to reduce the concentration of amine in the region of the receptor. Such studies therefore have to be carried out on denervated vessels or in conditions when this uptake is blocked by, for example, cocaine (Edvinsson & Owman 1977*a*). Another aspect of the neuronal uptake of noradrenaline is the prejunctional supersensitivity of the vascular receptors that develops after sympathetic denervation (Edvinsson *et al.* 1975*a*). Thus, already within three days of the operation, brain vessels become two or three times more sensitive to the contractile effect of noradrenaline than intact vessels, and a corresponding increase in sensitivity can be achieved after blockade of the neuronal uptake with cocaine. This is in good agreement with a neuromuscular interval of 80–100 nm (Verity 1971) as measured in pial arteries (Nelson & Rennels 1970). The rate at which this type of supersensitivity develops corresponds to the disappearance of noradrenaline from the degenerating nerves after denervation (Edvinsson *et al.* 1972*a*), showing that it is indeed directly related to the capacity of the perivascular plexus to take up and retain the transmitter and thereby terminate its effect in the region of the receptor. Several weeks after denervation, the sensitivity of the vascular receptors to noradrenaline becomes normalized even though no signs of reinnervation are seen, indicating that some type of post-junctional change in the receptors also occurs after sympathectomy. From an experimental point of view it should thus be noted that any kind of vascular reaction to, for example, noradrenaline can be observed after sympathetic denervation, depending on the time after operation at which the tests are performed (Owman *et al.* 1974).

Perivascular adrenergic nerves of intracerebral origin

Fluorescence histochemistry has shown that adrenergic nerves running in the brain parenchyma also have a close topographic association with many of the intracerebral arterioles (Csillik *et al.* 1971; Hartman *et al.* 1972; Edvinsson *et al.* 1973), and it has been suggested that these axons may constitute a second functional system supplying brain vessels with adrenergic vasomotor fibres.

The origin of these intracerebral adrenergic nerves was studied in rats (Lindvall *et al.* 1975). Bilateral lesions, about 1.5 mm in diameter, were produced electrolytically in the locus coeruleus. The animals were killed at least two weeks later, and various brain regions were analysed with the glyoxylic acid histofluorescence method after Vibratome sectioning (Lindvall & Björklund 1974*a*). The lesion destroyed all cell bodies within the locus coeruleus. Although the number of (non-sympathetic) adrenergic nerves with a vascular association was markedly reduced, a considerable number remained, particularly in the hypothalamus, in accordance with the fact that noradrenaline nerves in the brain originate from several other nuclei in the brain stem besides the locus coeruleus (cf. Ungerstedt 1971). Therefore, more extensive lesions were made using 6-hydroxydopamine which selectively destroys the catecholamine fibres. Thus, all ascending catecholamine nerves were lesioned by bilateral stereotaxic injection into the central tegmental tract in the caudal mesencephalon, and various brain regions were again studied by the glyoxylic acid method at least two weeks after the injection. This treatment resulted in a complete, or almost complete, disappearance of fluorescent noradrenaline nerves rostral to the injection site and, hence, also in the vicinity of cerebral arterioles. Thus, the perivascular nerves in question originate in the brain stem, but only partially from the locus coeruleus.

Electron microscope studies were done on cats to elucidate whether the perivascular cerebral catecholamine nerves really innervate the smooth musculature of brain arterioles (Lindvall *et al.* 1975). The perivascular sympathetic nerves were eliminated by unilateral or bilateral removal of the superior cervical ganglia, and the animals were killed 24 h or 4–21 days later. Pieces from numerous brain regions were fixed in glutaraldehyde–osmium for electron microscopy. Adjacent tissue pieces from all regions were processed according to the Falck–Hillarp fluorescence method (Björklund *et al.* 1972).

Fluorescence microscopy showed that all fluorescent perivascular sympathetic nerves had disappeared in all preparations taken later than 24 h after ganglionectomy. Arterioles in the glutaraldehyde–osmium-fixed preparations were first identified in 1–2 μm sections stained by the Giemsa method. Ultrathin sections from these regions were then stained in lead citrate for electron microscopy. One or several axons were found around the circumference of the arterioles, close to its outermost smooth muscle layer, in 66% of the arterioles analysed in unoperated cats (Cervós-Navarro & Matakas 1974). At 24 h after sympathectomy, several perivascular axons showed degenerative signs. At later stages no axons could be found in any of the arterioles. This indicates that sympathetic fibres are the only type of adrenergic nerves that innervate intracerebral arterioles in a conventional manner. In some instances it could be seen how the cerebral neuropil, containing axons with electron-dense vesicles, extended very close to arteriolar walls—though always with a thick intervening basement membrane—which might well correspond with the close vascular association of parenchymal nerves observed at the level of optical microscopy. If such axons influence the cerebral microcirculation functionally, we obviously have to accept an unconventional kind of neuro-vascular relation, in which very long diffusion distances for the adrenergic transmitter substance are involved.

Perivascular cholinergic nerves

The cholinergic innervation of the cerebrovascular bed has been investigated with the light microscope by the cholinesterase technique. The cholinergic nature of nerves can be established only after efficient irreversible inhibition of pseudocholinesterase, though important information can also be obtained after selective sympathetic and parasympathetic denervation. These prerequisites have been fulfilled only in the studies by Edvinsson *et al.* (1972*b*) and Denn & Stone (1976).

The distribution and density of the acetylcholinesterase-containing nerve plexus supplying the extracerebral arteries correspond very well with the organization of the adrenergic innervation. This has been directly confirmed by estimating the number of nerves in the perivascular plexus from the same vascular areas after either the formaldehyde or cholinesterase reaction (Edvinsson 1975). The choroid plexus system also receives a well-developed cholinergic nerve supply (Lindvall *et al.* 1977*a*). In the detailed histochemical study by de Sousa Pereira (1974) on dogs cholinesterase-positive fibres were absent from the arteries at the base of the brain supplied from the vertebral system, whereas stained fibres could be demonstrated rostrally to the posterior communicating arteries; adrenergic nerves, on the other hand, supplied the entire complex of arteries at the base of the brain contributing to and issuing from the circle of Willis.

Cholinesterase-positive nerve fibres have so far *not* been observed in association with intracerebral vessels (although these have a well-developed supply of adrenergic sympathetic nerves). Intracerebral microvessels in the brains of some animals, e.g. rabbit, show true acetylcholinesterase activity in the vessel wall proper (Hardebo *et al.* 1976). It is possible that reports of an intracerebral cholinergic vascular innervation may be based on mis-interpretations of the positive staining of the vessel wall itself, especially as seen in certain orientations of the plane of sectioning. The absence of cholinergic fibres around vessels within the brain is also supported by the lack of perivascular nerves visible by electron microscopy after sympathectomy (Lindvall *et al.* 1975). The acetylcholinesterase-containing nerve terminals around the pial vessels appear to be parasympathetic because they are not affected by excision of the superior cervical ganglia, which supply the brain vessels with adrenergic, sympathetic fibres. The parasympathetic nerves to the intracranial vessels seem to run in the facial nerve, turn off in the region of the geniculate ganglion, and continue in the greater superficial petrosal nerve to the plexus of the internal carotid artery, where they form synapses.

There is some evidence in the literature that the intracranial arteries are also supplied with afferent nerve fibres. They are considered to pass via the vertebral plexus along the posterior cerebral, basilar, cerebellar and vertebral arteries into the trigeminal, glossopharyngeal and possibly also vagus nerves. The amount of acetylcholinesterase in afferent (sensory) nerves appears to be so low that substantial staining is obtained only after prolonged incubation (Ehinger 1966). This would mean that acetylcholinesterase staining under normal conditions, such as those employed in the studies referred to, only reveals the efferent (parasympathetic) fibres.

Non-adrenergic nerve terminals can be distinguished at the electron microscope level by their empty (electron-lucent) synaptic vesicles of 50 nm, as seen in preparations fixed with potassium permanganate or after treatment with 5- or 6-hydroxydopamine (Iwayama *et al.* 1970; Nielsen *et al.* 1971*a*). All parts of the non-adrenergic axon closely follow the adrenergic fibres in pial vessels, and come in close contact with the vascular smooth muscle cells at the same distance as described above for the adrenergic nerves. The electron-microscopically visible non-adrenergic type of fibre remains after sympathectomy, and in view of the above-mentioned findings from the cholinesterase histochemistry (Edvinsson *et al.* 1972*b*), these fibres have been interpreted as being cholinergic nerve fibres.

Axo-axonal relationships

As mentioned above, the histochemical results demonstrated a close similarity between the distribution of adrenergic and cholinergic nerve terminals. This relationship was studied in further detail by using the same spread preparation from a brain vessel for the two chemical reactions consecutively (Edvinsson *et al.* 1972*b*): the preparation was first subjected to mild formaldehyde treatment to demonstrate the adrenergic nerve plexus; it was then photographed, treated for the demonstration of acetylcholinesterase during prolonged incubation, and re-photographed. The adrenergic and cholinergic nerve terminals in fact follow each other side by side in the meshes of the perivascular autonomic nerve plexus. This relationship could be confirmed in electron microscope studies, in which it was frequently seen that adrenergic or non-adrenergic (probably cholinergic) axon varicosities come in close apposition in the neuro-effector area, with a membrane-to-membrane distance of only 25 nm. Membrane thickenings were sometimes observed within circumscribed areas of the opposing membranes. Such appositions were found either between varicosities belonging to the same type of nerves, or between varicosities from an adrenergic and a cholinergic nerve. Axo-axonal relationships were even found in the terminal innervation region, i.e. the membranes of an adrenergic and a cholinergic varicosity were 25 nm apart, and both also innervated the smooth muscle cell from a distance of 80–100 nm. Similar arrangements between axons have been found in iris, heart and vas deferens. Apart from the pial system (see also Iwayama *et al.* 1970), a dual adrenergic and cholinergic innervation occurs in several vascular areas, for example in the heart. However, there are also regions, e.g. the mesenterium, in which the vessels are lacking a cholinergic nerve supply as evidenced by histochemical techniques. The dual vascular innervation is thus not as general a phenomenon as indicated by the study of Schenk & El Badawi (1968), in which no attempts were made to inhibit pseudocholinesterase: for this reason, the cholinesterase present in adrenergic nerves may also have been demonstrated under the conditions used.

There is experimental evidence from studies on the superfusion of tritiated noradrenaline during transmural electrical stimulation of the adrenergic nerves (Edvinsson *et al.* 1977) that the axo-axonal relationship corresponds to functional interaction between the two nerve systems, so that the cholinergic axon can inhibit the release of noradrenaline by a direct effect on the adjacent adrenergic axon terminal. Whether an interaction in the opposite direction is also operating is so far unknown; the ultrastructure of the relationship, anyhow, does not give us any clue to this question.

Peptidergic innervation

During our ultrastructural studies of cerebral vascular innervation in rats and cats (Nielsen *et al.* 1971*a*), we observed a third type of nerve which—from the appearance of the vesicles in the axon terminals—did not conform with either adrenergic or cholinergic nerves. These axons were characterized by the predominance of large vesicles, 85–200 nm in diameter, containing a moderately electron-dense core filling the entire vesicle. They resembled nerves designated as 'p-type' fibres because of the similarity of the large granular vesicles to those of the polypeptide-storing neurosecretory nerves. This led us to search for vasoactive peptides in perivascular nerves of the brain. A positive outcome was obtained with the immunohistochemical demonstration of vasoactive intestinal polypeptide (VIP) in perivascular nerves of the brain (Larsson *et al.* 1976). VIP is a potent hypotensive and vasodilatory agent which has been isolated from porcine small intestine. The molecular weight is about 3800.

Fibres containing VIP immunoreactivity were encountered in the adventitia or adventitia–media border in most of the pial vessels. Moderate numbers of single fluorescent fibres, or small fibre bundles, were seen to run along and close to the vertebral and basilar arteries, but none of the fibres seemed to reach the muscle layer. Only very few immunoreactive fibres were associated with the superior cerebellar arteries. However, a much richer supply was found in the anterior portion of the circle of Willis. Thus, a very well-developed plexus of fluorescent fibres with beaded (varicosed) appearance enclosed, for example, the anterior and middle cerebral arteries (and the small arteriolar branches derived from this area), being located mainly in the adventitia–media border. Occasionally, immunoreactive fibres have also been observed along small intracerebral vascular branches.

The VIP immunoreactive perivascular nerves in the brain were not affected by removal of the superior cervical ganglia, even long after operation. It is therefore assumed that the VIP-containing cell bodies recently found in these ganglia send their fibres to other regions; thus, the origin of the VIP nerves to the cerebral vascular bed is still not known.

It is suggested that the VIP-containing nerves represent a third system of nerve fibres, along with the adrenergic and cholinergic systems, which may have a vasodilatory function as evidenced by the dilatory action of VIP on isolated brain vessels of cats (Larsson *et al.* 1976). It is not unlikely that this type of nerve explains the non-adrenergic, non-cholinergic dilator effect observed in the pial arteries of the cat during transmural electrical stimulation of the nerves (Lee *et al.* 1975).

Innervation of contractile capillaries

Recent electron microscope evidence by Rennels & Nelson (1975) suggests that the brain capillaries are innervated: axon terminals were found in close approximation to the pericytes, and sometimes the terminals abutted directly on endothelial cells. These observations seem to have a particular relevance in view of our findings that the capillary walls contain immunohistochemically visible contractile proteins (Owman *et al.* 1977).

Sections from rat hypothalamus and cerebellum were prepared in a cryostat. They were incubated for 30 min at room temperature with specific, gammaglobulin-enriched rabbit antibodies and corresponding controls as follows: (*a*) antiserum raised against purified myosin from chicken gizzard smooth muscle, (*b*) antiserum to actin purified from acetone powder of chicken gizzard muscle, (*c*) antibody to the smooth muscle myosin previously adsorbed to chicken gizzard myosin, (*d*) the same antibody adsorbed to striated muscle (pectoralis) myosin, and (*e*) normal, non-immune rabbit gammaglobulin. After the preparations had been washed, fluorescein-labelled sheep anti-rabbit immunoglobulin was added.

Incubation of brain sections with specific antibodies against smooth muscle myosin, followed by fluorescein-labelled anti-gammaglobulin sera, gave intense fluorescence in the smooth muscle walls of pial arteries and arterioles. The fluorescent vessels issued branches into the hypothalamic and cerebellar parenchyma. The parenchyma contained a network of myosin-fluorescent capillaries; the fluorescence intensity in the capillary walls was lower than that of the precapillary vessels. The immunofluorescence was located in both pericytes and endothelial cells. The venules and veins also exhibited myosin fluorescence in their walls, of the same intensity as that seen in the capillary walls. Sections incubated with anti-actin showed a similar fluorescence distribution in the vessels, including the capillary walls. Incubation with myosin antibodies previously adsorbed to striated muscle myosin gave a more distinct fluorescence than that obtained with myosin antibodies alone, and the greenish background was reduced. Previous adsorption to smooth muscle myosin completely extinguished the fluorescence. Control sections incubated with either normal non-immune gammaglobulin or the second fluorescein-labelled antibody were completely negative.

The presence of actin and myosin has been confirmed in vessels of the adrenal gland, indicating that peripheral capillaries also have contractile properties. The findings seem to offer new aspects on the dynamics of flow and permeability, with particular regard to neurogenic control functions, in certain vascular beds.

ACKNOWLEDGEMENT

Supported by the Swedish Medical Research Council (grant No. 04X-732).

References

BENNETT, M. R. (1972) *Autonomic Neuromuscular Transmission*, Cambridge University Press, London

BEVAN, J. A. & BEVAN, R. D. (1973) Localized neurogenic vasoconstriction of the basilar artery. *Stroke 4*, 760–763

BJÖRKLUND, A. & LINDVALL, O. (1977) Anatomy of the catecholamine-containing projection systems of the brain stem reticular formation, in *Neurogenic Control of the Brain Circulation* (Owman, Ch. & Edvinsson, L., eds.), pp. 409–428, Pergamon Press, Oxford

BJÖRKLUND, A., FALCK, B. & OWMAN, CH. (1972) Fluorescence microscopic and microspectrofluorometric techniques for the cellular localization and characterization of biogenic amines, in *The Thyroid and Biogenic Amines* (Rall, J. E. & Kopin, I. J., eds.), pp. 318–368, North-Holland, Amsterdam

BJÖRKLUND, A., FALCK, B. & LINDVALL, O. (1975) Microspectrofluorometric analysis of cellular monoamines after formaldehyde or glyoxylic acid condensation, in *Methods in Brain Research* (Bradley, P. B., ed.), pp. 249–294, Wiley, Chichester

CERVÓS-NAVARRO, J. & MATAKAS, F. (1974) The innervation of cerebral arterioles in the cat. *Neurology 24*, 282–286

CHAN-PALAY, V. (1976) Serotonin axons in the supra- and subependymal plexuses and in the leptomeninges; their roles in local alterations of cerebrospinal fluid and vasomotor activity. *Brain Res. 102*, 103–130

COONS, A. H., CREECH, H. J., JONES, R. N. & BERLINER, E. (1942) The demonstration of pneumococcal antigen in tissues by the use of fluorescent antibody. *J. Immunol. 45*, 159–170

CSILLIK, B., JANCSÓ, G., TÓTH, L., KOZMA, M., KÁLMÁN, G. & KARCSU, S. (1971) Adrenergic innervation of hypothalamic blood vessels. A contribution to the problem of central thermodetectors. *Acta Anat. 80*, 142–151

DAHLSTRÖM, A. (1966) *The Intraneuronal Distribution of Noradrenaline and the Transport and Life-Span of Amine Storage Granules in the Sympathetic Adrenergic Neuron. A Histochemical and Biochemical Study*, pp. 1–44, Haeggström, Stockholm

DE LA TORRE, J. C. & SURGEON, J. W. (1976) A methodological approach to rapid and sensitive monoamine histofluorescence using a modified glyoxylic acid technique: the SPG method. *Histochemistry 49*, 81–93

DENN, M. J. & STONE, H. L. (1976) Cholinergic innervation of monkey cerebral vessels. *Brain Res. 113*, 394–399

DE SOUSA PEREIRA, J. M. M. (1974) *Circulacao Colateral do Cérebro nas Oclusoes da Carótida Interna. Estudo de Anátomo-Histoquimica, Cirurgia Experimental e Clinica*, pp. 1–294, Inova-Artes Gráficas, Porto

ECCLES, R. M. & Libet, B. (1961) Origin and blockade of the synaptic responses of curarized sympathetic ganglia. *J. Physiol. (Lond.) 157*, 484–503

EDVINSSON, L. (1975) Neurogenic mechanisms in the cerebrovascular bed. Autonomic nerves, amine receptors and their effects on cerebral blood flow. *Acta Physiol. Scand. Suppl. 427*, 1–35

EDVINSSON, L. & OWMAN, CH. (1977*a*) Pharmacological characterization of postsynaptic vasomotor receptors in brain vessels, in *Neurogenic Control of the Brain Circulation* (Owman, Ch. & Edvinsson, L., eds.), pp. 167–183, Pergamon Press, Oxford

EDVINSSON, L. & OWMAN, CH. (1977*b*) Characterization of the uptake of ^{3}H-noradrenaline into rabbit brain vessels and its relation to the degree of sympathetic nerve supply, in *Neurogenic Control of the Brain Circulation* (Owman, Ch. & Edvinsson, L., eds.), pp. 121–132, Pergamon, Oxford

EDVINSSON, L. & OWMAN, CH. (1977*c*) Sympathetic innervation and adrenergic receptors in intraparenchymal cerebral arterioles of baboon. *Acta Neurol. Scand. 56, Suppl. 64*, 304–305

EDVINSSON, L., OWMAN, CH., ROSENGREN, E. & WEST, K. A. (1972*a*) Concentration of noradrenaline in pial vessels, choroid plexus, and iris during two weeks after sympathetic ganglionectomy or decentralization. *Acta Physiol. Scand. 85*, 201–206

EDVINSSON, L., NIELSEN, K. C., OWMAN, CH. & SPORRONG, B. (1972*b*) Cholinergic mechanisms in pial vessels. Histochemistry, electron microscopy and pharmacology. *Z. Zellforsch. Mikrosk. Anat. 134*, 311–325

EDVINSSON, L., LINDVALL, M., NIELSEN, K. C. & OWMAN, CH. (1973) Are brain vessels innervated also by central (non-sympathetic) adrenergic neurons? *Brain Res. 63*, 496–499

EDVINSSON, L., HUGGEL, H. J., NIELSEN, K. C., OWMAN, CH. & PERISTIANY, J. G. (1974*a*) Histochemistry of autonomic nerves in wing vessels of *Pteropus giganteus* (Flying-fox), and the effects of denervation. *Cell Tiss. Res. 152*, 1–11

EDVINSSON, L., NIELSEN, K. C., OWMAN, CH. & WEST, K. A. (1974*b*) Adrenergic innervation of the mammalian choroid plexus. *Am. J. Anat. 139*, 299–308

EDVINSSON, L., AUBINEAU, P., OWMAN, CH., SERCOMBE, R. & SEYLAZ, J. (1975*a*) Sympathetic innervation of cerebral arteries: prejunctional supersensitivity to norepinephrine after sympathectomy or cocaine treatment. *Stroke 6*, 525–530

EDVINSSON, L., HÅKANSON, R., LINDVALL, M., OWMAN, CH. & SVENSSON, K.-G. (1975*b*) Ultrastructural and biochemical evidence for a sympathetic neural influence on the choroid plexus. *Exp. Neurol. 48*, 241–251

EDVINSSON, L., OWMAN, CH. & SJÖBERG, N.-O. (1976) Autonomic nerves, mast cells, and amine receptors in human brain vessels. A histochemical and pharmacological study. *Brain Res. 115*, 377–393

EDVINSSON, L., FALCK, B. & OWMAN, CH. (1977) Possibilities for a cholinergic action on smooth musculature and on sympathetic axons in brain vessels mediated by muscarinic and nicotinic receptors. *J. Pharmacol. Exp. Ther. 200*, 117–126

EHINGER, B. (1966) Cholinesterases in ocular and orbital tissues of some mammals. *Acta Univ. Lund Sect. II Med. Math. Sci. Rerum. Nat. 2*, 1–16

ELFVIN, L.-G. (1963) The ultrastructure of the superior cervical sympathetic ganglion of the cat. II. The structure of the preganglionic end fibres and the synapses as studied by serial sections. *J. Ultrastruct. Res. 8*, 441–476

FUXE, K. (1965) Evidence for the existence of monoamine neurons in the central nervous system. IV. Distribution of monoamine nerve terminals in the central nervous system. *Acta Physiol. Scand. Suppl. 64*, 37–85

FUXE, K., HÖKFELT, T. & UNGERSTEDT, U. (1968) Localization of indolealkylamines in CNS. *Adv. Pharmacol. 6*, 235–251

FUXE, K., OLSON, L. & ZOTTERMAN, Y. (eds.) (1974) *Dynamics of Degeneration and Growth in Neurons*, Pergamon Press, Oxford

GABELLA, G. (1976) *Structure of the Autonomic Nervous System*, Chapman & Hall, London

GOLDMAN, M. (1968) *Fluorescent Antibody Methods*, Academic Press, New York

HARDEBO, J. E., EDVINSSON, L., FALCK, B., LINDVALL, M., OWMAN, CH., ROSENGREN, E. & SVENDGAARD, N.-AA. (1976) Experimental models for histochemical and chemical studies of the enzymatic blood-brain barrier for amine precursors, in *The Cerebral Vessel Wall* (Cervós-Navarro, J. *et al.*, eds.), pp. 233–244, Raven Press, New York

HARTMAN, B. K., ZIDE, D. & UDENFRIEND, S. (1972) The use of dopamine β-hydroxylase as a marker for the central noradrenergic nervous system in rat brain. *Proc. Natl. Acad. Sci. U.S.A. 69*, 2722–2726

HILLARP, N.-Å. (1946) Structure of the synapse and the peripheral innervation apparatus of the autonomic nervous system. *Acta Anat. Suppl. 2*, 1–153

HÖKFELT, T. & LJUNGDAHL, Å. (1972) Application of cytochemical techniques to the study of suspected transmitter substances in the nervous system. *Adv. Biochem. Psychopharmacol. 6*, 1–36

HÖKFELT, T., FUXE, K. & GOLDSTEIN, M. (1975*a*) Applications of immunohistochemistry to studies on monoamine cell systems with special reference to nervous tissues. *Ann. N.Y. Acad. Sci. 254*, 407–432

Hökfelt, T., Kellerth, J.-O., Nilsson, G. & Pernow, B. (1975*b*) Experimental immunohistochemical studies on the localization and distribution of Substance P in cat primary sensory neurons. *Brain Res. 100*, 235–252

Holmstedt, B. (1957*a*) A modification of the thiocholine method for the determination of cholinesterase. I. Biochemical evaluation of selective inhibitors. *Acta Physiol. Scand. 40*, 322–330

Holmstedt, B. (1957*b*) A modification of the thiocholine method for the determination of cholinesterase. II. Histochemical application. *Acta Physiol. Scand. 40*, 331–357

Iwayama, T. (1970) Ultrastructural changes in the nerves innervating the cerebral artery after sympathectomy. *Z. Zellforsch. Mikrosk. Anat. 109*, 465–480

Iwayama, T., Furness, J. B. & Burnstock, G. (1970) Dual adrenergic and cholinergic innervation of the cerebral arteries of the rat. *Circ. Res. 26*, 635–646

Johansson, B., Ljung, B., Malmfors, T. & Olson, L. (1970) Prejunctional supersensitivity in the rat portal vein as related to its pattern of innervation. *Acta Physiol. Scand. Suppl. 349*, 5–16

Jonsson, G. (1971) Quantitation of fluorescence of biogenic monoamines demonstrated with the formaldehyde fluorescence method. *Prog. Histochem. Cytochem. 2*, 299–334

Kása, P. (1975) Histochemistry of choline acetyltransferase, in *Cholinergic Mechanisms* (Waser, P. G., ed.), pp. 271–281, Raven Press, New York

Koelle, G. B. (1963) Cytological distributions and physiological functions of cholinesterases, in *Cholinesterases and Anticholinesterase Agents* (Koelle, G. B., ed.) *(Handb. Exp. Pharmakol. Suppl. 15)*, pp. 187–298, Springer, Berlin

Langer, S. Z. (1970) The metabolism of ^{3}H-noradrenaline released by electrical stimulation from the isolated nictitating membrane of the cat and the vas deferens of the rat. *J. Physiol. (Lond.) 208*, 515–546

Larsson, L.-I., Edvinsson, L., Fahrenkrug, J., Hakanson, R., Owman, Ch., Schaffalitzky de Muckadell, O. & Sundler, F. (1976) Immunohistochemical localization of a vasodilatory polypeptide (VIP) in cerebrovascular nerves. *Brain Res. 113*, 400–404

Lee, T. J.-F., Su, C. & Bevan, J. A. (1975) Nonsympathetic dilator innervation of cat cerebral arteries. *Experientia (Basel) 31*, 1424–1426

Libet, B. (1970) Generation of slow inhibitory and excitatory postsynaptic potentials. *Fed. Proc. 29*, 1945–1956

Libet, B. & Owman, Ch. (1974) Concomitant changes in formaldehyde-induced fluorescence of dopamine interneurones and in slow inhibitory postsynaptic potentials of the rabbit superior cervical ganglion, induced by stimulation of the preganglionic nerve or by a muscarinic agent. *J. Physiol. (Lond.) 237*, 635–662

Libet, B. & Tosaka, T. (1970) Dopamine as a synaptic transmitter and modulator in sympathetic ganglia: a different mode of synaptic action. *Proc. Natl. Acad. Sci. U.S.A. 67*, 667–673

Lichtensteiger, W. (1969) Cyclic variations of catecholamine content in hypothalamic nerve during the estrous cycle of the rat, with a concomitant study of the substantia nigra. *J. Pharmacol. Exp. Ther. 165*, 204–215

Lindvall, O. & Björklund, A. (1974*a*) The glyoxylic acid fluorescence histochemical method: a detailed account of the methodology for the visualization of central catecholamine neurons. *Histochemistry 39*, 97–127

Lindvall, O. & Björklund, A. (1974*b*) The organization of the ascending catecholamine neuron systems in the rat brain as revealed by the glyoxylic acid fluorescence method. *Acta Physiol. Scand. Suppl. 412*, 1–48

Lindvall, M., Cervós-Navarro, J., Edvinsson, L., Owman, Ch. & Stenevi, U. (1975) Non-sympathetic perivascular nerves in the brain: origin and mode of innervation studied by fluorescence and electron microscopy combined with stereotaxic lesions and sympathectomy, in *Blood Flow and Metabolism in the Brain* (Harper, A. M. *et al.*, eds.), pp. 1.7–1.9, Churchill Livingstone, Edinburgh

LINDVALL, M., EDVINSSON, L. & OWMAN, CH. (1977*a*) Histochemical study on regional differences in the cholinergic nerve supply of the choroid plexus from various laboratory animals. *Exp. Neurol. 55*, 152–159

LINDVALL, M., EDVINSSON, L. & OWMAN, CH. (1977*b*) Histochemical, ultrastructural and functional evidence for a neurogenic control of cerebrospinal fluid production from the choroid plexus. *Acta Physiol. Scand. Suppl. 452*, 77–86

LORÉN, I., BJÖRKLUND, A., FALCK, B. & LINDVALL, O. (1976) An improved histofluorescence procedure for freeze-dried paraffin-embedded tissue based on combined formaldehyde-glyoxylic acid perfusion with high magnesium content and acid pH. *Histochemistry 49*, 177–192

LORÉN, I., BJÖRKLUND, A., FALCK, B. & LINDVALL, O. (1977) The use of magnesium ions for sensitive visualization of catecholamines and serotonin in the CNS. *Acta Physiol. Scand. Suppl. 452* 15–18

NELSON, E. & RENNELS, M. (1970) Neuromuscular contacts in intracranial arteries of the cat. *Science (Wash. D.C.) 167*, 301–302

NIELSEN, K. C. & OWMAN, CH. (1967) Adrenergic innervation of pial arteries related to the circle of Willis in the cat. *Brain Res. 6*, 773–776

NIELSEN, K. C., OWMAN, CH. & SPORRONG, B. (1971*a*) Ultrastructure of the autonomic innervation apparatus in the main pial arteries of rats and cats. *Brain Res. 27*, 25–32

NIELSEN, K. C., OWMAN, CH. & SPORRONG, B. (1971*b*) Sympathetic nervous control of pial arteries: tyramine-induced contraction of the isolated middle cerebral artery of the cat, in *Brain and Blood Flow* (Russell, R. W. R., ed.), pp. 244–247, Pitman Medical, London

OWMAN, CH. & FALCK, B. (1975) Functional approach to the histochemistry of catecholamines in peripheral sympathetic nerves, in *Golgi Centennial Symposium: Perspectives in Neurobiology* (Santini, M., ed.), pp. 415–436, Raven Press, New York

OWMAN, CH., EDVINSSON, L. & NIELSEN, K. C. (1974) Autonomic neuroreceptor mechanisms in brain vessels. *Blood Vessels 11*, 2–31

OWMAN, CH., EDVINSSON, L., HARDEBO, J. E., GRÖSCHEL-STEWART, U., UNSICKER, K. & WALLES, B. (1977) Immunohistochemical demonstration of actin and myosin in brain capillaries. *Acta Neurol. Scand. 56, Suppl. 64*, 384–385

PEASE, D. C. & MOLINARI, S. (1960) Electron microscopy of muscular arteries: pial vessels of the cat and monkey. *J. Ultrastruct. Res. 3*, 447–468

RENNELS, M. L. & NELSON, E. (1975) Capillary innervation in the mammalian central nervous system: an electron microscopic demonstration. *Am. J. Anat. 144*, 233–241

RICHARDSON, K. C. (1966) Electron microscopic identification of autonomic nerve endings. *Nature (Lond.) 210*, 756

ROSSIER, J., BAUMAN, A., RIEGER, F. & BENDA, P. (1975) Immunological studies on the enzymes of the cholinergic system, in *Cholinergic Mechanisms* (Waser, P. G., ed.), pp. 283–292, Raven Press, New York

SAMARASINGHE, D. D. (1965) The innervation of the cerebral arteries in the rat: an electron microscope study. *J. Anat. 99*, 815–828

SCHENK, E. A. & EL BADAWI, A. (1968) Dual innervation of arteries and arterioles. A histochemical study. *Z. Zellforsch. Mikrosk. Anat. 91*, 170–177

SERCOMBE, R., AUBINEAU, P., EDVINSSON, L., MAMO, H., OWMAN, CH., PINARD, E. & SEYLAZ J. (1975) Neurogenic influence on local cerebral blood flow. Effect of catecholamines or sympathetic nerve stimulation as correlated with the sympathetic innervation. *Neurology 25*, 954–963

STERNBERGER, L. A. (1974) *Immunocytochemistry*, Prentice-Hall Inc., N.J.

TRANZER, J. P. & THOENEN, H. (1967) Electronmicroscopic localization of 5-hydroxydopamine (3,4,5-trihydroxy-phenyl-ethylamine), a new 'false' sympathetic transmitter. *Experientia (Basel) 23*, 743–744

UNGERSTEDT, U. (1971) Stereotaxic mapping of the monoamine pathways in the rat brain. *Acta Physiol. Scand. Suppl. 367*, 1–48

VERITY, M. A. (1971) Morphologic studies of the vascular neuroeffector apparatus, in *Physiology and Pharmacology of Vascular Neuroeffector Systems* (Bevan, J. A. *et al.*, eds.), pp. 2–12, Karger, Basel

Discussion

Sandler: What correspondence is there between fluorescence observations and immunochemical studies of enzyme distribution? It is not safe to assume that a map of dopamine-β-hydroxylase (DBH) activity faithfully represents the distribution of noradrenaline. I suppose the enzyme should be called phenylethylamine-β-hydroxylase, rather than dopamine-β-hydroxylase, because phenylethylamine and the tyramines are all substrates for it. Similarly, phenylethylamine-*N*-methyltransferase (PNMT) will act on *any* phenylethanolamine, not only noradrenaline. This point is important because if such substances as octopamine do not have a specific storage apparatus (and they do not seem to), they could easily be ignored. There appears to be an extremely rapid turnover of octopamine. In human urine, for instance, there is as much *p*-hydroxymandelic acid as there is 4-hydroxy-3-methoxymandelic acid (M. Sandler *et al.*, unpublished). I am not saying that this all comes from the brain but what you are demonstrating in your fluorescence studies is storage ability, so the trace amines (Usdin & Sandler 1976), which may have a rapid turnover but little storage capacity, could easily be neglected.

Owman: I am aware of these pitfalls. There is no strict correspondence between the histochemically visible enzymes and the amines. The work I referred to has been carried out by T. Hökfelt and his co-workers (e.g. Hökfelt *et al.* 1975). There are examples also from the peripheral nervous system: in a study in collaboration with T. Hökfelt on Frankenhäuser's utero-vaginal ganglion we have found ganglion cells showing immunoreactive tyrosine hydroxylase activity without any histochemical evidence for the presence of noradrenaline (unpublished observations). On the other hand, PNMT immunofluorescence so far seems to correspond nicely with the presence of adrenaline–adrenergic nerve fibres. The demonstration of these fibres by the formaldehyde method is, however, somewhat difficult. Any discrepancy might be explained either on a purely technical basis or by the neuronal stores of other substrates for PNMT.

Heistad: Small vessels are certainly innervated with sympathetic nerves.

What is your estimate of the relative innervation of large and small arteries and of arterioles in the brain? Secondly, it would be useful to have direct evidence for a cholinergic response to nerve stimulation. Can you produce vasodilatation with field stimulation which is blocked by atropine?

Owman: The degree of innervation is related to the degree of innervation of the tributary vessels. In the vertebral system, innervation of the penetrating arteries is less well developed than in the carotid system; all of the small arteries are innervated. It is in the pre-capillary systems, such as the small arterioles, that there is a heterogeneous innervation (Edvinsson & Owman 1977). In some regions most of these small vessels are innervated, whereas in others only a few are supplied with adrenergic nerves (cf. Edvinsson & Owman 1977).

What I showed in my presentation was contractile responses of fully relaxed vessels. However, if a sympathectomized vessel is subjected to active tension, for example with 5-hydroxytryptamine, there is a dilatory response to electrical nerve stimulation. This response is not entirely inhibited by atropine. We suspect that some non-adrenergic, non-cholinergic nerve component might have been activated. It could well be a system corresponding to the vasoactive intestinal polypeptide (VIP) system. Other evidence from J. A. Bevan's group indicates that there might be this kind of unorthodox dilatory response (Lee *et al.* 1975).

Purves: You have shown that the large vessels at the base of the brain and the main afferent vessels have a very high density of fibres on them. Presumably a substantial number of these are actually *en passant* to more peripheral vessels?

Owman: The large vessels at the base of the brain are enclosed by a larger number of nerves than the intracerebral arterioles, but that takes into account only the *density* of the nerve plexus. If this plexus is then related to the underlying volume of smooth musculature, I would say that the true degree of innervation is similar in the extracerebral (pial) and intracerebral vessels. Then comes the question of whether there is innervation in the true sense or just passage of nerve fibres directed to other, more distally located areas. In the fluorescence microscope this can be distinguished by the fact that preterminals have a smooth outline whereas the terminals are varicosed. In regions such as the basal artery much of the plexus is composed of preterminal fibres whereas in other regions the nerve network consists mainly of terminals. This has some functional consequences, of course: one may find the same amount of noradrenaline in the two systems of vessels, yet they may be functionally very different with regard to the efficiency by which the perivascular nerves affect the vessel. If uptake studies of noradrenaline are carried out to demonstrate certain cellular properties of the adrenergic innervation, there is a much less efficient uptake in the basilar artery system than in other arteries containing the same amount of endogenous noradrenaline. This has been interpreted in various ways. The easiest interpretation is that this uptake is less efficient because preterminal rather than terminal fibres make up the plexus in the basilar artery.

Lübbers: There are different special inhibitors for the enzymes within the cells. Would this influence your results?

Owman: Such tissue inhibitors might influence the response during nerve stimulation. Histochemically, we are demonstrating a strictly intraneuronal distribution of the enzyme.

Lübbers: If the enzyme is in the cell in an inhibited form can you detect it at all?

Owman: The immunohistochemistry demonstrates the immunologically reactive enzyme molecule, whether active or inactive in a more functional sense. It is the *amount* of enzyme that is demonstrated, not its *activity*.

Siesjö: Those of us who are interested in how much the CBF increases and where it increases under various physiological conditions are trying to correlate that with the density of adrenergic and noradrenergic innervation. Can you distinguish between innervation from the peripheral sympathetic system and that from the locus coeruleus?

Owman: Yes, we can. The extrinsic and intrinsic nerves can be distinguished by fluorescence microscopy on the basis of differences in calibre, structure and distribution of the varicosities, etc. They also have an entirely different relationship to the vessel. In laboratory animals the two systems can be further separated by sympathectomy, for example, after which intracerebral adrenergic nerves remain unaffected.

Siesjö: We found that after amphetamine there is a very large increase in flow in the frontal cortex (Berntman *et al.* 1978). You showed sparse innervation in that area but could there be a dense innervation of the frontal cortex from the locus coeruleus?

Owman: Yes. The degree of sympathetic perivascular innervation in a given region is not related to whether vessels in this region are associated to a greater or slighter extent with intracerebral neurons. Vessels may be supplied by sympathetic nerves and yet have no particular relationship to the intracerebral adrenergic neuropil, and there are other vessels which have sympathetic nerves and which are also closely related to a number of intracerebral neurons. There is apparently a very complex neuroanatomical mixture of the two systems. If an adrenergic mechanism is diffusely activated pharmacologically —as with amphetamine, for example—the resultant effect on flow will reflect involvement of both the intrinsic and extrinsic systems.

As far as the frontal cortex is concerned, there is a dense supply of locus coeruleus neurons. Whether that represents also a true vascular innervation I don't know; but these nerves may have had an influence on flow without necessarily *innervating* the vessels (through the 'long-distance' diffusion of transmitter we have discussed previously) or, of course, through secondary effects by activation of *other* neuron systems.

Nilsson: To what extent is this pattern of nerves and receptors, which you have now described, specific to brain vessels as compared to other vascular beds?

Owman: The construction of the vascular neuroeffector apparatus is just the same in brain as in the periphery, but with regard to which part of the vascular bed is innervated, there are differences in the central nervous system and in the periphery. The large pial arteries, for example, correspond to the distributing arteries in the periphery, which are not well innervated and which are rather thick-walled. But these pial arteries are thin-walled and have an extensive innervation. They can be expected to respond well to nerve stimulation, whereas vessels of similar size in the periphery wouldn't.

There are marked quantitative and qualitative differences between the central and peripheral circulation in the character of the α and β receptors, and also other amine receptors (cf. Owman *et al.* 1978). For example, there are β_1-type receptors in the central circulation. In the peripheral vascular bed, only the coronary circulation has β_1 receptors. It is therefore dangerous to extrapolate from the peripheral circulation to the brain circulation in studies on neural and aminergic vascular responses.

Purves: It is difficult to think of another vascular bed with this unusual contact between cholinergic and sympathetic terminals. Is this so for example in the coronary circulation?

Owman: Yes, and the adrenergic–cholinergic axo-axonal relationship is found elsewhere too (Ehinger *et al.* 1970), but it is not a general phenomenon.

Heuser: In our own experiments with electrical transmural stimulation of the pial vessels (Linke & Heuser 1974) we often found spindle-like contractions of the pial vessels. That means that a central region was maximally constricted, whereas the adjacent regions of the vessels were dilated. Did you find any relationship between current intensity and change in vascular diameter?

Owman: We stimulated at supramaximum voltage routinely. The main dependence is therefore related to frequency. If you do not stimulate supramaximally you might activate only a part of the local plexus.

Sandler: You needn't apologise for making the whole picture more complex, Professor Owman, because that is the way it is. You talked about the different adrenergic receptors; both H_1- and H_2-receptors seem to be present in the cerebral vasculature too (Duckworth *et al.* 1976). There is even some evidence of thromboxane action on the cerebral vasculature (Ellis & Oates 1976), so things might be even more complex than you describe. Are any data available about the effects of catecholamine synthesis or metabolism inhibitors on cerebral blood flow?

Owman: Not that I am aware of.

Rosendorff: Some work we (Rosendorff 1972; Mitchell *et al.* 1975) did several years ago supports the idea that there are α and β receptors on cerebral vessels. We injected noradrenaline in doses ranging from 1 to 200 μg into the hypothalamus of the conscious rabbit and measured local cerebral blood flow in the hypothalamus by the clearance of ^{133}Xe. With the 1 μg dose the effect is vasodilatory. Flow increases by about 100%. Doses from 10–200 μg constrict the cerebral vessels. An intermediate dose of 2 μg produces an enormous scatter with a mean which does not significantly differ from control values. The 1 μg vasodilator effect could be blocked by the addition to the injectate of 20 μg of the β-blocker propranolol, while the vasoconstrictor effect of 40 μg noradrenaline could be blocked by the addition of the α-blocker phenoxybenzamine.

This suggests to us that noradrenaline has a dose-dependent effect when injected into the brain. The smallest dose activates β receptors and causes vasodilatation. Therefore presumably the β receptors have lower thresholds than the α receptors. The larger doses probably activate both β and α receptors but the net effect is of α-receptor-mediated vasoconstriction. This supports the idea that two types of receptors are present in cerebral vessels.

For many years we have been told that extracerebral vessels are more densely innervated than intraparenchymal vessels but from what you have told us today, Professor Owman, it is obvious that it is the density of the terminal varicosities that is functionally important. Is the density of terminal varicosities greater in intraparenchymal vessels than in extracerebral vessels?

Owman: That is very difficult to generalize. At the level of optical microscopy it is only possible to distinguish between innervated vessels and those that are not innervated. This means that a region with a well-developed perivascular nerve supply has a high proportion of its arterioles innervated, and a well innervated vessel is one with a high ratio of perivascular nerve terminals to the underlying volume of smooth musculature. From that I would say that several brain regions have a vascular innervation that is as well developed structurally—and hence probably also functionally with regard to efficient neurogenic vasomotor effects—as it is in the extracerebral (pial) vessels.

Rosendorff: You have stated in the past that the innervation of vessels in the brain doesn't fulfil the criteria for true vascular innervation. What are the criteria for true vascular innervation?

Owman: What we have stated refers to the perivascular *association* of adrenergic nerves of *intracerebral* origin. (I wouldn't like to call it innervation because, as you say, it does not fulfil the criteria.) The *sympathetic* adrenergic nerves *innervate* brain vessels in a true sense! The criteria are not very precise. They include a close relationship between the smooth muscle cell and the nerve terminal, whose Schwann cell sheath should be entirely, or at least partly, absent. The neuromuscular distance is a maximum 100 nm in the truly innervated vessels. Only a thin basement membrane separates the axon terminal and the smooth muscle cell; however, no membrane specializations are seen in any of the opposing membranes. Even with larger neuromuscular distances the transmitter may still diffuse fairly efficiently and produce a contraction. Such vessels, though, aren't considered as being *innervated* in the classical sense.

Rosendorff: What is the average distance in cerebral vessels which are innervated?

Owman: The sympathetic axon varicosities, from which the transmitter is released, are found at an average distance of 80 nm from the smooth muscle membrane. The intrinsic system of nerves from the locus coeruleus, for example, which do not have a classical close relationship with the vessels only reaches as close as some 1000 nm from the vascular wall and there is a thick intervening basement membrane. Sympathetic denervation abolishes all truly perivascular adrenergic nerves in the brain (Lindvall *et al.* 1975). So if we assume that the locus coeruleus neurons have an effect on the vessels, we have to assume that this is an unconventional effect through long-distance transmitter diffusion. That is certainly not impossible, especially when we are dealing with the central nervous system where the extracellular space has a very different composition compared with the periphery. Thus, the conditions for diffusion of the transmitter may be quite different in the central nervous system.

Because of the poor penetration of amines through the blood–brain barrier from brain to the circulation, high levels of transmitter released from the central monoamine neurons may rapidly build up in the perivascular space upon nerve activation before the transmitter is metabolized enzymically.

Moskowitz: Catecholamine metabolism in blood vessels does not appear to differ from that observed in other peripheral tissues except in two important ways: (*a*) enzymic degradation rather than neuronal re-uptake appears to be the major mechanism by which blood vessels dispose of the bulk of physiologically active catecholamines (Kalsner & Nickerson 1969); (*b*) blood vessels may exhibit some resistance to the pharmacological effects of certain systematically administered drugs (e.g. 6-hydroxydopamine and anti-nerve growth factor) (Spector *et al.* 1972). Is anything known about the dynamics of monoamine synthesis, storage, release and inactivation within nerve terminals surrounding brain blood vessels?

Owman: They pick up 6-hydroxydopamine given intraventricularly (i.e. if the blood–brain barrier is circumvented). The uptake mechanisms and the inactivation of the released noradrenaline seem to be the same as in peripheral vessels. If the vessels are denervated or if cocaine is given to inhibit re-uptake of the noradrenaline transmitter, the sensitivity of the vascular receptors to noradrenaline increases about threefold, which is the increase we would expect from peripheral vessels with a similar neuromuscular distance. A relationship has been established between the neuromuscular distance and the degree of receptor supersensitivity seen after blockade of the uptake (Verity 1971).

Plum: Have you any notion yet of the biological meaning of these observations?

Owman: From a functional point of view one would assume that vasodilatory mechanisms are more important in the brain than vasoconstriction, although there is a strange tendency among many to study primarily α-receptor activation. I am glad that Clive Rosendorff brought up the β receptors, which mediate dilatory effects. The cholinergic muscarinic receptors, the nicotinic receptors and the peptidergic receptors all mediate cerebral vasodilatation, and I would look upon this as a system for very rapid adjustments of flow. Bo Siesjö's evidence that such rapid adjustments can be demonstrated experimentally before 'metabolic' effects are seen would fit very well with some kind of neurogenic control mechanism. These functions are probably involved in reflex functions which are very difficult to elucidate properly. I would like to point out again the interesting reflex whereby external lighting conditions may, via a neuronal link, influence the cerebral vasculature directly. This kind of link may have a greater importance in lower animals, where seasonal and diurnal variations in other functions are more prominent than in the primates which are being studied most intensively. We also seem to be at the beginning of looking into some kind of physiological reflex mechanism in our studies on the neural influence on autoregulation, though at present we are only elucidating the pathophysiological extremes of such a reflex mechanism. The proper way to approach the problem would be to lead off action potentials from the perivascular nerve plexuses or the nerves going to the vessels during progressive increase in blood pressure, namely at the stage when cerebral blood flow is still constant. We might then see how there is an increasing sympathetic discharge to account for the progressive cerebral vasoconstriction, which suddenly fails at the breakthrough point when the brain vessels dilate.

Lübbers: Does denervation influence the capillary exchange properties?

Owman: Denervation could have that effect, as shown in Dr Edvinsson's presentation, but that would only explain part of the functional significance of the cerebrovascular innervation. There is a prominent innervation also of those parts of the vascular bed in which exchange wouldn't be very important, but where regulation of vascular resistance is the primary feature.

References

BERNTMAN, L., CARLSSON, C., HÄGERDAL, M. & SIESJÖ, B. K. (1978) Circulatory and metabolic effects in the brain induced by amphetamine sulphate. *Acta Physiol. Scand.*, in press

DUCKWORTH, J. W., LANCE, J. W., LORD, G. D. A. & MYLECHARANE, E. J. (1976) Histamine receptors in the cranial circulation of the monkey. *Br. J. Pharmacol. 58*, 444P

EDVINSSON, L. & OWMAN, CH. (1977) Sympathetic innervation and adrenergic receptors in intraparenchymal cerebral arterioles of baboon. *Acta Neurol. Scand. 56, Suppl. 64*, 304–305

EHINGER, B., FALCK, B. & SPORRONG, B. (1970) Possible axo-axonal synapses between peripheral adrenergic and cholinergic nerve terminals. *Z. Zellforsch. Mikrosk. Anat. 107*, 508–521

ELLIS, E. F. & OATES, J. A. (1976) Cerebral arterial smooth muscle contraction by thromboxane A_2 release from platelets. *Circulation 54, Suppl. 2*, 197

HÖKFELT, T., FUXE, K. & GOLDSTEIN, M. (1975) Applications of immunohistochemistry to studies on monoamine cell systems with special reference to nervous tissues. *Ann. N.Y. Acad. Sci. 254*, 407–432

KALSNER, S. & NICKERSON, M. (1969) Effects of reserpine in the disposition of sympathomimetic amines in vascular tissue. *Br. J. Pharmacol. 35*, 394–405

LEE, T. J.-F., SU, C. & BEVAN, J. A. (1975) Nonsympathetic dilator innervation of cat cerebral arteries. *Experientia (Basel) 31*, 1424–1426

LINDVALL, M., CERVÓS-NAVARRO, J., EDVINSSON, L., OWMAN, CH. & STENEVI, U. (1975) Non-sympathetic perivascular nerves in the brain: origin and mode of innervation studied by fluorescence and electron microscopy combined with stereotaxic lesions and sympathectomy, in *Blood Flow and Metabolism in the Brain* (Harper, A. M. *et al.*, eds.), pp. 1.7–1.9, Churchill Livingstone, Edinburgh

LINKE, A. & HEUSER, D. (1974) The influence of electrical stimulation and vasoactive substances on H^+ activity of the surface of pial vessels, in *Pathology of Cerebral Microcirculation* (Cervós-Navarro, J., ed.), pp. 121–129, W. de Gruyter, Berlin

MITCHELL, G., SCRIVEN, D. R. L. & ROSENDORFF, C. (1975) Adrenoreceptor in intracerebral resistance vessels. *Br. J. Pharmacol. 54*, 11–15

OWMAN, CH., EDVINSSON, L. & HARDEBO, J. E. (1978) Pharmacological *in vitro* analysis of amine-mediated vasomotor functions in the intracranial and extracranial vascular beds. *Blood Vessels 15*, 128–147

ROSENDORFF, C. (1972) The measurement of local cerebral blood flow and the effect of amines, in *Cerebral Blood Flow* (Meyer, J. S. & Schadé, J. P., eds.), pp. 115–156, Elsevier, Amsterdam

SPECTOR, S., TARVER, J. & BERKOWITZ, B. (1972) Effects of drugs and physiological factors in the disposition of catecholamines in blood vessels. *Pharmacol. Rev. 24*, 191–202

USDIN, E. & SANDLER, M. (eds.) (1976) *Trace Amines and the Brain*, Dekker, New York

VERITY, M. A. (1971) Morphologic studies of the vascular neuroeffector apparatus, in *Physiology and Pharmacology of Vascular Neuroeffector Systems* (Bevan, J. A. *et al.*, eds.), pp. 2–12, Karger, Basel

Evidence against H^+ and K^+ as main factors for the control of cerebral blood flow: a microelectrode study

JENS ASTRUP*, DIETER HEUSER+, NIELS A. LASSEN*, BENGT NILSSON, KARIN NORBERG and BO K. SIESJÖ

Brain Research Laboratory, University Hospital, Lund

Abstract The role of H^+ and K^+ in the control of cerebral blood flow was investigated in four previously studied conditions of cerebral hyperaemia in the rat: bicuculline-induced epileptic seizures, acute profound arterial hypoxia, amphetamine activation and insulin-induced hypoglycaemia. The extracellular activities of H^+ (pH_e) and K^+ (K_e^+) were measured by inserting pH glass electrodes and double-barrelled potassium electrodes miniaturized so that the normal response of the surrounding tissue was not seriously suppressed.

It was found that in addition to H^+ and K^+ other factors control cerebral hyperaemia, and in some conditions the mechanisms which initiate hyperaemia seem different from those maintaining hyperaemia. The hyperaemia in epileptic seizures and hypoxia was initiated in spite of a transient alkaline change in pH_e appearing initially during the phase of vasodilatation and increase in blood flow. This was due to outwash of tissue CO_2 which for epileptic seizures was aided by a drop in arterial P_{CO_2}. Later, severe tissue acidosis developed due to accumulation of lactic acid, and in status epilepticus and prolonged hypoxia acid pH_e is the possible mechanism by which vasoparalysis is maintained. The rise in K_e^+ at onset of seizures is likely to induce vasodilatation which as a local factor together with the concomitant increase in blood pressure may explain the initiation of hyperaemia. Blood pressure also increased in amphetamine activation but neither H^+ nor K^+ were involved as local vasodilators in this condition. That factors other than H^+ and K^+ are involved in the control of cerebral blood flow was further indicated by the measurements in hypoglycaemia in which hyperaemia was developed and maintained without relevant changes in pH_e, K_e^+ and blood pressure.

**Present address:* Department of Clinical Physiology, Bispebjerg Hospital, 2400 Copenhagen NV, Denmark

+*Present address:* Institute of Physiology, Tübingen, Germany

As shown by the microapplication technique, acid solutions cause dilatation and alkaline solutions cause constriction of pial arterioles (Elliott & Jasper 1949; Wahl *et al.* 1970; Kuschinsky *et al.* 1972; Betz *et al.* 1973). This proof of a pH effect on cerebral vessels supports the pH hypothesis of cerebral blood flow control proposed on the basis of a close correlation between cerebral blood flow (CBF) and brain extracellular pH. This has been demonstrated in a number of studies applying either variations in ventilation (Gotoh *et al.* 1961; Severinghaus 1964; Betz & Heuser 1967; Fencl *et al.* 1969) or ventriculocisternal perfusion (Siesjö *et al.* 1968; Pannier *et al.* 1972). That H^+ rather than CO_2 is the factor controlling the arteriolar tone was evidenced by studies of chronic hypercapnia and hypocapnia, during which CBF was found to correlate with the adaptive changes in cerebrospinal fluid pH rather than with arterial P_{CO_2} (Severinghaus *et al.* 1966; Agnoli 1968; McDowall & Harper 1968). In addition, it could be demonstrated, by stepwise induction of hypocapnia, that it was the arterial P_{CO_2} that governed the arteriolar tone (Severinghaus & Lassen 1967), probably by changing periarteriolar pH. This effect of arterial P_{CO_2} is due to the arteriolar vessel wall being readily permeable to CO_2 but not to H^+ and HCO_3^-, and thus acting as a fast CO_2 electrode (Lassen 1968). The role of pH in the adjustment of cerebral blood flow in hyper- and hypocapnia has been confirmed by many studies (see review by Betz 1972), and has only been brought into question by observations in severe hypocapnia. In severe hypocapnia vasoconstriction is largely maintained, although lactic acid accumulates in the tissue (Betz 1969; Kjällquist *et al.* 1969; Raichle *et al.* 1971).

It was suggested that the pH hypothesis of blood flow control, originally restricted to the conditions of hypercapnia and hypocapnia, might also explain the coupling between metabolism and flow in the metabolic control of cerebral blood flow (Siesjö *et al.* 1968; Lassen 1966; Betz & Heuser 1967; Skinhøj 1966). However, a correlation between perivascular pH and CBF has not yet been established in such conditions, but has merely been assumed to occur secondary to the changes in metabolic rate.

That such a correlation between extracellular pH and CBF may not generally exist is indicated by the published work, since the usual experimental findings in hypoxia and seizures have been an initial alkaline shift in brain surface pH which in time corresponded to the onset of hyperaemia (Dusser de Barenne *et al.* 1938; Jasper & Erickson 1941; Betz & Heuser 1967; Caspers & Speckmann 1972; Howse *et al.* 1974; Betz & Severinghaus 1975). Further, calculations of intracellular pH in the rat cortex from metabolic data have revealed a slight transient alkalosis within the first minute after acute profound arterial hypoxia (Norberg *et al.* 1975) or the onset of epileptic seizures (Chapmann *et al.* 1977), while marked vasodilatation occurred in the brain within that time.

However, the weight of these observations as conclusive evidence against the pH hypothesis of flow regulation had already been questioned. As stated by Howse *et al.* (1974), surface pH may not reflect perivascular pH, and MacMillan & Siesjö (1972) pointed out that the method of calculating pH from metabolic data is based on a steady-state assumption.

The present study attempts to correlate perivascular pH and cerebral blood flow (a preliminary report has already been published by Astrup *et al.* 1976). Brain extracellular pH (pH_e), which is assumed to reflect true perivascular pH closely, was measured by a glass pH electrode made small enough to insert into the cortical tissue. pH_e was measured in four different experimental conditions in which the time course and the magnitude of the cerebral hyperaemia were given by previous studies in this laboratory (Meldrum & Nilsson 1976; Nilsson *et al.* 1975; Carlsson *et al.* 1975; Norberg & Siesjö 1976). These four conditions were epileptic seizures evoked by bicuculline, amphetamine activation, acute profound arterial hypoxia and insulin-induced severe hypoglycaemia.

Simultaneously, the possible role of perivascular K^+ activity in the blood flow control was studied. Extracellular K^+ activity (K_e^+), assumed to reflect perivascular K^+ activity closely, was measured by double-barrelled K^+ electrodes inserted close to the pH electrodes in the cerebral cortex. Like H^+, K^+ acts as a potent vasodilator when applied on pial (Kuschinsky *et al.* 1972; Knabe & Betz 1972) and parenchymal (Caronna & Cameron 1975; Cameron *et al.* 1976) vessels. Since cellular K^+ is released into the extracellular space in a number of conditions in which hyperaemia occurs and in particular in conditions with activation—for example epileptic seizures (Futamachi *et al.* 1974) or local activation by afferent stimulation (Kriz *et al.* 1974)—K^+ seems well suited as a vasodilator in the local coupling between activation of function and metabolism and blood flow.

METHODS

Preparation of animals

Wistar rats were anaesthetized with halothane, 2.5%, and immobilized with tubocurarine, 2.5 mg/kg i.p., while tracheotomy was performed and catheters were placed in both femoral arteries and one femoral vein. Arterial blood pressure (BP) was monitored by an electro-manometer. EEG recordings were made from two gold-plated copper bolts screwed into the exposed skull bone. After operation halothane was switched off and anaesthesia was maintained with 70% N_2O and 30% O_2. Arterial P_{CO_2}, pH and P_{O_2} were regularly measured and the mechanical ventilation was adjusted to ensure normocapnia and normoxia. Rectal temperature was kept at about 37 °C by intermittent warming of the animal table. A piece of the parietal bone (3–4 mm in diameter) was removed and the exposed dura-arachnoid was pierced to let the electrodes through. The electrodes were inserted through the pool of cerebrospinal fluid (CSF) that accumulated under the operated area.

K^+ and pH electrodes

Double-barrelled glass capillaries with a tip diameter of about 2–5 μm were used as K^+ electrodes. We coated one barrel with silicon on the inside by allowing dichlor-dimethyl-silane vapour to diffuse into the proximal end for 45 s. The glass capillaries were subsequently baked for about 15 min at 100 °C; the reference barrel was filled with saline (NaCl 150 mmol/l) and the tip of the potassium barrel with K^+ exchange resin (Corning 477317). Filling was achieved by ejection of droplets of the fluids by long filling glass capillaries placed on the inside and moved as far out in the tip of the barrels as possible. Spontaneous filling occurred within seconds. The internal solution contained KCl 100 mmol/l and NaCl 50 mmol/l. New electrodes were prepared daily. Calibrations were done at room temperature in three isotonic solutions containing 3, 5 and 50 mmol/l KCl and 147, 145 and 100 mmol/l NaCl respectively and adjusted to 35 °C (assumed temperature of the exposed cortex) according to the Nernst equation. The pH electrodes were miniaturized conventional glass electrodes with a bulb-shaped pH-sensitive tip of about 80–100 μm in diameter (Gebert 1972; Heuser *et al.* 1975). Calibrations were done at room temperature using Radiometer standard buffers (pH at 35 °C 6.844 and 7.386). The electrodes were inserted to a depth of about 500 μm, with the pH electrode going into a stab wound made by a 50–70 μm glass capillary (Persson *et al.* 1976). The distance between the electrodes was less than 1 mm. Electrode potentials were recorded differentially, using the K^+ electrode reference as the common reference.

By replacing the electrodes with a 10^9 Ω resistor and injecting a square wave pulse into the system, we found that the capacitance of the connections was 235 pF. Repeating this with the electrodes replaced in series with the 10^9 Ω resistor, we found that the resistance of both types of electrodes was in the range of 10^8 to 10^9 Ω. Thus the electrical time constant of the recording system had a range of about 23 to 235 ms. Results in agreement with these figures were obtained when the electrodes were dipped in the calibration solution and the signal change was recorded from an open circuit. In this way the K^+ and pH electrodes were found to have time constants of 160–720 ms and 83–1280 ms, respectively (extreme ranges). Thus this simplified method using no capacitance feedback was sufficiently rapid to allow the measured pH_e and K_e^+ values to be correlated with the blood flow changes.

EXPERIMENTAL DESIGN

Four separate series were completed: (1) epileptic seizures released by bicuculline, 1.2 mg/kg i.v.; (2) amphetamine activation obtained by amphetamine sulphate, 2.5 mg/kg i.v.; (3) acute arterial hypoxia induced in one-minute periods by a switch to another respirator in which O_2 was partially replaced by N_2 (in this way arterial Po_2 was reduced to about 30 mmHg within 30 s); (4) hypoglycaemia induced by crystalline zinc-insulin, 10–15 iu/kg i.p. Experimental conditions (1), (2) and (3) were induced after a control period of 20 min. In hypoglycaemia the electrodes were inserted in the second hour after the insulin injection.

These four experimental models have been studied previously in this laboratory (Meldrum & Nilsson 1976; Nilsson *et al.* 1975; Carlsson *et al.* 1975; Norberg & Siesjö 1976). In epileptic seizures and in acute arterial hypoxia the concomitant changes in CBF were measured by the venous outflow method as described by Nilsson & Siesjö (1976). In amphetamine activation and in hypoglycaemia CBF was measured by the ^{133}Xe Kety & Schmidt (1948) technique as well as regionally by the [^{14}C]ethanol method (Eklöf *et al.* 1974). The experimental conditions in the present studies were matched to the earlier CBF studies so that we could obtain corresponding data for pH_e, K^+_e and blood flow.

RESULTS

Control state

The values of pH_e and K_e^+, of respiratory parameters of the arterial blood and of mean arterial blood pressure just before induction of experimental changes (in hypoglycaemia just after electrode insertion) are given in Table 1 and in part of Table 2.

Epileptic seizures

Fig. 1 combines the present pH_e and K_e^+ measurements with previous data for CBF, perfusion pressure (PP) and calculated cerebrovascular resistance (CVR) (Meldrum & Nilsson 1976). The increase of about eightfold in CBF

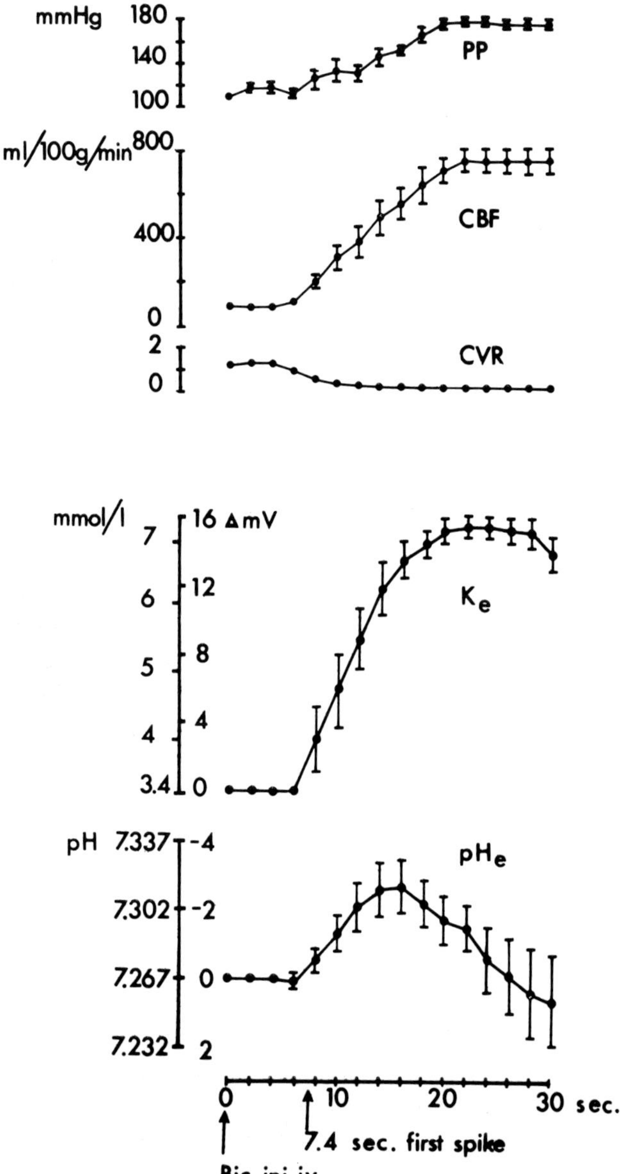

FIG. 1. Present measurements of pH_e and K_e^+ ($\bar{x} \pm$ S.E.M., $n = 6$) combined with measurements of cerebral blood flow (CBF), perfusion pressure (PP) and cerebrovascular resistance (CVR) obtained previously (Meldrum & Nilsson 1976). Epileptic seizures.

TABLE 1

Brain extracellular pH (pH_e) and K^+ activity (K_e^+), respiratory parameters in the arterial blood, and mean arterial blood pressure: control state before induction of seizures or hypoxia

$\bar{x} \pm$ S.E.M.	*Epileptic seizures* $n = 6$	*Acute arterial hypoxia* $n = 5$
pH_e	7.32 ± 0.03	7.39 ± 0.09
K_e^+(mmol/l)	3.3 ± 0.30	2.9 ± 0.18
P_{CO_2} (mmHg)	36.5 ± 1.5	34.9 ± 0.7
pH	7.348 ± 0.021	7.383 ± 0.010
P_{O_2} (mmHg)	129 ± 7	121 ± 13
BP (mmHg)	153 ± 3	138 ± 8

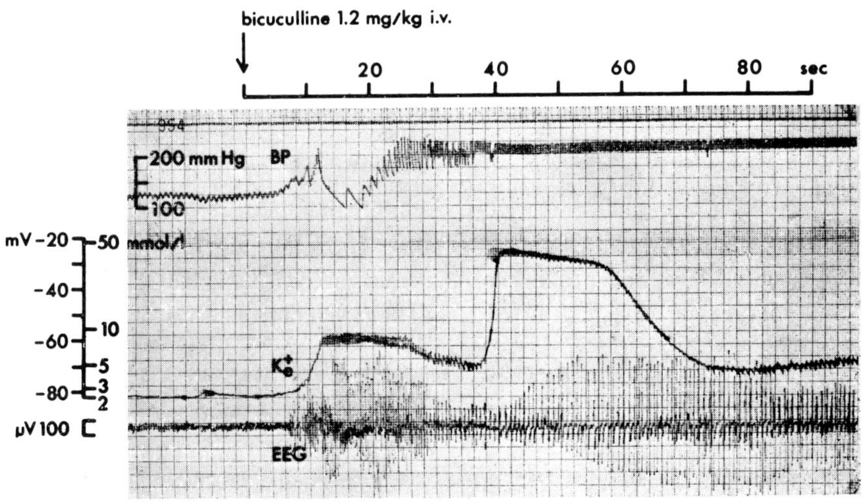

FIG. 2. Release of seizures by bicuculline, 1.2 mg/kg i.v. A spreading depression regularly appeared within the first minute. Cardiac arrhythmias usually occurred before the stable rise in blood pressure. Note the immediate rise in K_e^+ at onset of seizures.

is caused by an almost maximal vasodilatation in combination with the rise in perfusion pressure. Fig. 1 shows that vasodilatation occurs while the pH electrode is indicating extracellular alkalosis and extracellular K^+ activity is rapidly increasing. The synchrony between the appearance of seizures on the EEG and the rise in K_e^+ is shown in Fig. 2. In this model of epilepsy a 'spreading depression' is regularly released within the first minute, and cardiac arrhythmias are regularly present initially (Fig. 2). The transient alkalosis lasting for about 30 s is most probably due to an initial net removal of acid in the form of carbonic acid from the brain tissue surrounding the electrode tip ('CO_2 outwash'). The basis for this explanation is the increase of about eightfold in CBF in combination with a consistent spontaneous drop in arterial P_{CO_2} from 35.9 ± 0.9 to 31.8 ± 1.1 mmHg ($\bar{x}$ ± S.E.M., $n = 8$) as measured 20 s after the bicuculline injection. In the 20 s after onset of the seizures extracellular brain pH is presumably dominated by this CO_2 outwash, since pH_e consistently indicated alkalosis. After about 20 s the alkaline pH_e is converted into a progressive severe acidosis. This is in accordance with tissue analyses showing progressive lactic acid accumulation (Chapmann *et al.* 1977).

Amphetamine activation

Within 5 min of the amphetamine injection CBF had increased about threefold, as indicated by previous studies using the [^{14}C]ethanol method (Carlsson *et al.* 1975). Mean arterial blood pressure (MABP) increased 11%, while pH_e and K_e^+ did not change (Table 2).

Acute profound arterial hypoxia

In these experiments arterial P_{O_2} fell to about 30 mmHg within 15–30 s while arterial P_{CO_2} and pH did not change significantly (Table 3). After 15 s MABP increased 12%, on average, but fell to control levels after 60 s, at

TABLE 2

Brain extracellular pH (pH_e) and K^+ activity (K_e^+), respiratory parameters in the arterial blood (P_{O_2} excluded because only sporadic measurements were obtained) and mean arterial blood pressure (MABP). No 'vasodilatory' changes in pH_e or K_e^+ during the time of observation.

$\bar{x}$ ± S.E.M.	*Amphetamine activation* $n = 5$	$n = 5$	*Hypoglycaemia* $n = 6$	$n = 6$
	Control state	*After 5 min*	*Time of insertion*	*Before EEG flat*
pH_e	7.36 ± 0.05	7.36 ± 0.004	7.39 ± 0.003	7.43 ± 0.04
K_e^+ (mmol/l)	3.8 ± 0.06	3.8 ± 0.06	3.7 ± 0.4	3.2 ± 0.3
P_{CO_2} (mmHg)	41.5 ± 4.2	43.1 ± 3.3	38.2 ± 1.9	33.9 ± 1.6
pH	7.368 ± 0.055	7.337 ± 0.050	7.303 ± 0.021	7.287 ± 0.006
MABP (mmHg)	140 ± 4	156 ±	148 ± 6	142 ± 10

TABLE 3

Arterial P_{O_2}, P_{CO_2} and pH and mean arterial blood pressure in 16 one-minute episodes of acute arterial hypoxia in five animals. P_{CO_2} and pH were measured only at 30 s and only on seven occasions due to difficulties with rapid sampling of sufficient amounts of blood.

$\bar{x} \pm$ S.E.M. n	*Control*	*15 s*	*30 s*	*45 s*	*60 s*
P_{O_2}	121 ± 6 $n = 16$	38 ± 1,5 $n = 14$	31 ± 0.6 $n = 16$	30 ± 0.8 $n = 10$	26 ± 0.7 $n = 16$
BP	142 ± 4 $n = 16$	159 ± 3.5 $n = 16$	151 ± 3 $n = 16$	146 ± 3 $n = 16$	142 ± 2 $n = 16$
P_{CO_2}	34.4 ± 0.9 $n = 16$	—	34.2 ± 1.5 $n = 7$	—	35.1 ± 2 $n = 7$
pH	7.370 ± 0.011 $n = 11$	—	7.403 ± 0.010 $n = 7$	—	7.391 ± 0.008 $n = 7$

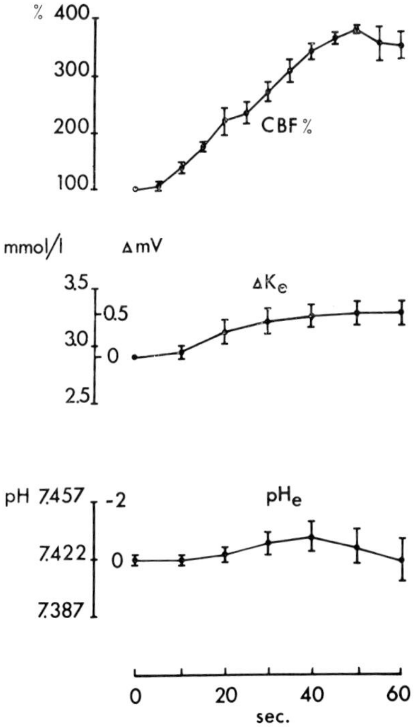

FIG. 3. Present measurements of pH_e and of changes in K_e^+ ($\triangle K_e^+$) ($\bar{x} \pm$ S.E.M., $n = 5$) combined with the relative changes in CBF (CBF%) obtained previously (Nilsson *et al.* 1975). Acute arterial hypoxia. (Reproduced, with permission, from Astrup *et al.* 1976.)

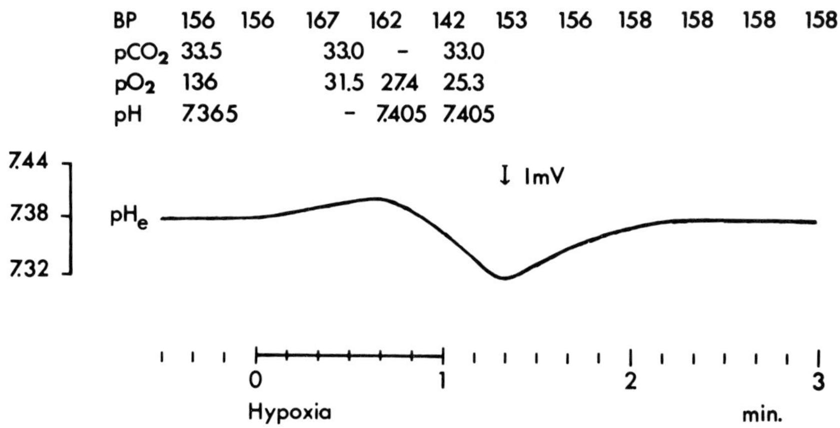

FIG. 4. pH_e, BP and respiratory parameters of arterial blood during a 1-min episode of acute hypoxia. Note the initial transient alkaline shift in pH_e.

the end of the hypoxic period, while CBF had increased fourfold at that time, as previously reported (Nilsson *et al.* 1975). The electrodes indicated a slight transient extracellular alkalosis and a modest increase in K_e^+ (Fig. 3). Of 16 episodes of acute arterial hypoxia in 5 animals alkalosis was seen in 12 ($0.1 > P > 0.05$, sign test). In the remaining four episodes of hypoxia (two animals), acidosis occurred after 10–15 s in three and after 30 s in one episode. This acidosis could tentatively be explained as an increase in arterial P_{CO_2} induced unintentionally when the respirators were switched on. This was indicated by the increases in arterial P_{CO_2} of 2.1, 0.9, 0.5 and 0.3 mmHg respectively, in these four cases. These increases in arterial P_{CO_2}, although small, tend to counteract the flow-conditioned CO_2 outwash which supposedly occurred in most cases. During this CO_2 outwash tissue P_{CO_2} approximates to arterial P_{CO_2}, leading to a drop in tissue P_{CO_2} and a net removal of acid as carbonic acid from the brain tissue. As in the bicuculline-induced seizures, this may explain the transient alkalosis regularly shown by the pH_e measurements. After 60 s the accumulation of lactic acid causes tissue acidosis which is transient if normoxia is re-established after 60 s (Fig. 4) but progressive if hypoxia is continued (Fig. 5). If complete ischaemia is induced by cardiac arrest, pH_e turns acidotic without an initial alkalotic swing (Fig. 6). This finding supports the suggestion that the initial transient alkalosis observed in acute hypoxia as well as in the model of epilepsy is associated with the increase in blood flow. K_e^+ was measured in only 10 of the 16 episodes of hypoxia because the K^+ electrode failed in one animal. In nine episodes a

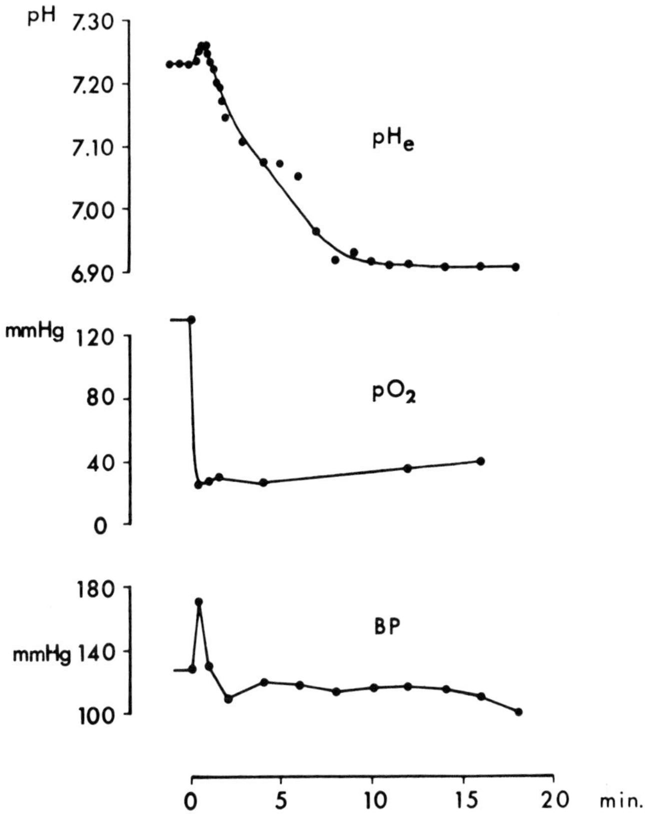

FIG. 5. pH$_e$, arterial P_{O_2} and BP during a 17-min episode of hypoxia. Note the initial transient alkaline shift in pH$_e$ and the subsequent development of severe acidosis.

reversible slight increase in K_e^+ was recorded (Morris 1974) while no changes occurred in one case ($P = 0.05$, sign test). In cardiac arrest cellular K^+ is progressively released, as shown by the rise in K_e^+ in Fig. 6.

Hypoglycaemia

The electrodes were inserted 89 ± 21 min ($\bar{x}$ ± S.E.M., $n = 6$) before the appearance of an isoelectric EEG. At the time of insertion the EEG showed predominantly slow waves (EEG group 3–4, Lewis *et al.* 1974*b*). As seen from Table 2, tissue acidosis could not be detected at the time of insertion and did not develop during the time of observation, which continued until an isoelectric EEG appeared and massive amounts of cellular K^+ were

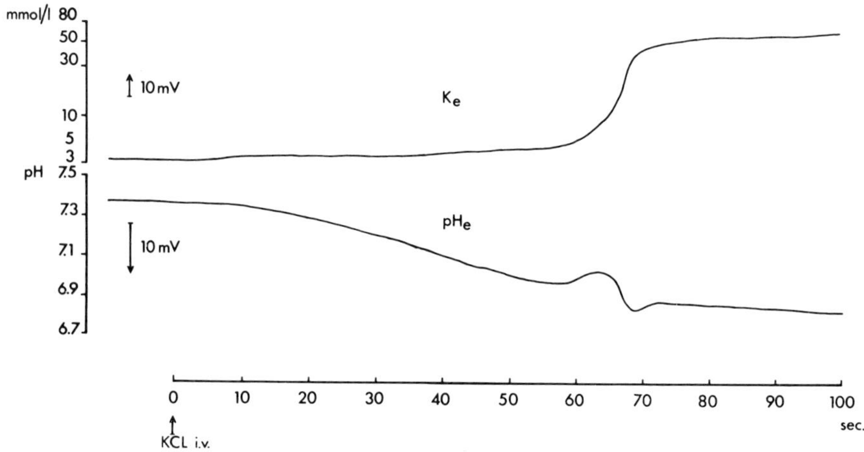

FIG. 6. pH_e and K_e^+ during complete ischaemia after cardiac arrest induced by saturated KCl, about 1 ml i.v. The transient alkaline shift in pH_e as seen in hypoxia (Figs. 4 and 5) is absent in ischaemia due to the cessation of blood flow. The artifact seen on the pH_e trace at the time of the massive release of K^+ is explained by the spatial separation between the pH electrode and its reference (in the K^+ electrode).

released, as previously reported (Astrup & Norberg 1976*a*). As in this previous study, K_e^+ remained low until the massive K^+ release occurred in the terminal state. MABP and arterial P_{O_2}, P_{CO_2} and pH also remained fairly constant (Table 2). That no tissue acidosis could be recorded agrees well with the previous metabolic studies, showing net depletion of lactic acid due to the profound glucose depletion (Lewis *et al.* 1974*a*). These observations thus support the previous conclusion that the twofold increase in cortical blood flow occurring in this experimental condition is not caused by tissue acidosis or by an increase in perivascular K^+ activity (Norberg & Siesjö 1976; Astrup & Norberg 1976*b*).

DISCUSSION

If we assume that the extracellular activities of H^+ and K^+ in the cortex are truly reflected by the pH_e and K_e^+ measurements, the present study strongly suggests that the initiation of hyperaemia at onset of activation or hypoxia is not controlled by a profuse release of either H^+ or K^+ by the neuronal tissue. Such a control mechanism includes as one step a diffusion of these ions along a concentration gradient generated at the site of release through the extracellular space to the blood vessels. Thus, if they are to confirm this view, measurements of extracellular H^+ and K^+ activities as provided by the present study should reveal an increase in extracellular H^+ or K^+ activity which in time should correlate with the onset of hyperaemia. Betz & Heuser (1967), using simultaneous measurements of local blood flow and perivascular surface pH, have provided such evidence in hypocapnia and hypercapnia, while surface pH measurements as mentioned in the introduction have indicated that alkalosis occurs initially during the development of hyperaemia in such conditions as seizures and arterial hypoxia (Dusser de Barenne *et al.* 1938; Jasper & Erickson 1941; Betz & Heuser 1967; Caspers & Speckmann 1972; Howse *et al.* 1974; Betz & Severinghaus 1975). This study largely confirms these results, although its purpose was to make extracellular measurements in the tissue with miniaturized electrodes.

Whenever electrodes are experimentally inserted in brain tissue a major concern must be the extent to which such procedures actually disrupt the structure and function of the surrounding tissue. The ideal condition, which is a local measurement of the performance of intact reactive tissue, may never be obtained with such invasive techniques, although this is attempted by miniaturization. In the present study this problem applies especially to the pH recording technique, due to the large size of the pH electrodes. The K^+ electrodes have tip diameters of a few microns and from earlier data obtained with this technique it seems reasonable to accept that it yields reliable absolute and dynamic measurements of extracellular K^+ activity (Lux 1974). Since the pH electrodes used in this study had an outer diameter of about 100 μm and were inserted in a previously made stab wound of about 50–75 μm, the tissue is damaged and its function and vasoreactivity are locally disturbed; local extravasion and occasional haemorrhage have probably also occurred (Persson *et al.* 1976). Furthermore, a pool of CSF might regularly have accumulated between the electrode and the tissue because of the respiratory movements of the brain surface, even though these are small in the rat and usually not visible in the stereomicroscope. From these considerations the transient alkalosis recorded at onset of hyperaemia may be considered erroneous if there is a layer of non-reactive damaged tissue between the surrounding intact tissue and the pH electrode tip. The metabolism of this shell of damaged tissue is presumably low and does not respond to the induced experimental conditions. When hyperaemia develops in the surrounding intact tissue, CO_2 is washed out and pH_e transiently increases in the damaged tissue and at the pH electrode tip, until sufficient amounts of the lactic acid accumulating during the seizures and during hypoxia have diffused into the area 'seen' by the pH electrode. On this argument the onset of hyperaemia in seizures and in acute hypoxia may still be caused by immediate acidosis in intact tissue, which in the experimental invasive condition is not 'seen' by the electrodes. This argument applies in seizures and hypoxia, in which the transient alkaline shifts in pH were followed by tissue acidosis; it does not apply in amphetamine activation and hypoglycaemia, in which tissue acidosis does not occur.

We attempted to evaluate tissue damage at the site of electrode insertion by autoradiography with the [^{14}C]deoxyglucose technique (Reivich *et al.* 1975). Bicuculline-induced seizures are of special interest since a layer of non-reactive tissue around the site of insertion would be maximally elucidated in contrast to the hyperactive tissue in the immediate surroundings. After seizures were induced, 25 μCi of [^{14}C]deoxyglucose (New England Nuclear, 25 μCi dissolved in 0.5 ml ethanol: water, 9:1, with 1.0 ml Krebs' solution added before injection) was injected i.v. and the animals were killed after 45 min. Autoradiograms were made of 20 μm thick slices cut tangentially in steps of 100 μm from the cortical surface at the site of electrode insertion. Two pH electrodes were inserted (diameters 300 and 100 μm). A total of 35 autoradiograms were developed from one animal with seizures and one control animal. Exposure time was nine days. As a result, 'insertion holes' of between 700 and 200 μm in diameter (cross-section) were observed corresponding to electrode diameters of 300 and 100 μm, respectively. The 'holes' were sharply defined against the surrounding stained tissue, indicating that no state of reduced metabolic activity was present beyond the holes. Similar results were obtained in seizures and in the control state. The distinction between grey and white matter was clearly visible on the deep sections. By extrapolating these data to the experimental conditions we conclude that holes of about 160–200 μm are produced by the insertion of the pH electrodes with a tip diameter of 80–100 μm (Fig. 7). This means that there is a 40–50 μm layer of metabolically inactive tissue between the intact tissue and the pH electrode. These observations correspond well with the microscopic appearance of an experimental stab wound made with a 50 μm glass capillary in the rat cortex (Persson *et al.* 1976). Within the first hours such a lesion appears as a slightly enlarged hole essentially free of substance. With an intravascular tracer such as Evans' blue–albumin, fluorescence was seen in the cell bodies and the neuropil at 200–300 μm from the centre, the staining being most intense close to the hole. On the basis of these findings the time required for diffusion of lactic acid, in amounts sufficient to oppose the CO_2 outwash, can be estimated by the diffusion equation, if unrestricted diffusion from a 1 mmol/l source accumulated in the surrounding tissue and a diffusion coefficient of 0.7×10^{-5} s^{-1}, are assumed. To oppose a change in extracellular pH of 0.50 (i.e. about 0.7×10^{-7} mol/l H^{+} as lactic acid), which is an over-estimate of

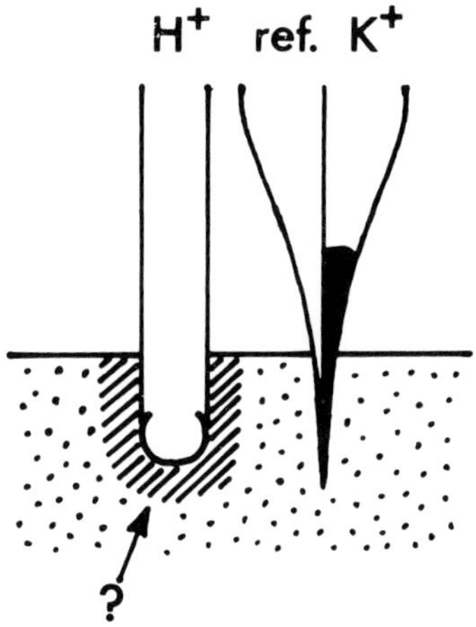

FIG. 7. Inserted pH and K^+ electrodes. Assumed layer of damaged tissue around the pH electrode.

the CO_2 outwash effect, a diffusion time of about 0.1 s appears sufficient if a 100 μm layer of damaged tissue surrounding the pH electrode is considered. Calculations which cover the experimental conditions of gradual changes in tissue P_{CO_2} and in lactic acid content can hardly be applied. However, this simple estimate indicates that although lactic acid diffuses more slowly than CO_2, the delay in development of extracellular acidosis of 30–60 s found experimentally can hardly be accounted for by a delay in lactic acid diffusion through a 100 μm layer of damaged non-reactive tissue, even though the diffusion is restricted by the structure of the tissue.

Experience with the pH_e recording technique is in favour of its use for local measurements in the brain. Firstly, severe acidosis is only occasionally recorded immediately after insertion. Of 22 consecutive insertions (this study), two gave initial pH_e values below 7.20 (7.08 and 7.14), six were between 7.20 and 7.30 and 14 above 7.30. With the exception of the hypoglycaemic group, pH_e in the control state was regularly slightly below arterial pH. The difference was 0.058 ± 0.015 ($\bar{x} \pm$ S.E.M., $n = 16$). Secondly, it has previously been demonstrated that insertion of electrodes leaves the blood–brain barrier functionally intact with respect to H^+ and HCO_3^-. This is shown by an *acidotic* pH_e change when bicarbonate is injected intravenously (Heuser *et al.* 1975). This indicates that an inserted pH electrode does more than merely reflect changes in plasma pH due to extravasation at the insertion site.

Altogether we consider that the available information concerning the reliability of the pH electrode technique as an indicator of true extracellular pH to be in favour of the technique. From these arguments it seems justified to consider the pH_e and K_e^+ recordings obtained in this study in any discussion of the role of extracellular H^+ and K^+ in the local adjustment of cerebral blood flow.

That extracellular alkalosis, although transient, consistently occurs at onset of seizures and acute hypoxia—conditions during which lactic acid massively accumulates and severe tissue acidosis rapidly develops—appears controversial and deserves careful discussion. In epileptic seizures and in hypoxia all the evidence points to an accumulation of lactic acid, already detectable while the pH electrode in the present experiments was showing extracellular alkalosis (Duffy *et al.* 1972; Bolwig & Quistorff 1973; Howse *et al.* 1974; Norberg *et al.* 1975; Chapmann *et al.* 1977). This experimental finding necessarily implies a removal of acids which initially exceeds the lactic acid production. As already mentioned, evidence indicates that there is CO_2 outwash, i.e. a net removal of tissue carbonic acid as CO_2 by the perfusing blood. In bicuculline-evoked seizures this is conditioned by the enormous increase in blood flow in combination with a substantial spontaneous drop in arterial P_{CO_2}. In acute arterial hypoxia the accumulation of lactic acid is considerably less intense than in the model of epilepsy (cf. Norberg *et al.* 1975; Chapmann *et al.* 1977) and a sufficient CO_2 outwash is supposedly provided solely by a large increase in blood flow since no significant drop in arterial P_{CO_2} was observed. This interpretation of the initial extracellular alkalosis as a CO_2 outwash which initially exceeds the lactic acid production has direct quantitative support from previous observations, made in this laboratory, that total tissue CO_2 falls enough to produce a temporary alkaline shift in the calculated intracellular pH in seizures and acute hypoxia (Siesjö *et al.* 1975; Chapmann *et al.* 1977). In amphetamine intoxication no net accumulation of lactic acid has been found (Carlsson *et al.* 1975) and in hypoglycaemia no lactic acid is produced, due to lack of substrate (Lewis *et al.* 1974*a*). Thus the present pH measurements confirm previous metabolic data obtained in these four different experimental conditions.

Extracellular K^+ may be causally related to the hyperaemia at onset of seizures since K_e^+ rises two- to threefold during the phase of vasodilatation. If mock CSF of varying K^+ content is applied locally on pial arterioles the strongest vasodilating effect is obtained with a K^+ activity of three- to fourfold higher than normal (Kuschinsky *et al.* 1972). Such experiments inevitably include some dilution of the applied solutions, and it may well be that the observed two- to threefold increase in K_e^+ at onset of seizures is of optimum vasodilatory effect. This applies to pial arterioles but is also likely to apply to parenchymal vessels (Caronna & Cameron 1975; Cameron *et al.* 1976).

We are thus inclined to conclude that extracellular K^+ contributes to the hyperaemia at onset of seizures and probably also in local activation.

The data presented indicate that there are different modes of *initiating* and *maintaining* cerebral hyperaemia. This study has confirmed previous evidence and suggestions that extracellular K^+ acts as a vasodilator initiating hyperaemia in seizures. In seizures, acute arterial hypoxia and amphetamine intoxication local mechanisms are aided by systemic hypertension increasing the perfusion pressure and forcing the arterioles to dilate. In maintaining the hyperaemia extracellular H^+ seems important in seizures and in profound arterial hypoxia. But hyperaemia may be initiated and maintained by other mechanisms, as illustrated by the normal or alkaline pH_e and the normal K_e^+ recordings in amphetamine activation and hypoglycaemia. In conclusion, it is tempting to extend the concept put forward by Moskalenko (1975) of a multifactorial control mechanism for cerebral blood flow: that is, the brain seems to have at its disposal several potent and independent local vasodilatory mechanisms, including H^+ and K^+, which, together with the perfusion pressure that is influenced to a large extent by the systemic blood pressure, control cerebral blood flow. These partially identified mechanisms may apply in different combinations, each covering the variety of metabolic and functional states of the brain.

ACKNOWLEDGEMENTS

The technical assistance of Mrs Lena Barnekow, Brain Research Laboratory, Lund, and of Mrs Eck, Institute of Physiology, Tübingen, is gratefully acknowledged.

References

AGNOLI, A. (1968) Adaptation of CBF during induced chronic normo-oxic respiratory acidosis. *Scand. J. Clin. Lab. Invest. Suppl. 102*, VIIID

ASTRUP, J. & NORBERG, K. (1976*a*) Potassium activity in cerebral cortex in rats during progressive severe hypoglycemia. *Brain Res. 103*, 418–423

ASTRUP, J. & NORBERG, K. (1976*b*) CBF increase in hypoglycemia but no brain acidosis and normal extracellular K^+, in *Cerebral Vessel Wall* (Cervós-Navarro, J. *et al.*, eds.), pp. 157–163, Raven Press, New York

ASTRUP, J., HEUSER, D., LASSEN, N. A., NILSSON, B., NORBERG, K. & SIESJÖ, B. K. (1976) Evidence against H^+ and K^+ as the main factors in the regulation of cerebral blood flow during epileptic discharges, acute hypoxia amphetamine intoxication, and hypoglycemia. A microelectrode study, in *Ionic Actions on Vascular Smooth Muscle* (Betz, E., ed.), pp. 110–115, Springer, Berlin

BETZ, E. (1969) Influence on cerebrospinal fluid pH on the regulation of cerebral circulation. *Int. Anesthesiol. Clin. 7*, 525–537

BETZ, E. (1972) Cerebral blood flow: its measurement and regulation. *Physiol. Rev. 52*, 595–630

BETZ, E. & HEUSER, D. (1967) Cerebral cortical blood flow during changes in acid-base equilibrium in the brain. *J. Appl. Physiol. 23*, 726–733

BETZ, E. & SEVERINGHAUS, J. W. (1975) Comment, in *Brain Work* (Ingvar, D. H. & Lassen, N. A., eds.) *(Alfred Benzon Symp. 8)*, p. 124, Munksgaard, Copenhagen

BETZ, E., ENZENROSS, H. G. & VLAHOV, V. (1973) Interaction of H^+ and Ca^{++} in the regulation of local pial vascular resistance. *Pflügers Arch. Eur. J. Physiol. 343*, 79–88

BOLWIG, T. G. & QUISTORFF, B. (1973) *In vivo* concentration of lactate in the brain of conscious rats before and during seizures: a new ultra-rapid technique for the freeze-sampling of brain tissue. *J. Neurochem. 21*, 1345–1348

CAMERON, I. R., CARONNA, J., MILLER, R. & LINTON, R. A. F. (1976) The action of K^+ at the cerebral vessels, in *Ionic Actions on Vascular Smooth Muscle* (Betz, E., ed.), pp. 92–96, Springer, Berlin

CARLSSON, C., HÄGERDAL, M. & SIESJÖ, B. K. (1975) Influence of amphetamine sulphate on cerebral blood flow and metabolism. *Acta Physiol. Scand. 94*, 128–129

CARONNA, J. & CAMERON, I. R. (1975) The effect of local changes in bicarbonate and potassium concentrations on hypothalamic blood flow, in *Cerebral Circulation and Metabolism* (Langfitt, T. W. *et al.*, eds.), pp. 52–54, Springer, New York

CASPERS, H. & SPECKMANN, E. J. (1972) Cerebral Po_2, Pco_2 and pH: changes during convulsive activity and their significance for spontaneous arrest of seizures. *Epilepsia 13*, 699–725

CHAPMANN, A. G., MELDRUM, B. S. & SIESJÖ, B. K. (1977) Cerebral metabolism during prolonged epileptic seizures in rat. *J. Neurochem. 28*, 1025–1035

DUFFY, T. E., NELSON, S. R. & LOWRY, O. H. (1972) Cerebral carbohydrate metabolism during acute hypoxia and recovery. *J. Neurochem. 19*, 959–977

DUSSER DE BARENNE, J. G., MARSHALL, C. S., MCCULLOCH, W. S. & NIMS, L. F. (1938) Observations on the pH of the arterial blood, the pH and the electrical activity of the cerebral cortex. *Am. J. Physiol. 124*, 631–636

EKLÖF, B., LASSEN, N. A., NILSSON, L., NORBERG, K., SIESJÖ, B. K. & TORLÖF, P. (1974) Regional cerebral blood flow in the rat measured by the tissue sampling technique; a critical evaluation using four indicators, C^{14}-antipyrine, C^{14}-ethanol, H^3-water and xenon^{133}. *Acta Physiol. Scand. 91*, 1–10

ELLIOTT, K. A. C. & JASPER, H. H. (1949) Physiological salt solutions for brain surgery: studies of local pH and pial vessel reactions to buffered and unbuffered isotonic solutions. *J. Neurosurg. 6*, 140–152

FENCL, V., VALE, J. R. & BROCH, J. A. (1969) Respiration and cerebral blood flow in metabolic acidosis and alkalosis in humans. *J. Appl. Physiol. 27*, 67–76

FUTAMACHI, K. J., MUTANI, R. & PRINCE, D. A. (1974) Potassium activity in rabbit cortex. *Brain Res. 75*, 5–25

GEBERT, G. (1972) Die Messung von Na^+, K^+ and H^+ Aktivitäten im Gewebe mit Glasmikroelektroden. *Arzneim.-Forsch. 26*, 379–385

GOTOH, F., TAZAKI, Y. & MEYER, J. S. (1961) Transport of gases through brain and their extravascular vasomotor action. *Exp. Neurol. 4*, 48–58

HEUSER, D., ASTRUP, J., LASSEN, N. A. & BETZ, E. (1975) Brain carbonic acid acidosis after acetazolamide. *Acta Physiol. Scand. 93*, 385–390

HOWSE, D. C., CARONNA, J. J., DUFFY, T. E. & PLUM, F. (1974) Cerebral energy metabolism, pH and blood flow during seizures in the cat. *Am. J. Physiol. 227*, 1444–1451

JASPER, H. & ERICKSON, T. C. (1941) Cerebral blood flow and pH in excessive cortical discharge induced by metrazol and electrical stimulation. *J. Neurophysiol. 4*, 333–347

KETY, S. S. & SCHMIDT, C. F. (1948) The nitrous oxide method for the quantitative determination of cerebral blood flow in man: theory, procedure and normal values. *J. Clin. Invest. 27*, 476–480

KJÄLLQUIST, Å., NARDINI, M. & SIESJÖ, B. K. (1969) The regulation of extra- and intracellular acid-base parameters in the rat brain during hyper- and hypocapnia. *Acta Physiol. Scand. 76*, 485–494

KNABE, U. & BETZ, E. (1972) The effect of varying extracellular, K^+, Mg^{2+} and Ca^{2+} on the diameter of pial arterioles, in *Ionic Actions on Vascular Smooth Muscle* (Betz, E., ed.), pp. 83–85, Springer, Berlin

KRIZ, N., SYKOVÁ, E., UJEC, E. & VYKLICKÝ, L. (1974) Changes of extracellular potassium concentration induced by neuronal activity in the spinal cord of the cat. *J. Physiol. (Lond.) 238*, 1–15

KUSCHINSKY, W., WAHL, M., BOSSE, O. & THURAU, K. (1972) Perivascular K^+ and pH as determinants of local pial arterial diameter in cats: a microapplication study. *Circ. Res. 31*, 240–247

LASSEN, N. A. (1966) The luxury-perfusion syndrome and its possible relation to acute metabolic acidosis localised within the brain. *Lancet 2*, 1113–1115

LASSEN, N. A. (1968) Brain extracellular pH: the main factor controlling cerebral blood flow. *Scand. J. Clin. Lab. Invest. 22*, 247–251

LEWIS, L. D., LJUNGGREN, B., NORBERG, K. & SIESJÖ, B. K. (1974*a*) Changes in carbohydrate substrates, amino acids and ammonia in the brain during insulin-induced hypoglycemia. *J. Neurochem. 23*, 659–671

LEWIS, L. D., LJUNGGREN, B., RATCHESON, R. A. & SIESJÖ, B. K. (1974*b*) Cerebral energy state in insulin-induced hypoglycemia, related to blood glucose and to EEG. *J. Neurochem. 23*, 673–679

LUX, H. D. (1974) The kinetics of extracellular potassium: relation to epileptogenesis. *Epilepsia 15*, 375–393

MACMILLAN, V. & SIESJÖ, B. K. (1972) Intracellular pH of the brain in arterial hypoxemia, evaluated with the CO_2 method and from the creatine phosphokinase equilibrium. *Scand. J. Clin. Lab. Invest. 30*, 117–125

MCDOWALL, D. G. & HARPER, A. M. (1968) CBF and CSF pH in the monkey during prolonged hypocapnia. *Scand. J. Clin. Lab. Invest. Suppl. 102*, VIIIE

MELDRUM, B. & NILSSON, B. (1976) Cerebral blood flow and metabolic rate early and late in prolonged epileptic seizures induced in rats by bicuculline. *Brain 99*, 523–542

MORRIS, M. E. (1974) Hypoxia and extracellular potassium activity in guinea-pig cortex. *Can. J. Physiol. Pharmacol. 52*, 872–882

MOSKALENKO, Y. Y. (1975) Regional cerebral blood flow and its control at rest and during increased functional activity, in *Brain Work* (Ingvar, D. H. & Lassen, N. A., eds.) *(Alfred Benzon Symp. 8)*, pp. 343–351, Munksgaard, Copenhagen

NILSSON, B. & SIESJÖ, B. K. (1976) A method for determining blood flow and oxygen consumption in the rat brain. *Acta Physiol. Scand. 96*, 72–82

NILSSON, B., NORBERG, K., NORDSTRÖM, C. H. & SIESJÖ, B. K. (1975) Influence of hypoxia and hypercapnia on CBF in rats, in *Blood Flow and Metabolism in the Brain* (Harper, A. M. *et al.*, eds.), pp. 9.19–9.23, Churchill Livingstone, Edinburgh

NORBERG, K. & SIESJÖ, B. K. (1976) Oxidative metabolism of the cerebral cortex of the rat in severe insulin-induced hypoglycemia. *J. Neurochem. 26*, 345–352

NORBERG, K., QUISTORFF, B. & SIESJÖ, B. K. (1975) Effects of hyperoxia of 10–45 seconds duration on energy metabolism in the cerebral cortex of unanesthetized and anesthetized rats. *Acta Physiol. Scand. 95*, 301–310

PANNIER, I. L., WEYNE, J., DEMEESTER, G. & LEUSEN, I. (1972) Influence of changes in acid-base composition of the ventricular system on cerebral blood flow in cats. *Pflügers Arch. Eur. J. Physiol. 333*, 337–351

PERSSON, L., HANSSON, H. A. & SOURANDER, P. (1976) Extravasation, spread and cellular uptake of Evans Blue-labelled albumin around a reproducible small stab-wound in the rat brain. *Acta Neuropathol. 34*, 125–136

RAICHLE, M. E., POSNER, J. B. & PLUM, F. (1971) Cerebral blood flow during and after hyperventilation, in *Brain and Blood Flow* (Ross Russell, R. W., ed.), pp. 223–228, Pitman, London

Reivich, M., Sokoloff, L., Kennedy, C. & Des Rosiers, M. (1975) An autoradiographic method for the measurement of local glucose metabolism in the brain, in *Brain Work* (Ingvar, D. H. & Lassen, N. A., eds.) *(Alfred Benzon Symp. 8)*, pp. 377–384, Munksgaard, Copenhagen

Severinghaus, J. W. (1964) Cerebral blood flow in chronic hypoxia. *Acta Anaesthesiol. Scand. Suppl. 15*, 96

Severinghaus, J. W. & Lassen, N. A. (1967) Step hypocapnia to separate arterial from tissue P_{CO_2} in the regulation of cerebral blood flow. *Circ. Res. 20*, 272–278

Severinghaus, J. W., Chiodi, H., Eger, E. I., Brandstater, B. & Hornbein, T. F. (1966) Cerebral blood flow in man at high altitude: role of cerebrospinal fluid pH in normalization of flow in chronic hypocapnia. *Circ. Res. 19*, 274–282

Siesjö, B. K., Kjällquist, D., Ponten, U. & Zwetnow, N. (1968) Extracellular pH in the brain and cerebral blood flow. *Brain Res. 30*, 93–98

Siesjö, B. K., Johannsson, H., Norberg, K. & Salford, L. (1975) Brain function, metabolism and blood flow in moderate and severe arterial hypoxia, in *Brain Work* (Ingvar, D. H. & Lassen, N. A., eds.) *(Alfred Benzon Symp. 8)*, pp. 101–125, Munksgaard, Copenhagen

Skinhøj, E. (1966) Regulation of cerebral blood flow as a single function of the interstitial pH in the brain: a hypothesis. *Acta Neurol. Scand. 42*, 604–607

Wahl, M., Deetjen, P., Thurau, K., Ingvar, D. H. & Lassen, N. A. (1970) Micropuncture evaluation of the importance of the perivascular pH for the arteriolar diameter on the brain surface. *Pflügers Arch. Eur. J. Physiol. 316*, 152–163

Discussion

Rapoport: Wade Marshall and I measured pH at the pia-arachnoid surface of the cat cortex during spreading cortical depression, and found only a slight acidic shift in the later part of the process, although blood flow is reported to increase markedly (Rapoport & Marshall 1964; Marshall 1965). In animals forced to breathe N_2, and which therefore should have an initial increase in cerebral blood flow, a pH change was not recorded at the pia-arachnoid surface of the brain even when anoxia was sufficiently severe to depolarize the cortex (Marshall 1965). Although cortical pH may not reflect rapid intracerebral changes, the findings are consistent with your conclusion that changes in flow can occur independently of large pH changes.

The alkaline shift that you record during convulsive behaviour agrees, as you say, with findings of McCulloch and his colleagues (Dusser de Barenne *et al.* 1937). However, these authors used an intercerebral pH electrode that destroyed the integrity of the blood–brain barrier, as witnessed by an alkaline response of their electrodes to intravenous $NaHCO_3$ (cf. Rapoport 1964). An alkaline change during epileptic activity, despite a broken vascular integrity, suggests that the change is independent of capillary permeability limitations and is due, as you suggest, to rapid exchange of diffusible CO_2 between blood and brain.

Are you sure that the alkaline shift that you measure, which is of the order of 0.03 pH units, is a true pH change? Could an apparent change be caused by a cortical temperature change or a hydrostatic pressure change that acted on the pH or reference electrode, or a change in junctional potential at the reference electrode?

Astrup: We must consider the possibility of error in these measurements. We should also remember that the old studies may have errors of this kind. We have done a few calculations and some extra experiments to look at the tissue damage and I think we are measuring the right thing. A very large shift in temperature would be needed to give the kind of change in potential that you mentioned. Dr Heuser's electrode has a pH on the inside of about 7.5 and on the outside of about 7.3. Its offset potential is about 20–40 mV. This potential is proportional to the absolute temperature so even if the temperature changes by a few degrees on the surface during hyperaemia one would not see any changes in electrode potential.

Rapoport: What change in temperature could produce a change of 0.03 pH units in your records?

Astrup: With this kind of electrode that would be a very high temperature change (about 10–12 °C). With a more conventional electrode with 0.1 N-HCl on the inside there would be a pH on the inside of 1 and on the outside of 7. Measuring over 6 pH units with a sensitivity of about 50 mV/unit gives a potential of about —300 mV to start off with. That would be very liable to temperature changes. But with our technique temperature is not a critical factor. It is the same with the potassium electrodes. Shifts in d.c. potential between reference and ground could be easily recognized as symmetrical potential changes in potassium and pH since these electrodes are using the same reference.

Lübbers: Where do you have your reference electrode?

Astrup: It is in the double barrel of the potassium electrode.

Rapoport: You may have different degrees of injury potential, some of which can be accelerated by diffusion of KCl from the KCl electrode.

Astrup: We don't use KCl electrodes. The reference electrodes were filled with isotonic saline.

Rapoport: If the electrode is filled with isotonic saline, the diffusion potential —the junction potential—may change significantly at the reference electrode.

Astrup: Certainly there is a junction potential but it is not causing any trouble. There are junction potentials of a few millivolts at the tip of the reference, but that would only change substantially if there was a change in the outside sodium concentration, which doesn't change much in these conditions.

Rubio: What is the tip size of your reference electrode?

Astrup: One hole in the double-barrelled potential electrode measures about 2 μm.

Lübbers: In regard to the behaviour of the H^+ activity during and after electrical stimulation we get the same results as Dr Astrup. But one cannot conclude that flow is dependent on pH just because they follow a parallel course, since other factors may be involved. Our pH electrodes are about the same size as our microplatinum electrodes. We know from histological measurements that, in brain, puncture by the micro Pt electrodes does not disturb the microcirculation of the anaesthetized animal. This is a critical point which must be investigated for each experimental situation.

Astrup: There is no doubt that with inserted electrodes we have damage, but if we had significant damage then we would see acidotic pH values after insertion.

Purves: The values you showed were variable: one was 7.26 and the other was 7.42.

Astrup: Occasionally we get acidotic values and this may indicate occasional damage or haemorrhage.

Lübbers: What is the mean value you get for brain tissue?

Astrup: The extracellular measurements are about 0.06 pH units below arterial pH on average. Out of 22 consecutive insertions we found only two that gave initial values below 7.2. Six were between 7.2 and 7.3 and 14 were above 7.3, but slightly below the arterial values.

We could test how significant the extravasation was around the electrode by injecting bicarbonate into the systemic circulation. This would initially release a little CO_2 in the blood, thereby increasing the CO_2 tension in the brain tissue. If the blood–brain barrier is functionally intact around the pH electrode, the barrier around would make it a CO_2 electrode leading to an immediate acid pH shift, in spite of an alkaline shift in plasma pH. This is actually what we see with these electrodes (Heuser *et al.* 1975). So extravasation is occurring around the electrode but the blood–brain barrier remains functionally intact.

Rapoport: When I measured pH at the pia-arachnoid surface of the brain, I found that excessive pressure caused by the electrodes could modify the normal acidic response to intravenous $NaHCO_3$. In order to accept that barrier integrity in curarized animals was unaffected, I required that the acidic response remain for at least 1 min after injection of $NaHCO_3$ (Rapoport 1964). How long did the acidic response last after you injected bicarbonate?

Astrup: About one minute.

Silver: My experience has been with microelectrodes, both with a double barrel and a single barrel, with anaesthetized rats and cats. In hypoxia, we always see a slight alkaline shift initially (when the blood flow increases), but in acute *ischaemia* the pH always becomes acidotic.

Purves: So the two stimuli that you have tried are acute hypoxia and some form of seizure of electrical stimulation. Is it your interpretation that there is a disproportionate rise in blood flow?

Silver: Yes. With our rather unreliable lactate electrode, we can sometimes see an increase in lactate at the end of the period when the pH is still going up. I am, therefore, almost sure that CO_2 washout is the answer. However, the lactate electrodes are still very much a toy for us.

Purves: It seems clear that more slender electrodes give approximately the same results.

Siesjö: I would like to come back to the general problem of flow increase in hypoxia and emphasize what we mean when we say that flow may increase dramatically at a time when there is still alkalosis in the tissue. From data on maximal glycolytic capacity of brain tissue we can easily calculate that if lactic acid production is maximally stimulated, less than 2 μmol/g of lactate is formed in 10 s, and less than 5 μmol g in 30 s. During such short periods, any acidotic effect can be counteracted just by reducing P_{CO_2}. In some early experiments we estimated the increase in CBF in hypoxia from arteriovenous differences in oxygen content (Borgström *et al.* 1975). We lowered arterial P_{O_2} to about 25 mmHg and simultaneously hyperventilated the animals so as to reduce the P_{CO_2} by 10–15 mmHg. Simple calculations show that there couldn't have been any acidosis in the tissue at the time when CBF was increasing rapidly (see also Nilsson *et al.* 1975). On the contrary there should have been a period of substantial alkalosis, yet we see this increase in flow.

Plum: Dr Siesjö's pretty experiment seems conclusively to prove that cerebral vasodilatation can occur without a fall in pH, so that hydrogen ion cannot be the universal messenger from metabolism to the vascular receptor. Any further arguments from electrodes must be taken as inconclusive. Since brain is a compartmental tissue the argument always was possible that the electrode wasn't in the (acid?) compartment responsible for the signal. These present experiments seem to make that an untenable view.

Negative experiments none the less leave behind their own difficulties in interpretation. Under many circumstances, increased hydrogen ion content, associated with either an increase in CO_2 or an increase in lactate in the tissue, has appeared tightly coupled to vasodilatation. Do the present findings imply some final common intermediary for which the hydrogen ion represents only one of the stimuli? Or does the vascular receptor directly respond to multiple agents? Accepting that during both hypoxia and hypoglycaemia the blood flow rises so greatly that total hydrogen ion content falls, one must postulate a stimulus so strong that it produces vasodilatation during the equivalent of relative hypocapnia. The worst problem at the moment seems to be that no definitive experiments seem possible until someone emerges with a better candidate for the putative metabolic to vascular transmitter.

Purves: It may be worth recalling that we really know very little in strict quantitative terms about the sensitivity of vascular smooth muscle to hydrogen ion. An attempt to determine this was made by Wahl *et al.* (1970) in experiments in which bicarbonate solutions were applied close to pial vessels and as pH was reduced, the pial vessels dilated. However, the changes in pH were very large, that is between about pH 5 and pH 8 and of course this is orders greater than the changes in interstitial fluid pH that we have been discussing. So it is uncertain whether the changes that have actually been observed could be responsible for alterations in the calibre of blood vessels and, hence, of blood flow.

Astrup: Professor Lübbers, what kind of internal solution did you use in your pH electrodes?

Lübbers: Mostly we are trying to get to the same pH in the internal solution as we expect to measure. The asymmetrical potential in the electrode is small.

Heuser: That may depend on the cable capacity. With large back-off potentials, e.g. when there is an internal filling solution of pH 1 or 2, there will be a long response time of the pH electrode. We solved this problem by using amplifiers with neutralization of capacitance and internal filling solutions for our pH electrodes, which are close to the physiological pH range.

Purves: How accurate are your absolute values for the pH of interstitial fluid?

Heuser: It depends on the kind of reference cell we use. We made a lot of efforts to come close to the absolute pH values. We used different kinds of reference electrodes, but still we have not been very successful. At the moment we use pH calibration solutions, originally described by Maas (1971). They permit us to work with NaCl-filled reference electrodes, giving junction potentials which are similar to those filled with 3 M-KCl. The second problem is that there may be pH gradients between the surface and the different layers of the cortical tissue.

References

Borgström, L., Johannsson, H. & Siesjö, B. K. (1975) The relationship between arterial P_{O_2} and cerebral blood flow in hypoxic hypoxia. *Acta Physiol. Scand. 93*, 423–432

Dusser de Barenne, J. G., McCulloch, W. S. & Nims, L. F. (1937) Functional activity and pH of the cerebral cortex. *J. Cell. Comp. Physiol. 10*, 277–289

HEUSER, D., ASTRUP, J., LASSEN, N. A. & BETZ, E. (1975) Brain carbonic acid acidosis after acetazolamide. *Acta Physiol. Scand. 93*, 385–390

MAAS, A. H. J. (1971) pH determination in body fluids using a cell with an isotonic sodium chloride bridge. *J. Appl. Physiol. 30*, 248–250

MARSHALL, W. H. (1965) Quelques problèmes de neurophysiologie général du cerveau. *Actual. Neurophysiol. Ser. 6*, 43–54

NILSSON, B., NORBERG, K., NORDSTRÖM, C.-H. & SIESJÖ, B. K. (1975) Influence of hypoxia and hypercapnia on CBF in rats, in *Blood Flow and Metabolism in the Brain* (Harper, M. *et al.*, eds.), pp. 9.19–9.23, Churchill Livingstone, Edinburgh

RAPOPORT, S. I. (1964) Cortical pH and the blood-brain barrier. *J. Physiol. (Lond.) 110*, 238–249

RAPOPORT, S. I. & MARSHALL, W. H. (1964) Measurement of cortical pH in spreading cortical depression. *Am. J. Physiol. 206*, 1177–1180

WAHL, M., DEETJEN, P., THURAU, K., INGVAR, D. H. & LASSEN, N. A. (1970) Micropuncture evaluation of the importance of perivascular pH for the arteriolar diameter on the brain surface. *Pflügers Arch. Eur. J. Physiol. 316*, 152–163

The significance of cortical extracellular H^+, K^+ and Ca^{2+} activities for regulation of local cerebral blood flow under conditions of enhanced neuronal activity

DIETER HEUSER

Institute of Physiology I, University of Tübingen

Abstract Experiments with the microperfusion technique have shown that changes in activity of several ion species can influence the tone of the cerebral vessel walls (Knabe & Betz 1972; Kuschinsky *et al.* 1972). Consequently, these ions can be regarded as possible information mediators from the neuronal tissue to the cells of cerebral vascular smooth muscle, which adjust cerebral blood flow to the metabolic demands of the tissue. In order to elucidate the role of H^+, K^+ and Ca^{2+} in initiating and maintaining functional hyperaemia in the cerebral cortex, 23 cats were anaesthetized with pentobarbital (Nembutal 25 mg/kg). Local H^+, K^+ and Ca^{2+} activities were continuously monitored with ion-selective microelectrodes implanted in the cortical tissue (500 μm). Local cerebral blood flow (CBF) was recorded qualitatively and continuously with heated thermocouples. D.c. potential, mean arterial blood pressure (MABP) and end-expiratory CO_2 concentration were recorded simultaneously. Functional hyperaemia was induced by direct electrical stimulation of the cerebral cortex or by injection of bicuculline (1.2 mg/kg i.v.). The result was an immediate increase in cortical CBF, with increased local extracellular potassium ($\triangle K^+$: + 2.4 and + 3.8 mequiv./l) and diminished Ca^{2+} activity ($\triangle Ca^{2+}$: — 0.6 and — 1.2 mequiv./l). Measurements of local extracellular pH showed transient shifts to alkaline pH values or no change at all before a distinct tissue acidosis developed ($\triangle$pH: — 0.2 and — 0.36). Shifts in d.c. potential were always in a negative direction. The variations in the time course of the recorded parameters support the hypothesis that onset and maintenance of cerebral functional hyperaemia after epileptic seizures or direct electrical stimulation of the cortex cannot be regarded as a function of changes in activity of a single ion species.

The regulatory mechanisms of cerebral vascular resistance which provide a blood supply to the brain sufficient to meet the metabolic demands of the tissue have not yet been identified completely. Despite many experimental results, which support the pH hypothesis of metabolic control of cerebral blood flow (CBF), it has been shown by more recent investigations that activity changes of other cations, namely K^+, Ca^{2+} and Mg^{2+} as well as of certain anions (e.g. Cl^-), can also influence the diameter of pial vessels (Betz *et al.* 1977; Knabe & Betz 1972). This information was obtained with the perivascular perfusion technique (Baez 1966; Kuschinsky *et al.* 1972), in which the perivascular space of single vessels on the cortical surface is perfused with mock cerebrospinal fluid (CSF) of varying ionic composition. Simultaneously the variations of the pial vascular diameters are observed and documented. Though this technique provided much information about the reactivity of pial vessels to various stimuli, it was not possible to elucidate the significance for the regulation of cerebrovascular resistance of ionic shifts in the perivascular space, since this technique does not give information about the extent of changes in ion activity in physiological and pathophysiological conditions. The use of ion-selective microelectrodes has now filled the gap in this field of vascular research. The potentiometric determination of several ion species permits continuous recording not only of ion activities in exactly defined areas of cerebral extracellular space, but also of their dynamic variation during changes in cerebral blood flow and metabolism. Thus it could be demonstrated (Astrup *et al.* 1976) that during hypoxia, in severe hypoglycaemia, and in amphetamine intoxication, there was no obvious direct relationship between changes in CBF and local extracellular H^+ activity. These results were obtained with glass pH-microelectrodes with tip diameters of 80–100 μm. Consequently, the possibility of tissue damage during the implantation procedure should be considered. The purpose of the present investigation was to extend the measurements to Ca^{2+} as a possible information carrier with regard to induction of cerebral functional hyperaemia and to minimize tissue damage during the implantation procedure, and possibly erroneous measurements, by using pH-microelectrodes of a smaller diameter (8–10 μm).

METHODS

Experiments were done with 23 cats, weighing 2.1–2.9 kg. The animals were anaesthetized with pentobarbital (Nembutal, 25–30 mg/kg i.p.) and artificially ventilated (N_2O 60–70%/O_2 30–40%) under relaxation with gallaminetriethiodide (Flaxedil, 5 mg/kg). Mean arterial blood pressure (MABP) was measured with a Statham transducer connected to a measuring bridge (Hellige, Freiburg). The end-tidal concentration of CO_2 was monitored continuously with an URAS-analyser (Hartmann & Braun, Frankfurt), and body temperature was kept constant by a thermostat table. Through a 6–15 mm borehole in the parietotemporal region, visually intact cortex was exposed after parts of the dura mater had been removed with a microknife.

For measurements of local H^+, Ca^{2+} and K^+ we used microelectrodes implanted 500 μm into the cortical tissue under stereomicroscopical control so that the distances between the sensitive sites and the microreference (filled with NaCl) was only a few micrometres. The pH electrode was a glass microelectrode, built using a modification of the technique originally described by Hinke (1967). The sensitive tip was made from Titan glass (Ingold, Frankfurt); its diameter varied between 5 and 10 μm, and its length was between 10 and 40 μm. Calibration was performed at 34 °C in 'physiological' buffer solutions containing NaCl (Maas 1971) in order to minimize junction potentials at the tip of the reference cell. Extracellular Ca^{2+} and K^+ activities were measured with liquid ion-exchanger microelectrodes, originally described by Walker (1971). Calibration was done in mock CSF with different concentrations of K^+ and Ca^{2+}. Total ionic strength was kept constant by varying the Na^+ concentration so that approximately identical activity coefficients were maintained in CSF and calibration solutions. The potentials were measured against a NaCl reference in the direct vicinity of the sensitive sites by means of high-impedance differential amplifiers with capacitance neutralization. Mobile suspensions of the electrodes were used in some experiments in order to allow the electrodes to follow the respiration-induced excursions of the cortical surface. Changes in d.c. potential were recorded from the 'micro-reference' in the cortical tissue against a NaCl 'macroreference' buried deep in the neck muscles. Qualitative local CBF was recorded by means of heated thermocouples placed on the cortical surface. In the first experimental series (11 cats), functional hyperaemia was induced by epileptic seizures after intravenous injection of bicuculline (1.2 mg/kg). In the second group (12 cats), direct electrical stimulation of the cerebral cortical tissue was achieved by two chlorinated silver wires placed on either side of the measuring devices at a distance of about 3–5 mm. The wires were connected to a stimulator (Stimulator T, Hugo Sachs, Freiburg) via a stimulus isolation unit. Amplitude, frequency and stimulation duration were varied systematically; pulse duration was always 1 ms.

RESULTS

In cats epileptic seizures induced by intravenous injection of bicuculline (1.2 mg/kg) lead to an immediate increase in CBF and to a less dramatic increase in MABP. End-expiratory CO_2 increases transiently, whereas d.c. potential always shifts in a negative direction. These results are in accordance with previous experiments on rats, showing a dramatic increase in CBF and a decrease in local cerebrovascular resistance (Meldrum & Nilsson 1976).

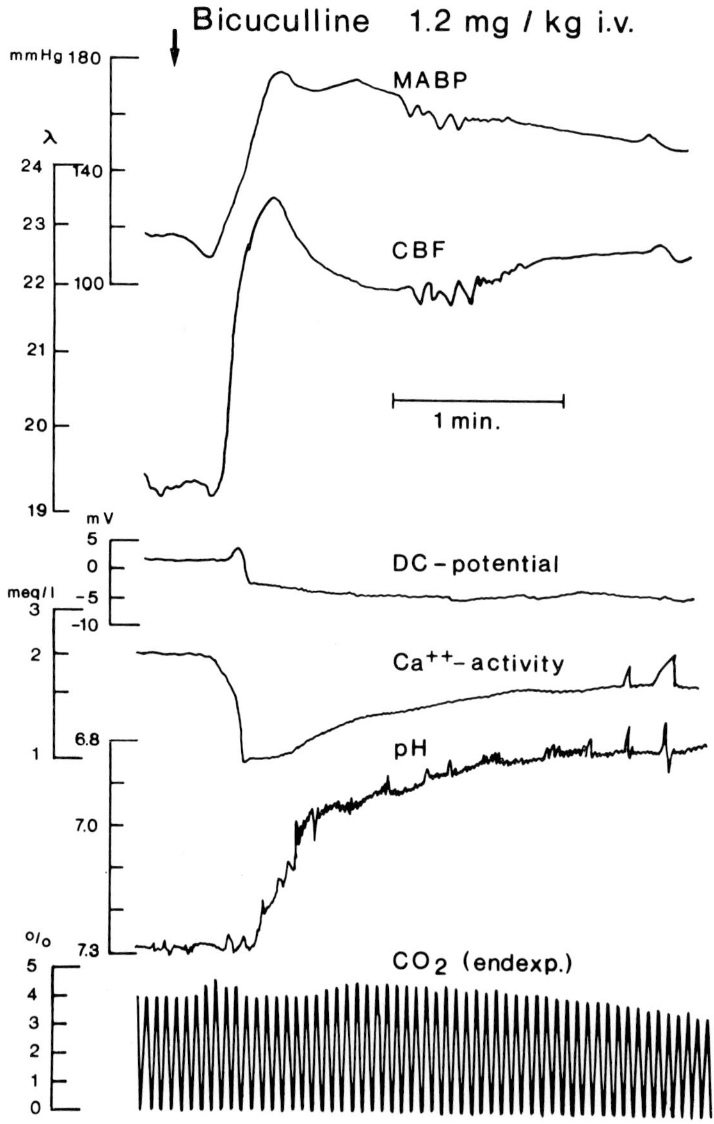

FIG. 1. Time course of changes in extracellular Ca^{2+}, pH and CBF during epileptic seizures induced by bicuculline (1.2 mg/kg i.v.) in a cat. (Original recording.)

Local Ca^{2+} activity decreases rapidly, returning to the initial values after 2–3 min. Changes in extracellular potassium were earlier investigated in rats (Astrup *et al.* 1976). Control measurements with cats also showed an identical

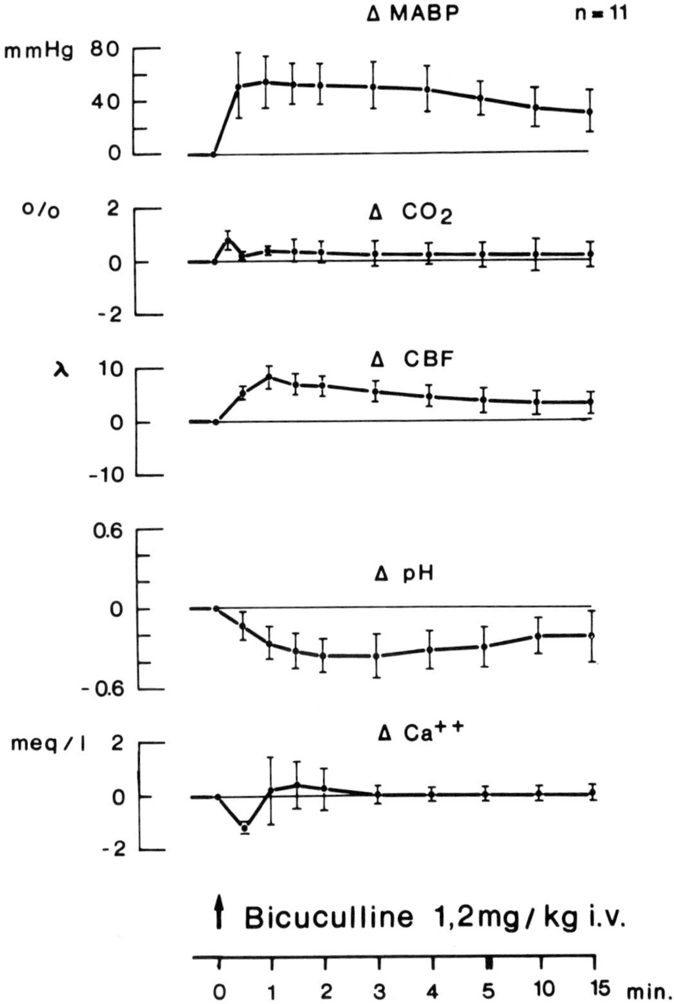

FIG. 2. Mean values (± S.D.) of the measured parameters in 11 cats during epileptic seizures induced by bicuculline (1.2 mg/kg i.v.).

rapid increase in potassium (ΔK^+ + 3.8 mequiv./l ± 0.2) to that in rats, so we did not repeat the K^+ measurements systematically in cats. Extracellular pH fails to show the initial transient shift in the alkaline direction that was seen in the earlier experiments in rats. A distinct acidosis develops, starting about 15–20 s after the onset of the increase in flow. The time course of the

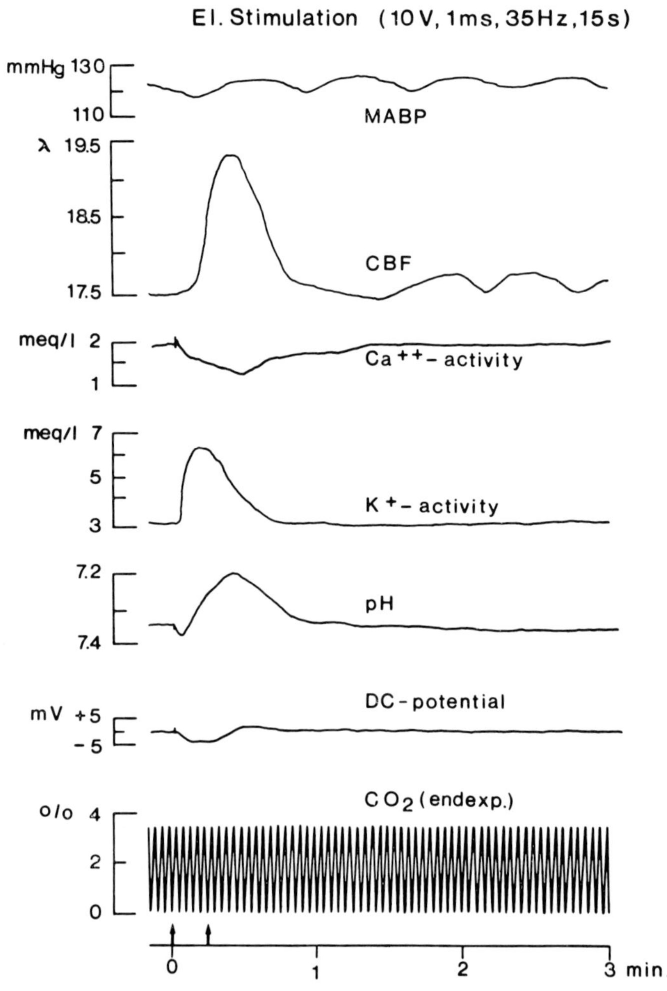

FIG. 3. Time course of changes in local extracellular Ca^{2+}, K^{+}, H^{+} activities and cerebral blood flow in cats during electrical stimulation of the cerebral cortex in one experiment.

variations in the individual parameters in one experiment is shown in Fig. 1, while mean values (± S.D.) are presented in Fig. 2. The latter summarizes results obtained in 11 cats. The initial values of the single parameters and the extent of their maximal deviation during seizures are shown in Table 1.

Local electrical stimulation of the cerebral cortex leads to an increase in CBF accompanied by a decrease in cerebrovascular resistance, as demonstrated

TABLE 1

Initial values and maximal changes of the measured parameters in 11 cats during epileptic seizures induced by bicuculline (1.2 mg/kg i.v.).

	pH	Ca^{2+} *(mequiv./l)*	K^{+} *(mequiv./l)*	*MABP (mm Hg)*	CO_2 *(%)*
Initial value (± S.D.)	7.18 (± 0.126)	2.2 (± 0.46)	3.1 (± 0.3)	132 (± 16)	4.2 (± 0.47)
Maximal change (± S.D.)	−0.36 (± 0.17)	−1.26 (± 0.28)	+ 3.8 (± 0.2)	+ 67 (± 19.6)	+ 0.93 (± 0.83)

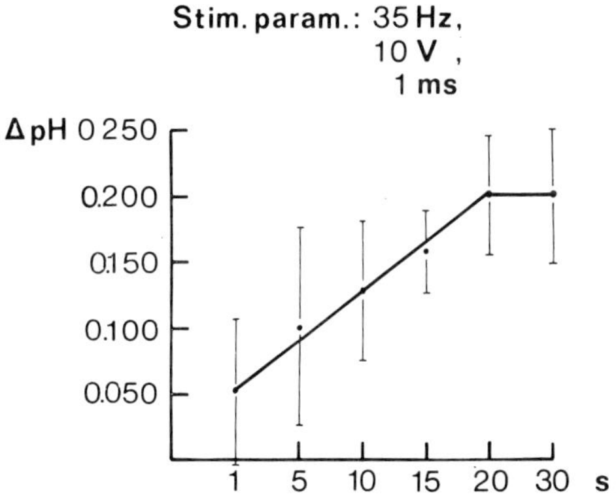

FIG. 4. Correlation between extent of local extracellular acidosis (△pH) and stimulation duration in the cerebral cortex. Maximum value is reached after 20 s.

by the constancy of MABP. A concomitant d.c. potential shift in the negative direction is regularly observed and is independent of stimulation polarity. Local K^+ activity increases immediately, reaching maximal values at 6–7 mequiv./l, whereas Ca^{2+} activity decreases significantly. Extracellular pH shows a biphasic response, starting with a transient but consistent alkalosis followed by a distinct shift in the acid direction (Fig. 3). The time courses of changes in cerebral flow and measured ion activities are similar to each other and vary with stimulation time. First deviations can be observed when stimulation has lasted 1 s; maximal changes are reached at stimulation times between 20 and 30 s (Fig. 4). The threshold of stimulation for the occurrence of the

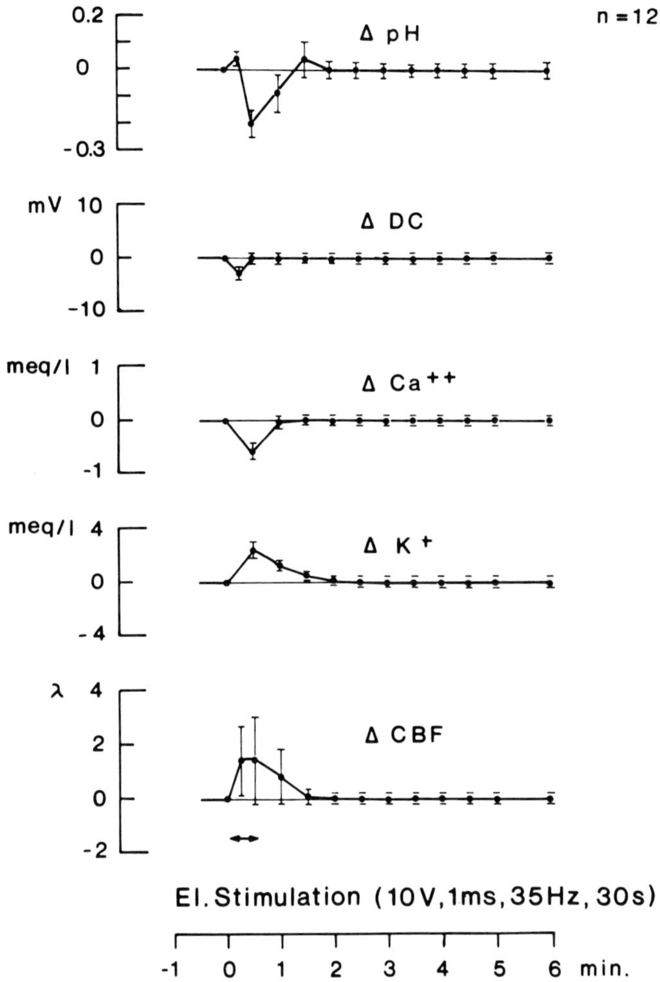

FIG. 5. Mean values (± S.D.) of the measured parameters in 12 cats during and after electrical stimulation of the cerebral cortex (stimulation parameters: 10 V, 1 ms, 35 Hz, 30 s).

reactions described was between 4 and 5 V amplitude and 10 and 15 Hz; pulse duration was always 1 ms. Changes in MABP as well as in end-expiratory CO_2 content could not be detected. Fig. 3 shows the variation in the measured parameters in one typical experiment in which stimulation lasted 15 s. The mean values (± S.D.) are shown in Fig. 5. Initial values as well as the maximal changes in the measured parameters are given in Table 2.

TABLE 2

Initial values and maximal changes of the measured parameters in 12 cats during and after direct electrical cortical stimulation (10 V, 1 ms, 35 Hz, 30 s)

	pH	*Ca^{2+} (mequiv./l)*	*K^+ (mequiv./l)*	*D.C. (mV)*
Initial value (± S.D.)	7.24 (± 0.13)	2.0 (± 0.04)	3.8 (± 0.14)	10.0 (± 2.8)
Maximal change (± S.D.)	—0.20 (± 0.05)	—0.60 (± 0.14)	+ 2.35 (± 0.35)	—2.5 (± 0.7)

DISCUSSION

The results confirm the existence of a decrease in cerebrovascular resistance after activation of central nervous structures. This has been pointed out recently in rats (Meldrum & Nilsson 1976) as well as in cats (Leniger-Follert & Lübbers 1976). But the mechanism which triggers the onset of CBF increase has not yet been identified. The development of local hypoxia has been excluded by direct Po_2 measurements with microelectrodes during electrical stimulation (Leniger-Follert & Lübbers 1976), where the Po_2 exactly followed the increase in microflow. Changes in H^+ activity also seem to be of less importance in the initial phase since there is either no change or even transient alkalosis at onset of CBF increase. In bicuculline-induced seizures this has been confirmed by metabolic data (Chapmann *et al.* 1978) which indicate that transient alkalosis occurs during vasodilatation in rats. In both kinds of neuronal activation local extracellular K^+ and Ca^{2+} activities are changed to the degree which has been demonstrated to have dilating effects on cerebral vessels (Knabe & Betz 1972; Kuschinsky *et al.* 1972). The nearly identical time course of changes in CBF, K^+, Ca^{2+} and also, at a later phase, in H^+ under electrical stimulation is obvious. Likewise, during bicuculline-induced seizures Ca^{2+} and K^+ seem to be essential information carriers from the activated nerve cells to the vascular smooth muscles, triggering the adjustment of CBF to the enhanced metabolic activity of the tissue. For the maintenance of cerebral vasodilatation, however, K^+ and H^+ seem to be more important. The conclusion to be drawn from these experimental data is that it is not possible to correlate onset and maintenance of cerebral functional hyperaemia to the extracellular changes in activity of a single ion species. Certainly K^+, Ca^{2+} and H^+ ions are important factors among these regulatory mechanisms, and the mode of their interaction has been discussed recently (Betz & Csornai 1977). Besides these ionic effects, other trigger mechanisms, e.g. changes in the adenosine concentration, must also be taken into account, and their mode of interaction with the changes in activity of several ion species should be a topic for further investigation.

ACKNOWLEDGEMENTS

I wish to thank Professor W. Simon (Eidgenössische Technische Hochschule, Zürich, Switzerland) for supplying the liquid Ca^{2+} exchanger, Professor E. Betz for encouraging me to complete this work; and Mrs Christa Eck for expert and dedicated technical assistance.

References

Astrup, J., Heuser, D., Lassen, N. A., Nilsson, B., Norberg, K. & Siesjö, B. K. (1976) Evidence against H^+ and K^+ as the main factors in the regulation of cerebral blood flow during epileptic discharges, acute hypoxemia, amphetamine intoxication and hypoglycemia. A microelectrode study, in *Ionic Actions on Vascular Smooth Muscle* (Betz, E., ed.), pp. 110–115, Springer, Berlin

Baez, S. (1966) Recordings of microvascular dimensions with an image-splitter television microscope. *J. Appl. Physiol. 21*, 299–301

Betz, E. & Csornai, M. (1977) Ionic actions on cerebral vessels. *Int. J. Neurol.*, in press

Betz, E., Karlitzky, G. & Heuser, D. (1977) The effect of pial perivascular chloride on the diameters of small pial arteries, in *Cerebral Function Metabolism and Circulation* (Ingvar, D. H. & Lassen, N. A., eds.), pp. 390–391, Munksgaard, Copenhagen

Chapmann, A. G., Meldrum, B. S. & Siesjö, B. K. (1978) Cerebral metabolic changes during prolonged epileptic seizures in rats. *J. Neurochem.*, in press

Hinke, J. A. M. (1967) Cation-selective microelectrodes for intracellular use, in *Glass Electrodes for Hydrogen and other Cations* (Eisenmann, G., ed.), pp. 464–477, Arnold, London

Knabe, U. & Betz, E. (1972) The effect of varying extracellular K^+, Mg^{++} and Ca^{++} on the diameter of pial arterioles, in *Vascular Smooth Muscle* (Betz, E., ed.), pp. 83–85, Springer, Berlin

Kuschinsky, W., Wahl, M., Bosse, G. & Thurau, W. (1972) Perivascular potassium and pH as determinants of local pial arterial diameter in cats. *Circ. Res. 31*, 240–247

Leniger-Follert, E. & Lübbers, D. W. (1976) Behavior of microflow and local Po_2 of the brain cortex during and after direct electrical stimulation. *Pflügers Arch. Eur. J. Physiol. 366*, 39–44

Maas, A. H. J. (1971) pH determination in body fluids using a cell with an isotonic sodium chloride bridge. *J. Appl. Physiol. 30*, 248–250

Meldrum, B. & Nilsson, B. (1976) Cerebral blood flow and metabolic rate early and late in prolonged epileptic seizures induced in rats by bicuculline. *Brain 99*, 523–542

Walker, J. L. (1971) Ion specific liquid ion exchanger microelectrodes. *Anal. Chem. 43*, 89A–93A

Discussion

Nilsson: For the understanding of physiological mechanisms it is important to establish to what extent we can extrapolate from various types of experimental stimulation to physiological activation. Have you used other methods of activation?

Heuser: No.

Purves: Can you tell us how far these changes in calcium or potassium are likely to affect smooth muscle quantitatively?

Heuser: No. It has been shown that an increase in potassium causes vasodilatation (Kuschinsky *et al.* 1972) whereas an increase in Ca^{2+} leads to constriction of pial arteries (Betz *et al.* 1973). But the small changes seen in our experiments have not been correlated with variations in vascular diameter. They are not small in respect to shifts in intracellular Ca^{2+} activity, which are necessary for the interaction of the contractile proteins.

Lübbers: There are many nerves around and I wonder whether potassium could work by stimulating intrinsic nerves, producing dilatation?

Heuser: We cannot rule that out.

Astrup: A more physiological method is stimulation of peripheral nerves. This evokes potentials in the central nervous system and increases extracellular K^+ (Kriz *et al.* 1974; Krnjevic & Morris 1974).

Plum: A curious thing about these activation experiments, whether with epilepsy or peripheral stimulation, is that not only is a rise in pH and a decrease in H^+ concentration associated with a rise in P_{O_2}, but also at the same time there is a steady increase in lactic acid and a small but steady increase in pyruvate. This implies that there is an impediment in the oxidation of pyruvate in the citric acid cycle and a new metabolic steady state which I have not seen satisfactorily explained. But at least in the stimulation experiments the rise in lactate is linked in time to the vasodilatation. This is why we and others concluded that the hydrogen ion was the stimulus to vasodilatation. Williamson & Jamieson (1966) showed the same increase in lactate in heart muscle and Brauer *et al.* (1970) showed it in the superior cervical ganglion.

Sokoloff: It is difficult to explain the changes in the levels of intermediates when a pathway consisting of a long series of consecutive chemical reactions, such as those involved in the conversion of glucose into the intermediates of the Krebs cycle, shifts from one steady state to a new steady state. There is frequently a shift in the position of the rate-limiting steps and the concentrations of all the intermediates are readjusted. One could explain the changes in the concentrations of the intermediates if the rate-limiting steps were known.

Jöbsis: If a skeletal muscle is stimulated from rest there is a sudden outpouring of lactate. This was considered for some time as indicating that hypoxia occurred before the microcirculation adjusted. By observing NADH in these cells we have shown that there is no signal whatsoever of hypoxia. Typically this is a steady-state disturbance, apparently with the glycolytic chain stimulated faster. Pyruvate cannot enter sufficiently rapidly into the Krebs cycle. The result is that it goes to lactate (Jöbsis & Stainsby 1968).

Plum: But this happens at submaximal rates, which means that the rate limit can't be on pyruvate entry into the citric acid cycle.

Jöbsis: There must be activation of the Krebs cycle because after a while the glycolytic and Krebs cycle turnover rates are matched again. There is a temporary imbalance.

Sokoloff: One should not consider only maximal rates in dealing with a chain of sequential reactions. Even if a given step has a capacity for a higher maximal rate, its substrate concentrations can still rise when the whole pathway is changed to a new steady state at a higher rate. Indeed, it may well be that the rate of that step is increased because its substrates have risen to higher concentrations. Readjustment of the substrate concentrations is a major mechanism by which new steady-state rates are achieved.

For example, even though the pyruvate oxidase system has a capacity for a much higher rate than the rate at which it is actually operating, an increased concentration of pyruvate may still occur and, in fact, be necessary to increase the rate of pyruvate oxidation. The pyruvate concentration may remain high even with the increased pyruvate metabolism. This would occur, for example, if the rate-limiting step were switched from the phosphofructokinase step to the pyruvate oxidase step. It is not a matter of maximal rates; it is a matter of the location of the rate-limiting steps.

Pickering: The model Dr Heuser is studying is a very difficult one. There are two apparently simpler models. One is work hyperaemia of skeletal muscle and the other is the reactive hyperaemia that occurs after circulation to a limb has been arrested and then released. Is the mechanism of vasodilatation in those two circumstances known?

Purves: I would think those models are more difficult and just as much a subject of controversy.

Heuser: These models were studied with ion-selective electrodes (Gebert 1976; Hirche *et al.* 1976). There was an increase in K^+ and H^+ activities during functional hyperaemia, which means that the mechanism could be the same. In the brain there are changes in three kinds of ions, which are able to induce relaxation of vascular smooth muscle cells. The problem is that variations in their activities occur with different time constants.

Rubio: Evidence that several mechanisms may regulate blood flow has been demonstrated in skeletal muscle in the dog. In these experiments stimulation of the motor nerves to a hindlimb to induce exercise hyperaemia shows that venous potassium release is accelerated at the same time as the hyperaemic response. As the hyperaemic response continues, adenosine concentrations in the skeletal muscle increase and potassium levels in the venous effluent decrease. In these studies changes in venous osmolality and phosphate, which have also been suggested as possible mediators of the hyperaemic response, were not observed. Thus, it appears that potassium is raised as a result of the initial activity of a tissue and that more sustained exercise gives rise to production of adenosine (Bockman *et al.* 1976). With respect to reactive hyperaemia, if in the same dog hindlimb preparation one occludes the artery to a contracting muscle and collects the venous blood after the release of the occlusion one will find that both adenosine and potassium are greatly increased, indicating that they play a role in the dilatory response (Dobson *et al.* 1971).

Pickering: Are they increased enough to account for the increased blood flow?

Rubio: Yes.

Siesjö: I agree with Dr Sokoloff that when one finds increases in pyruvate concentrations one may have to assume that nature increases the glycolytic rate more than the citric acid cycle requires. It is more difficult to interpret increases in lactate concentrations since, at any given pyruvate concentration, lactate may increase by two mechanisms. First, if glycolytic rate is increased there will also be increased production of NADH which has to be reoxidized in the mitochondria after the operation of a shuttle system for reducing equivalents. This may well be rate-limiting, hence markedly increased glycolytic rates could lead to lactate accumulation via an increase in the $NADH/NAD^+$ ratio. Second, even if this ratio does not increase, acidosis would cause lactate accumulation via its effect on the equilibrium of lactate dehydrogenase (EC 1.2.1.22).

Does physiological stimulation, as opposed to pathophysiological stimulation such as seizure or direct electrical stimulation, really lead to perturbation of levels of lactate and pyruvate in tissue? In steady-state situations where we increase metabolic flux and blood flow in the tissue by, for example, hyperthermia (Carlsson *et al.* 1976) or immobilization stress (Berntman *et al.* 1976), there is no such perturbation. The tissue metabolites remain essentially unchanged, which would indicate that the tissue just sets the metabolic rate at a higher level. Is it known whether a physiological stimulus from the periphery perturbs the metabolism?

Plum: During local penicillin seizures in rat, lactate rises in the mirror focus from a control level of 1.41 ± 0.08 to 3.92 ± 0.52 (Collins 1976). Perhaps this provides an equivalent situation to peripheral stimulation.

Siesjö: Are there comparable data for more physiological stimulation?

Purves: Has anybody done this with the kind of precision you are asking about? You are talking about a very early transient shift. It is clear that these experiments with microelectrodes are very difficult to do. Have you any other kind of information about potassium or calcium ions in the first fraction of a second after electrical stimulation, Professor Silver?

Silver: If cells are *driven* either electrically or via a peripheral stimulus, extracellular potassium rises in about 30–100 ms. With *hypoxia*, potassium activity doesn't rise by more than 1 or 2 mV at 15–20 s. Then it very slowly increases over a minute or two to about 5 mV. Blood flow increases enormously in that time. This degree of increase in blood flow certainly can't be produced by injecting that amount of potassium. It is only in the later state of hypoxia when the membrane potential starts to fail that there is a major rise in extracellular potassium to the concentrations that have been shown by extravascular injection to affect flow.

In our experience, any chloride shift is very slight until the borderline of irreversible hypoxia is reached. The only time when I have seen massive reversible changes in chloride is in spreading depression. With a triple-barrelled electrode measuring potassium, chloride and d.c. changes, we could see strict separation of the three parameters (R. do Carmo, H. Martins-Ferreira and I. A. Silver, 1976, unpublished work). However, the blood flow changes did not seem to be particularly related to any of those three things.

Astrup: I think the reason why you don't see an initial immediate rise in potassium in the hypoxia experiments may be because you used barbiturate anaesthesia. With lighter anaesthesia one can see general activation just at the moment hypoxia is getting around the brain. There is an immediate increase in potassium, though it is not very great.

Silver: Initially in hypoxia we actually see a very small decrease in extracellular potassium when the hypoxia first hits. This seems to go with a very short-lived hyperpolarization of the membrane lasting 5–10 s. Then the potential falls to below normal and we see the slow rise in extracellular potassium. This occurs with both methane (in cats) and barbiturate (cats) anaesthesia.

Lübbers: What about the flow?

Silver: I can't tell you how that correlates with the potassium except that the initial increase in local flow may start during the hyperpolarization phase.

References

BERNTMAN, L., CARLSSON, C., HÄGERDAL, M. & SIESJÖ, B. K. (1976) Cerebral metabolic state after discontinuation of nitrous oxide supply in artificially ventilated rats. *Acta Physiol. Scand. 98*, 248–256

BETZ, E., ENZENROSS, H. G. & VLAHOV, V. (1973) Interaction of H^+ and Ca^{++} in the regulation of local pial vascular resistance. *Pflügers Arch. Eur. J. Physiol. 343*, 79–88

BOCKMAN, E. L., BERNE, R. M. & RUBIO, R. (1976) Adenosine and active hyperemia in dog skeletal muscle. *Am. J. Physiol. 230*, 1531

BRAUER, B., BÜCHER, T. & DOLIVO, M. (1970) Redox transitions of cytochromes and pyridine nucleotides upon stimulation of an isolated rat ganglion. *FEBS (Fed. Eur. Biochem. Soc.) Lett. 8*, 297–300

CARLSSON, C., HÄGERDAL, M. & SIESJÖ, B. K. (1976) The effect of hyperthermia upon consumption and upon organic phosphates, glycolytic metabolites, citric acid cycle intermediates and associated amino acids in rat cerebral cortex. *J. Neurochem. 26*, 1001–1006

COLLINS, R. C. (1976) Metabolic response to focal penicillin seizures in rat: spike discharge vs. afterdischarge. *J. Neurochem. 27*, 1473–1482

DOBSON, J. G. JR., RUBIO, R. & BERNE, R. M. (1971) Role of adenine nucleotides, adenosine and inorganic phosphate in the regulation of skeletal muscle blood flow. *Circ. Res. 29*, 375

GEBERT, G. (1976) Tissue electrolytes and blood flow in skeletal muscle, in *Ion and Enzyme Electrodes in Biology and Medicine* (Kessler, M. *et al.*, eds.), pp. 376–380, Urban & Schwarzenberg, Munich

HIRCHE, H., STEINHAGEN, C., HOSSELMANN, J., MANTHEY, J. & BOVENKAMP, U. (1976) The interstitial pH of the isolated skeletal muscle of the dog at rest and during exercise, in *Ion and Enzyme Electrodes in Biology and Medicine* (Kessler, M. *et al.*, eds.), pp. 372–375, Urban & Schwarzenberg, Munich

JÖBSIS, F. F. & STAINSBY, W. N. (1968) Oxidation of NADH during contractions of circulated mammalian skeletal muscle. *Respir. Physiol. 4*, 292–300

KRIZ, N., SYKOVÁ, E., UJEC, E. & VYKLICKY, L. (1974) Changes of extracellular potassium concentration induced by neuronal activity in the spinal cord of the cat. *J. Physiol. (Lond.) 238*, 1–15

KRNJEVIC, K. & MORRIS, M. E. (1974) Extracellular accumulation of potassium evoked by activity of primary afferent fibres in the cuneate nucleus and dorsal horn of cats. *Can. J. Physiol. Pharmacol. 52*, 852–871

KUSCHINSKY, W., WAHL, M., BOSSE, O. & THURAU, K. (1972) The dependency of the pial arterial and arteriolar resistance on the perivascular H^+ and K^+ concentrations, in *Cerebral Blood Flow and Intracranial Pressure* (Fieschi, C., ed.), Karger, Basel

WILLIAMSON, J. R. & JAMIESON, D. (1966) Metabolic effects of epinephrine in the perfused rat heart. *Mol. Pharmacol. 2*, 191–205

Production, metabolism and possible functions of adenosine in brain tissue *in situ*

RAFAEL RUBIO, ROBERT M. BERNE and H. RICHARD WINN

Department of Physiology, University of Virginia School of Medicine, Charlottesville, Virginia

Abstract Adenosine and H^+ may act synergistically to regulate cerebral blood flow because adenosine production is enhanced under various experimental conditions associated with an imbalance between oxygen supply and oxygen need. Direct application of adenosine dilates the pial vessels, but changes in cerebral vascular resistance are not observed when adenosine is infused intra-arterially. This is because adenosine does not readily cross the blood–brain barrier. The studies reported here show that in dogs the adenosine released into the interstitium is partly reincorporated into adenine nucleotides via an adenosine kinase (EC 2.7.1.20) reaction (salvage pathway) and partly degraded to inosine and hypoxanthine. However, in contrast to other tissues, the accumulation of inosine and hypoxanthine in brain tissue proceeds at a rate slower than that of adenosine because one of the degradative enzymes, namely purine-nucleoside phosphorylase (EC 2.4.2.1) is located only in the vessel wall, which is not readily permeable to adenosine. Thus, the slow access of adenosine to its degradative enzymes delays the appearance of its products, inosine and hypoxanthine.

Certain organs such as the brain, heart, eye, skeletal muscle and kidney display strong intrinsic regulatory mechanisms of blood flow (Schmidt *et al.* 1945; Eckenhoff *et al.* 1947; Bill 1975; Haddy & Scott 1975; Shipley & Study 1951). The evidence available indicates that in these organs parenchymal tissue signals the arteriolar smooth muscle to dilate or constrict to meet its blood requirements for any given level of activity. This coupling mechanism appears to be mediated by the release of vasoactive metabolites from the parenchymal cells. It also appears that multiple metabolites rather than a single one may be responsible for the observed vascular adjustments. Furthermore, the importance of a specific metabolite may vary with the vascular bed. In brief, the problem of determining the critical vasoactive regulatory processes and establishing their link with cell metabolism will not be easily solved, because of the many factors that probably act in concert, and because the interrelationships of these factors will have to be determined quantitatively. Therefore, one of the main goals of studies on metabolic control of blood flow should be to thoroughly characterize the release and fate of the various possible candidates considered in the mediation of blood flow control. For several years we have focused our attention on the characterization of the release and metabolism of adenosine by various organs. The present study reports our results in brain tissue *in situ*.

STUDIES ON ADENOSINE, LACTATE AND PYRUVATE PRODUCTION

To determine whether adenosine levels are directly related to changes in vascular conductance, we measured adenosine levels in tissue under various physiological conditions known to be associated with changes in brain vascular resistance. In addition, the production of lactate, the main H^+ donor, was measured to see whether adenosine and lactate could act in concert as regulators of cerebral blood flow. Ideally, when blood flow regulation is being studied, experimental conditions should allow independent alteration of variables that in turn do not trigger changes in other variables that also alter vascular resistance. Arterial pressure, P_{O_2}, P_{CO_2} and brain oxygen consumption are variables that affect brain arteriolar tone and indirectly each other through circulatory, respiratory and metabolic changes. Furthermore, under normal conditions brain blood flow correlates well with oxygen consumption (Schmidt *et al.* 1945) and the oxygen consumption in turn is proportional to neuronal electrical activity (Davies & Remond 1947; Larrabee & Bronk 1952; McIlwain & Joanny 1963). Controlled neuronal electrical stimulation could be the means of approaching the ideal situation in which oxygen consumption is kept constant when changes in brain vascular resistance are induced by changes in either arterial pressure, P_{O_2} or P_{CO_2} that are also known to affect neuronal activity (Krnyevic *et al.* 1965; Lennox *et al.* 1938; Schmidt *et al.* 1945). In the experiments described below, neuronal activity was controlled by electrical stimulation at a constant rate throughout the experimental period.

In these studies rats were anaesthetized with pentobarbital and bilateral craniotomies were performed. Ventilation was maintained constant (tidal volume 5 ml, rate 60/min). The brain was stimulated electrically by a pair of electrodes placed on the dura and stimulation consisted of square-wave pulses of 5–10 V, 3 ms duration and 30 Hz. Variations in arterial pressure were produced by bleeding the animal and variations in arterial P_{O_2} and P_{CO_2} were produced by ventilating the animals with different gas mixtures containing variable amounts of O_2 or CO_2. In the latter case, O_2 was maintained at about 20% and in all experiments the difference was made up with N_2.

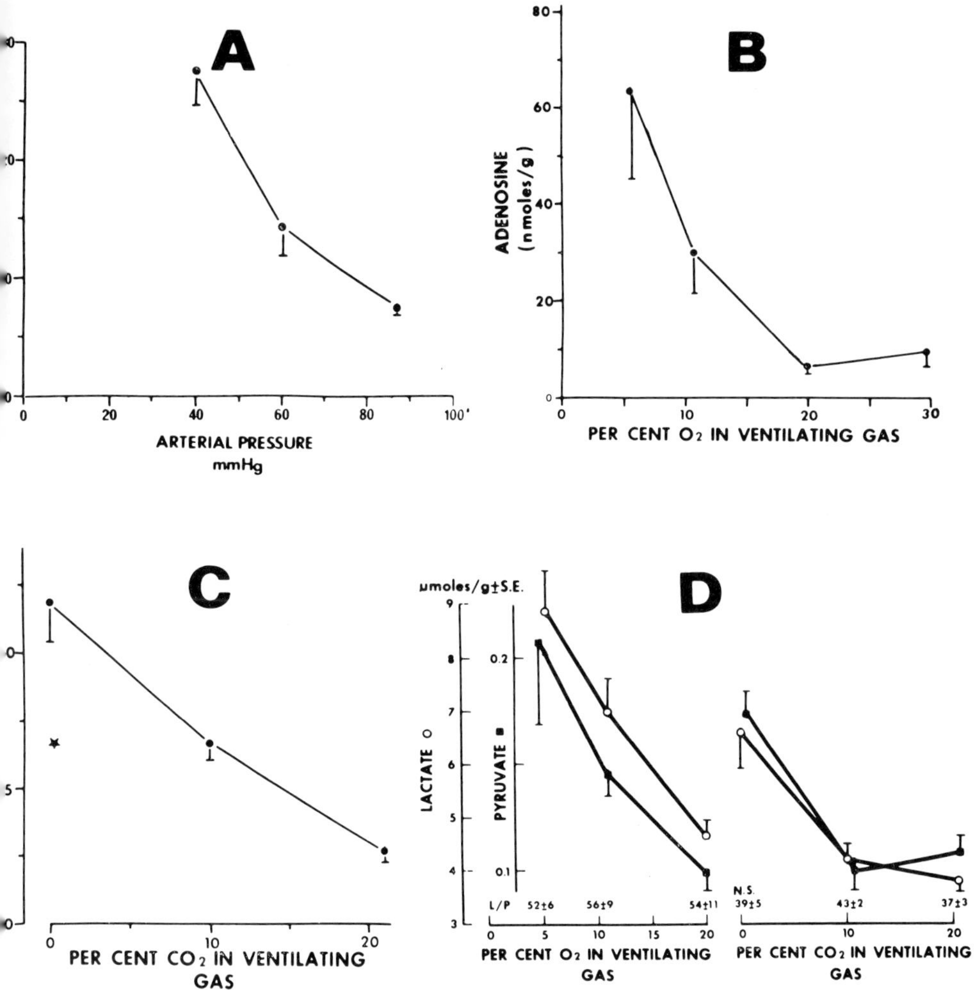

FIG. 1. Increases in concentrations of adenosine (A–C), lactate and pyruvate (D) in brain tissue produced by lowering either systemic arterial pressure, P_{O_2} or P_{CO_2}. Ventilation rate in A, B and left side of D was 60/min. Ventilation rate in C and right side D was 100/min. In C the star represents the levels of adenosine when animals were ventilated with air at a rate of 60/min, i.e. hyperventilation increased adenosine (C) and lactate and pyruvate levels (D, right) above control levels. However these levels were reduced when the percentage of CO_2 in the ventilating gas was increased. In D lactate/pyruvate (L/P) ratios remained constant. (Reproduced, with permission, from Rubio *et al.* 1975.)

TABLE 1

Effect of different rates of brain electrical stimulation and ischaemia on cerebral levels of adenosine, inosine and hypoxanthine

Rat brain: effect of electrical stimulation

Rate Stim. (Hz)	*Adenosine (nmol/g* ± S.E.*)*	*Inosine (nmol/g* ± S.E.*)*	*Hypoxanthine (nmol/g* ± S.E.*)*
0	5.4 ± 0.7	20.0 ± 3.6	28.2 ± 3.5
15	10.5 ± 1.5 $P < 0.02$	24.4 ± 4.0	27.9 ± 1.8
30	13.0 ± 1.2 $P < 0.02$	22.0 ± 1.5	34.7 ± 1.6

Dog brain: effect of ischaemia

Ischaemia (min)	*Adenosine (nmol/g* ± S.E.*)*	*Inosine (nmol/g* ± S.E.*)*	*Hypoxanthine (nmol/g* ± S.E.*)*
0	11.4 ± 1.2	11.5 ± 5.0	43.7 ± 10.9
1	28.4 ± 5.7	27.6 ± 13.8	52.6 ± 15.3
2	59.3 ± 22.5	25.6 ± 12.5	59.9 ± 15.0
3	90.5 ± 17.3	38.5 ± 11.5	46.1 ± 8.8
5	130.8 ± 35.0	51.8 ± 19.8	46.2 ± 12.7

At the end of a 5-min experimental period, the brain tissue was frozen *in situ* with small bone rongeurs precooled in liquid N_2. The frozen tissue was homogenized in ice-cold perchloric acid and centrifuged; the supernatant fraction was neutralized and enzymically assayed for adenosine, inosine, hypoxanthine, lactate and pyruvate.

These studies showed that brain adenosine levels increased significantly when arterial pressure ($P < 0.04$) or arterial P_{O_2} ($P < 0.01$) were reduced (Fig. 1A and 1B respectively). However, an increase in P_{O_2} of the ventilating gas mixture from 21 to 30% did not produce changes in brain adenosine levels (Fig. 1B). Changes in arterial P_{CO_2} also affected brain adenosine levels (Fig. 1C). A decrease in arterial P_{CO_2} induced by increasing the ventilation rate from 60/min (star in Fig. 1C) to 100/min raised adenosine levels twofold (first experimental point at 0% CO_2). However, addition of CO_2 to the ventilating gas mixtures at a respiratory rate of 100/min reduced adenosine levels to values below control (Fig. 1C). Finally, adenosine levels in brain tissue were also a function of the frequency of cortical stimulation; with an increase in the frequency of stimulation, the adenosine levels rose (Table 1).

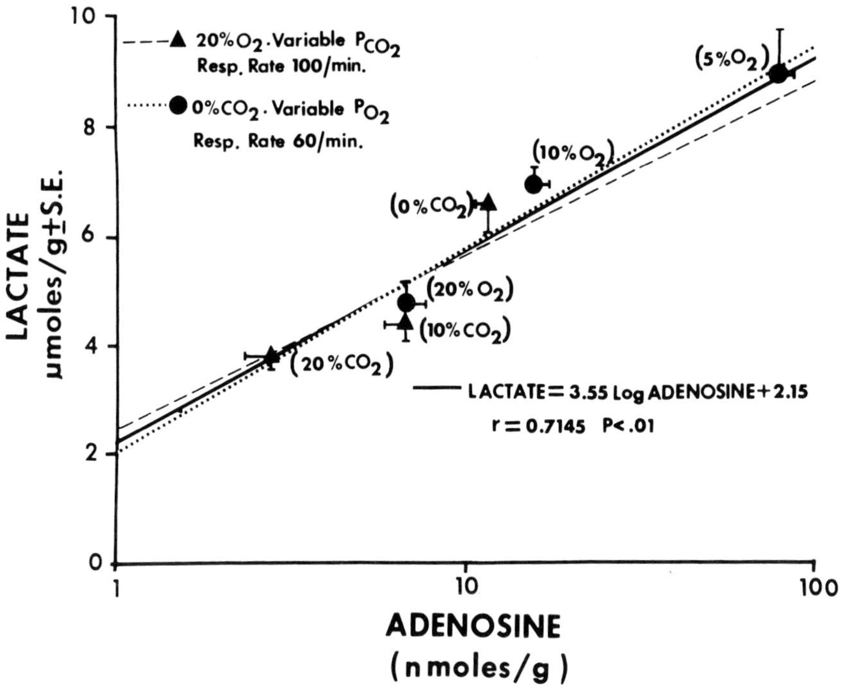

FIG. 2. Relationship between adenosine and lactate levels in brain when either arterial P_{O_2} or P_{CO_2} were varied. Since the plotted values for adenosine and lactate were indistinguishable a single regression line (solid line) was used to represent the data. (Reproduced, with permission, from Rubio & Berne 1975.)

Lactate and pyruvate levels in tissue also increased as arterial P_{O_2} or P_{CO_2} was reduced (Fig. 1D) in a fashion similar to that of adenosine. In these experiments the lactate-to-pyruvate ratios remained constant. However, in contrast to adenosine levels in tissue (Fig. 1C), further increases in the P_{CO_2} of the ventilating gas, up to 21% CO_2, slightly reduced the lactate levels (Fig. 1D right). The relationship between adenosine and lactate levels is illustrated in Fig. 2. A semilogarithmic plot of the changes in adenosine and lactate levels induced when either arterial P_{O_2} or P_{CO_2} were independently varied were not significantly different from each other. These results indicate that a 10-fold increase in adenosine is paralleled by an increase of 3.55 μmol lactate (Fig. 2).

Possible role of adenosine in control of brain blood flow

If adenosine were involved in the control of the cerebral vasculature, a correlation would be expected between the cerebral adenosine concentration and either blood flow, vascular conductance or oxygen supply (flow $\times$ O_2/ml blood), which in turn are all a function of arteriolar diameter. The three curves obtained for cerebral blood flow when either arterial pressure, arterial P_{O_2} or P_{CO_2} was independently varied are different (Harper 1966; Harper & Glass 1965; McDowall 1966; Rapela & Green 1964) and are depicted in Fig. 3A. Similarly, the curves relating vascular conductance (Fig. 3B) to these three independent variables are also different; however, for brain adenosine levels they are of similar shape (Fig. 1A, B and C), as depicted in the inserts in Fig. 3. Therefore, it is not possible to establish a unique correlation between either cerebral blood flow or vascular conductance and cerebral adenosine levels. However, with respect to oxygen supply, the three curves (Fig. 3C) show the same trend: oxygen supply increases as the independent variable increases. Thus, an inverse relationship is expected between oxygen supply and adenosine levels (Fig. 3D). However, the curve(s) relating oxygen supply and adenosine have to be defined between specific limits. For instance, in the cases in which arterial pressure or P_{O_2} are varied, the oxygen supply starts at zero and terminates at a fixed value, since further increases in pressure or P_{O_2} above their normal values do not cause any greater increase in cerebral blood flow or blood oxygen content (Fig. 3C). In fact brain adenosine levels do not change when the ventilating gas changes from one containing 20% O_2 to one containing 30% O_2 (Fig. 1B). With either decreases or increases in P_{CO_2}, the limits of oxygen supply are about 0.6 times normal or twice normal (Harper & Glass 1965), respectively, and these limits are associated with levels of adenosine higher and lower than control values (Fig. 1C). The representation of the relation between brain adenosine and oxygen supply will most probably be a family of curves, and the configuration of a given curve will probably depend on the means of changing the oxygen supply and the degree of interplay of other factors such as H^+, K^+, osmolality and myogenic and neurogenic factors.

As the interplay of a number of factors is most probably involved in the regulation of blood flow, a hypothesis unifying all these concepts is required. This is particularly true for the brain, where changes in cerebrospinal fluid H^+, a powerful vasodilator, are not always associated with changes in cerebral vascular conductance (Hernandez-Perez & Anderson 1976; Betz 1968; McDowall & Harper 1970). Thus, in view of our results with adenosine (another powerful vasodilator), we propose the following unifying hypothesis. This hypothesis, which will have to be modified as additional basic information

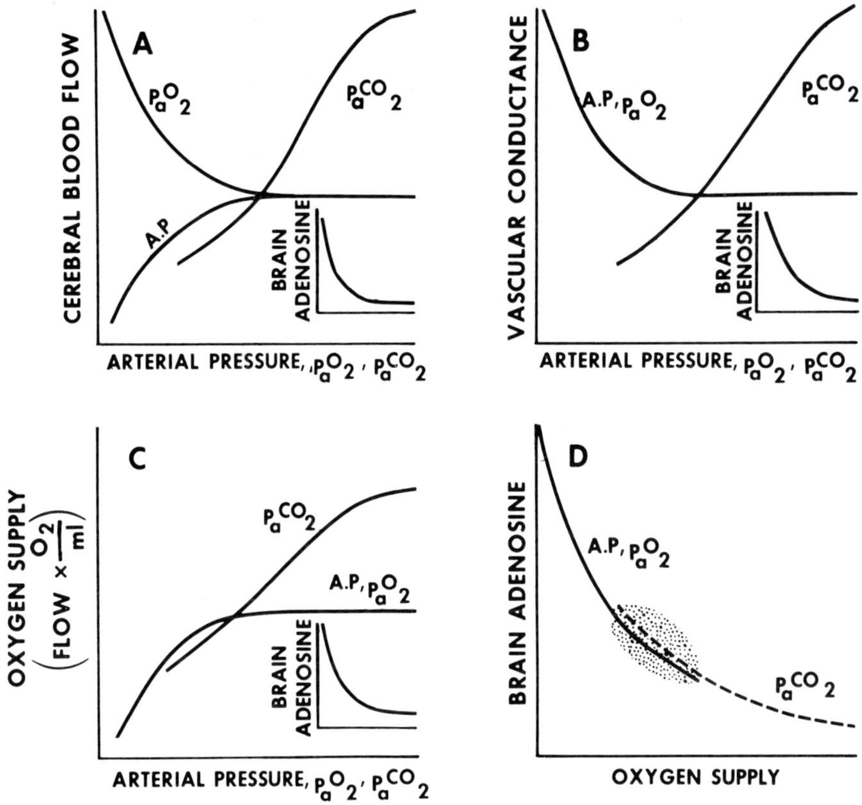

FIG. 3. Schematic relationships between cerebral blood flow (A), vascular conductance (B), oxygen supply $\left(\text{blood flow} \times \frac{O_2}{\text{ml blood}}\right)$ (C) and adenosine levels in brain tissue (inserts) when either arterial pressure, Pa_{O_2} and Pa_{CO_2} (abscissae) were varied. In B and C the curves obtained when arterial pressure and Pa_{O_2} were varied are represented by the same curve, for simplicity. In D the possible relation between brain adenosine level and oxygen supply is shown. The different points representing the adenosine-oxygen supply relationship when arterial pressure, Pa_{O_2}, Pa_{CO_2} and neuronal discharge all varied simultaneously within physiological ranges are shown by the shaded area, i.e. the brain adenosine–oxygen supply relationship is most probably represented by a family of curves. For further discussion see text.

is acquired, is illustrated in Fig. 4. In this scheme a series of interdependent variables—H^+ (arising mostly from lactate), adenosine, cerebral blood flow, O_2 supply and O_2 consumption—are considered. The H^+ and adenosine production are dependent upon the balance of inhibitory (O_2 supply, indicated by a minus sign) and stimulatory factors (O_2 consumption, indicated by a

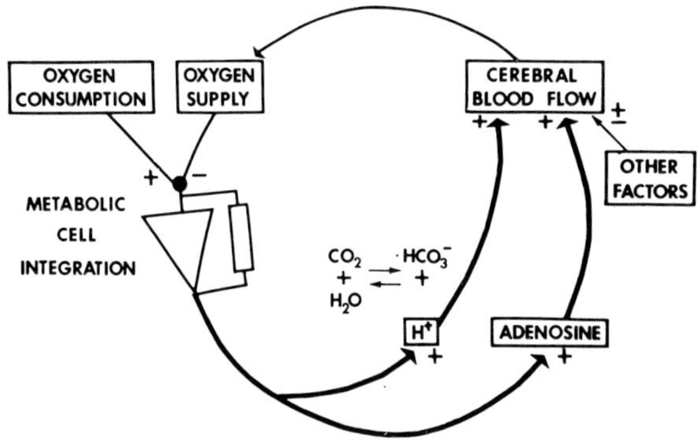

FIG. 4. Diagram to illustrate the interplay of H^+, adenosine, and other factors such as oxygen consumption and oxygen supply in the metabolic regulation of cerebral blood flow. See text for discussion. (Reproduced, with permission, from Rubio *et al.* 1975.)

plus sign). These two opposite signals represent the inputs to the integrator of the cell metabolic processes. In addition to its metabolic source, H^+ also arises from exogenous CO_2. A decrease in O_2 supply (produced by lowering either arterial pressure, P_{CO_2} or P_{O_2}) would exert less inhibition on the H^+ and adenosine-generating systems, thereby increasing their concentration. The increased levels of these two substances would act synergistically to increase blood flow and tend to restore cerebral oxygen balance. Similar results would be obtained if cerebral oxygen consumption were increased by an increase in neuronal activity. However, an increase in arterial P_{CO_2} through an increase in H^+ would increase the brain O_2 supply, thereby decreasing the levels of endogenous H^+ and adenosine. This decrease in concentration of these vasodilators would tend to buffer the vasodilator effects of exogenous H^+. Other factors (myogenic, neurogenic, potassium and osmolality) may have to be integrated into this scheme.

EFFECTS OF ADENOSINE ON BRAIN VASCULATURE

Application of adenosine to exposed pial vessels elicits a marked dilatation of the small arteries and arterioles (Fig. 5). The pial vessels show a high degree of sensitivity to adenosine and a graded effect is observed for increasing concentrations of adenosine between the range of 10^{-8} to 10^{-3} M (Berne *et al.* 1974; Wahl & Kuschinsky 1975). However, when adenosine was administered by continuous intra-arterial infusion, no detectable change in vessel diameter was noted even when concentrations as high as 0.5 mM were reached. Similarly,

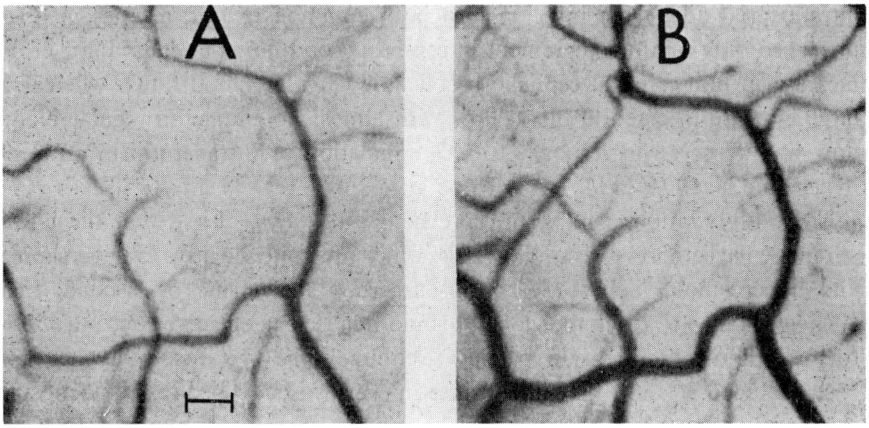

FIG. 5. Dilatation of cat pial arterial vessels induced by adenosine. A, control. B, 15 s after topical application of adenosine dissolved in cerebrospinal fluid. Bar = 100 μm. (Reproduced, by permission of the American Heart Association, from Berne *et al.* 1974.)

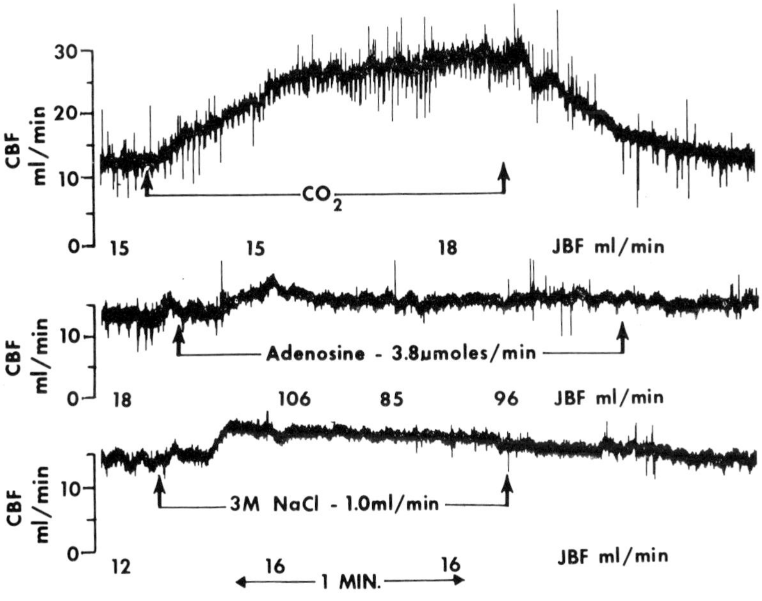

FIG. 6. Negligible effect of continuous infusion of adenosine into both common carotid arteries on cerebral blood flow (CBF) compared with the effect of 10% CO_2 inhalation or hypertonic saline infusion in the dog. In contrast jugular blood flow (JBF ml/min) is increased fivefold by adenosine. (Reproduced, by permission of the American Heart Association, from Berne *et al.* 1974.)

intra-arterial adenosine infusion into both common carotid arteries in dogs produced only a minor increment in cerebral blood flow but caused a fivefold increase in non-cerebral cephalic blood flow (jugular blood flow), whereas a large increase in cerebral blood flow with almost no change in jugular blood flow was observed in response to CO_2 inhalation or intracarotid infusion of hypertonic NaCl (Fig. 6).

These observations can be interpreted in two ways. First, that the intraparenchymal cerebral resistance vessels (which are quite sensitive to hypercapnia and hyperosmolar solutions) are insensitive to adenosine or, second, that adenosine failed to reach the vascular smooth muscle in effective concentrations because of the blood–brain barrier. Although the first possibility has not been excluded it is not very likely since in every vascular bed tested adenosine is vasoactive, and intraparenchymal brain vessels are probably no exception. We believe the second explanation is the more plausible because direct application of adenosine to the pial vessels caused them to dilate whereas administration of supramaximal concentrations of adenosine via the intravascular route was without effect (Berne *et al.* 1974). Additional evidence that adenosine is largely blocked by the blood–brain barrier was obtained from studies in which cerebrospinal fluid was sampled during intra-arterial administration of uniformly labelled adenosine and cerebral venous blood was sampled after injection of labelled adenosine into the cerebrospinal fluid. Essentially no radioactivity was recovered in the cerebrospinal fluid during infusion of [U–^{14}C]adenosine into both internal carotid arteries of the dog at a rate of 600 000 counts/min for about 10 min (a total of 6 000 000 counts). Furthermore, when 300 000 counts/min of [U–^{14}C]adenosine were added to the cerebrospinal fluid, a maximum of 150 counts/(min ml) of cerebral venous blood were measured. Finally, our studies in rats showed that when labelled adenosine was infused into the right common carotid artery and samples of blood, heart, brain and skeletal muscle were obtained about 1.5 min after infusion was begun, the total number of counts per gram of brain was not significantly different from that per gram of heart, despite the fact that the brain received the highest concentration of radioactive adenosine. With intracarotid infusion of labelled inosine, the difference in the counts in these two organs was large (Table 2); the reason for this difference is not known.

However, when the [U–^{14}C]adenosine was administered intravenously and presumably all tissues received an equal number of counts/ml blood in the form of [U–^{14}C]adenosine and [U–^{14}C]inosine (formed by adenosine degradation in the blood), the number of counts in brain was 20- to 30-fold lower than in heart and about equal to that observed in skeletal muscle (Table 2). Hence, it appears that some adenosine can cross the blood–brain barrier, but the

TABLE 2

Partial distribution of radioactivity, in counts/(min g), after intracarotid and intravenous infusion of [U–^{14}C]adenosine or [8–^{14}C]inosine in the rat

Tissue	*Intravenous infusion*[a] [*U*–^{14}*C*]*adenosine* *mean* ± S.E.	*Intracarotid infusion*[a] [*U*–^{14}*C*]*adenosine*[b] *mean* ± S.E.	[*8*–^{14}*C*]*inosine*[b] *mean* ± S.E.
Blood	6894 ± 1252	8419 ± 2000	3103 ± 308
Heart	8185 ± 884	4316 ± 194	1409 ± 198
Brain	357 ± 44	5091 ± 730	482 ± 90
Skeletal muscle	447 ± 24	1162 ± 272	523 ± 74

[a]Three rats in every group.
[b]Each rat received 945 800 counts/min of [U–^{14}C]adenosine and 287 300 counts/min of [8–^{14}C]inosine in a volume of 0.1 ml over a period of 25 s either intra-arterially or intravenously. Tissue samples were taken 1.5–6 min before isotope injections.

transfer is small relative to that in the heart; with inosine the difference between the two organs is even greater. After intravenous injection of the isotope, the counts in skeletal muscle were lower than those in the heart and of the same order of magnitude as those found in brain (Table 2). This dissimilarity between heart and skeletal muscle can be attributed to their differences in blood flow: 2–4 ml/(min · 100 g) for resting muscle and 80 ml/(min · 100 g) for cardiac muscle. Brain blood flow is about 55 ml/(min · 100 g tissue).

METABOLISM OF ADENOSINE

Incorporation of adenosine into adenine nucleotides

Our studies indicate that the adenosine released by brain tissue is rephosphorylated and suffers only minor degradation. When labelled adenosine was incubated in dog cerebrospinal fluid at 37 °C for 10 min, none was degraded and when it was added to the cerebrospinal fluid of anaesthetized dogs considerable radioactivity remained in the cerebrospinal fluid and was incorporated into brain tissue. Furthermore, chromatographic analysis showed that in brain tissue 86% of the total radioactivity corresponded to adenine nucleotides and 14% to adenosine, inosine and hypoxanthine (Berne *et al.* 1974). In contrast, in the cerebrospinal fluid the reverse was true. These results indicate that the brain, like the heart (Wiedmeier *et al.* 1972), is capable of avidly incorporating adenosine into adenine nucleotides. Since little adenosine is lost by blood washout because of the blood–brain barrier, the brain is unique because nucleotide degradation and resynthesis via an adenosine kinase (EC 2.7.1.20) (the salvage pathway) occur within a closed system (brain and cerebrospinal fluid), hence brain nucleotides are preserved. This retention of adenosine and its products in brain is to be contrasted with its behaviour in tissues like heart, skeletal muscle, lung, kidney and liver, in which some of the adenosine and its degradative products, inosine and hypoxanthine, are washed away and degraded by the perfusing blood (Rubio *et al.* 1972; Bockman *et al.* 1976; Mentzer *et al.* 1975; Berne & Rubio 1974).

In an attempt to shed light on whether the adenosine molecule is directly incorporated into nucleotides or is first degraded to adenine or hypoxanthine (after deamination to inosine), we added uniformly labelled [^{14}C]adenosine to the cerebrospinal fluid by means of convexity–cisternal perfusion and determined the relative specific activities in substrate and nucleotides. The rationale behind these experiments is as follows. Both the ribose and base moieties contribute to the total radioactivity of uniformly labelled adenosine. If adenosine is directly phosphorylated, its specific activity (SA) in the nucleotides will be lowered by dilution with the non-labelled adenosine moieties of the adenine nucleotides. However, the ratio of the specific activity of the perfused nucleoside (SA nucleoside = SA base + SA ribose) to that of its base moiety (SA base) is expected to be the same as the relative specific activity of nucleoside and base moiety $\left(\frac{\text{SA base} + \text{SA ribose}}{\text{SA base}} = 1 + \frac{\text{SA ribose}}{\text{SA base}}\right)$ from the brain nucleotides. However, if the ribose moiety is split from the nucleoside, it will be greatly diluted by unlabelled ribose and essentially only the base moiety of the infused [U–^{14}C]adenosine will be incorporated into the adenine nucleotides. The ratio of the nucleoside to base of cerebral adenine nucleotides would then yield a value of 1.0 $\left(1 + \frac{\text{SA ribose}}{\text{SA base}} = 1 + 0 = 1\right)$.

The results of these experiments have shown that the ratio of SA nucleoside/SA base in brain nucleotides was 1.70 ± 0.07, which compares rather well with the SA value of 1.76 obtained from the infused [U–^{14}C]adenosine. Thus, the brain incorporates adenosine into adenosine nucleotides by direct phosphorylation, as does the heart (Wiedmeier *et al.* 1972).

Degradation of adenosine into inosine and hypoxanthine

Breakdown of adenosine into inosine and hypoxanthine in brain differs somewhat from that occurring in other tissues. For example, degradation of adenine nucleotides via adenosine formation in tissues such as lung, kidney, liver and heart (ventricle and atrium) occurs with an accumulation of inosine and hypoxanthine that proceeds at a rate equal to or faster than that of adenosine (Rubio *et al.* 1972, 1973; Bockman *et al.* 1975; Thomas *et al.* 1975). However, in brain, significant increases in adenosine levels are followed by smaller or negligible increases in inosine, and particularly in hypoxanthine (Table 1). This suggests that in tissues other than brain, the nucleosides adenosine and inosine have ready access to their corresponding degradative enzymes: adenosine deaminase (EC 3.5.4.4) which deaminates adenosine to inosine and which in turn is transformed into hypoxanthine and ribose-1-phosphate by purine-nucleoside phosphorylase (EC 2.4.2.1). The restriction of purine-nucleoside phosphorylase to the capillary wall in cardiac tissue was suspected because of the greater proportion of inosine and hypoxanthine with respect to adenosine in the intravascular than in the extravascular compartments. The relationship of the concentration of adenosine (Ado) to that of its degradative products inosine (In) and hypoxanthine (Hyx) in cardiac tissue (extravascular compartment) gave ratios of Hyx:Ado:In of 0.6:1:1.2, whereas in cardiac venous effluents (intravascular compartment) these ratios were 6:1:6 (Rubio *et al.* 1972). In order to demonstrate that purine-nucleoside phosphorylase was largely concentrated in the capillary wall, we developed a histochemical technique for this enzyme. The reversible reaction catalysed

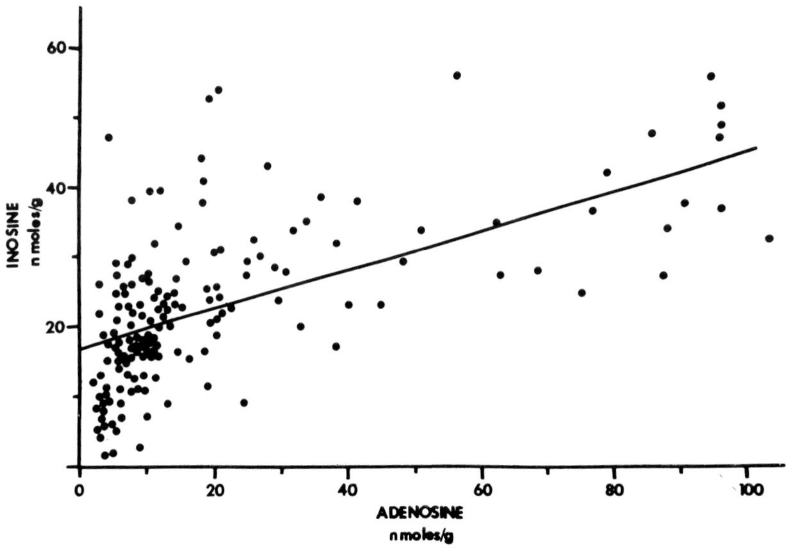

FIG. 7. Relationship between brain adenosine and inosine levels. Regression line, inosine $= 0.28 \times$ adenosine $+ 16.78$; $r = 0.56$, $n = 163$, $P < 0.01$.

by the enzyme is: inosine + inorganic phosphate ⇄ hypoxanthine + ribose-1-phosphate. Thin frozen sections of glutaraldehyde-fixed tissue were incubated in a medium containing ribose-1-phosphate and hypoxanthine and the released inorganic phosphate was trapped with lead. Incubation in a medium containing only ribose-1-phosphate without hypoxanthine was used as a control to rule out the possibility of non-specific hydrolysis of ribose-1-phosphate (Rubio *et al.* 1972; Rubio 1974). With the aid of electron microscopy, purine-nucleoside

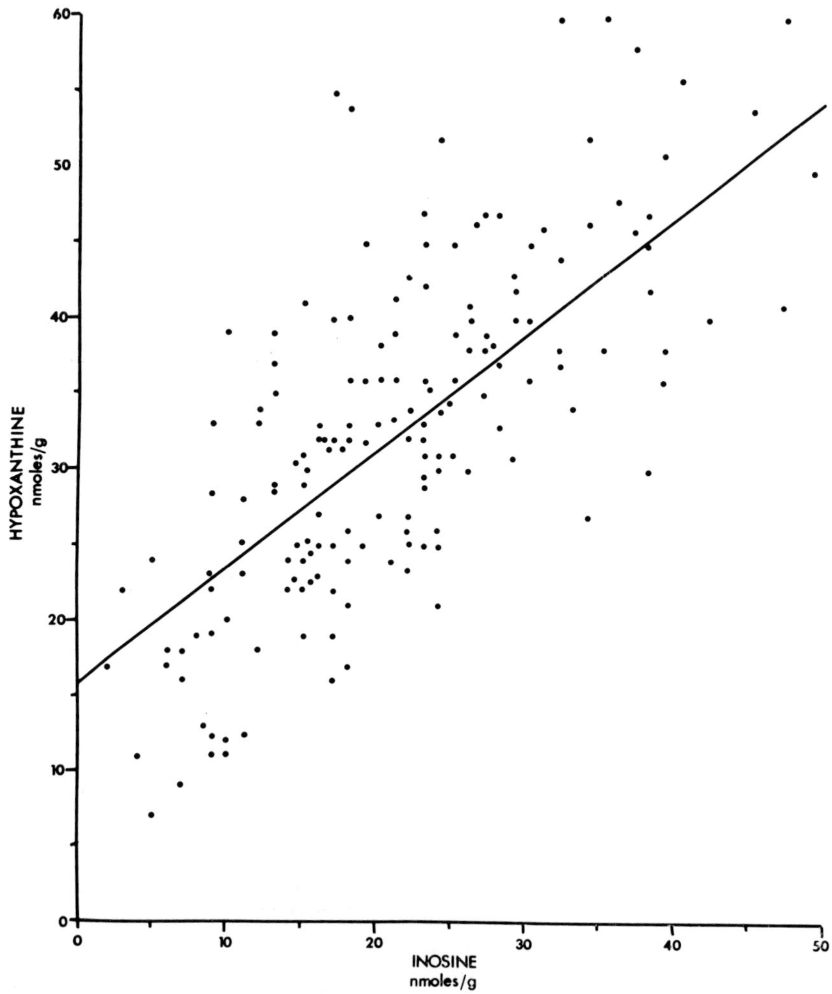

FIG. 8. Relationships between brain inosine and hypoxanthine levels. Regression line, hypoxanthine = 0.79 × inosine + 15.64; $r = 0.72$, $n = 160$, $P < 0.01$.

phosphorylase activity was detected in the cytoplasm of endothelial cells and pericytes but not in parenchymal or smooth muscle cells. Adenosine deaminase, an ubiquitous enzyme catalysing the formation of inosine from adenosine, has been found in large vessel walls and we are not aware of any histochemical technique for demonstrating the presence of this enzyme. These findings

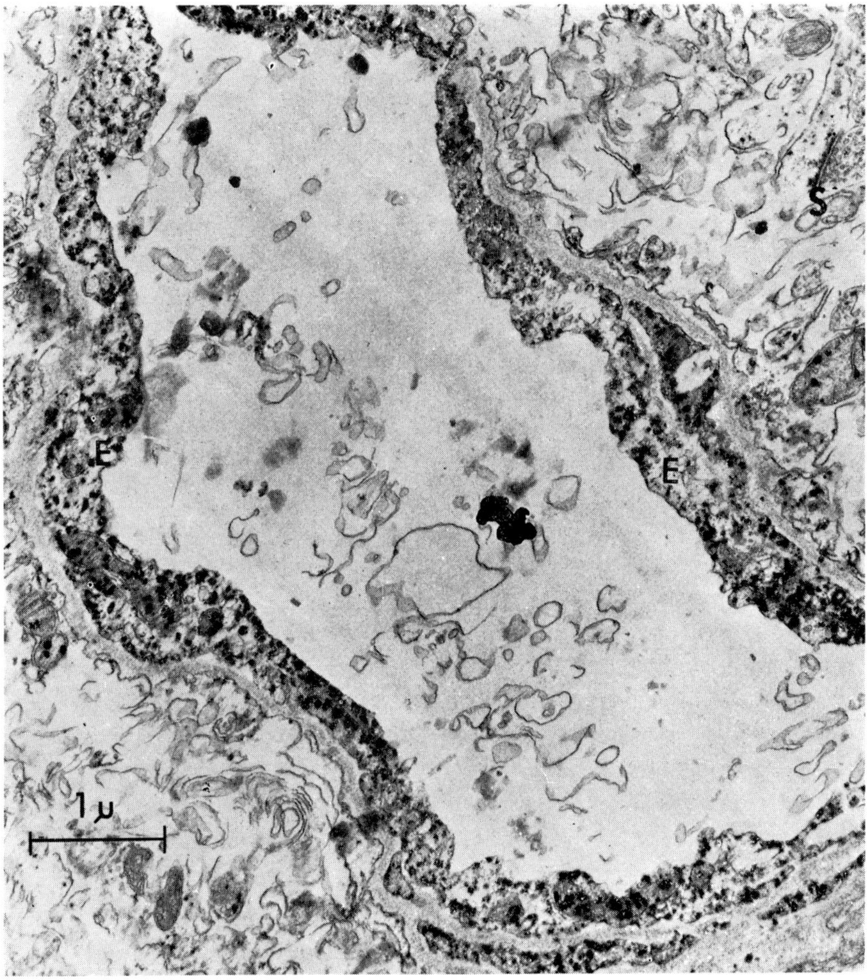

FIG. 9. Localization of purine-nucleoside phosphorylase activity in wall of brain capillary. Section from rat brain incubated in a medium containing hypoxanthine, ribose-1-phosphate and Pb^{2+}. Purine-nucleoside phosphorylase activity is evidenced by precipitated lead phosphate. Symbols: E, endothelium; S, synapse.

suggest that adenosine released from myocardial parenchymal cells has the highest concentration in the interstitial fluid and that it is degraded to inosine and hypoxanthine as it passes through the vessel walls. These studies have been extended to other organs such as lung, skeletal muscle, liver and kidney (Mentzer *et al.* 1975; Rubio 1974), with identical results.

In brain tissue, accumulation of inosine and hypoxanthine is lower than that of adenosine (Table 1 and Figs. 7 and 8). In our studies on rat brain

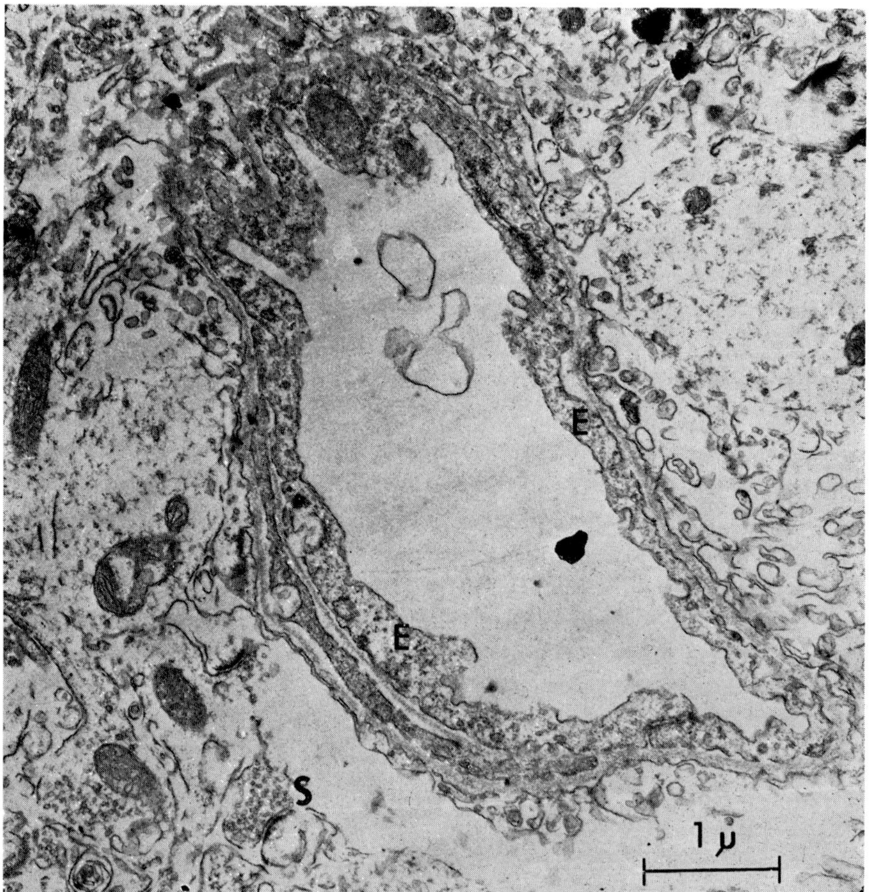

FIG. 10. Lack of enzyme activity when a section of brain tissue was incubated in a medium containing ribose-1-phosphate and lead without hypoxanthine. Purine-nucleoside phosphorylase requires both ribose-1-phosphate and hypoxanthine for activity. Thus, activity shown in Fig. 9 is not due to a non-specific hydrolysis of ribose-1-phosphate.

under the various experimental conditions, we observed that adenosine levels in brain tissue correlated with those of inosine (Fig. 7). These data can be represented by the straight line: In $=$ 0.28 Ado $+$ 16.78 ($r = 0.56$, $n = 163$, $P < 0.01$), i.e. adenosine tends to accumulate 3.57 times faster than inosine. The correlation of inosine levels with hypoxanthine levels is shown in Fig. 8. The data can also be represented by a straight line: Hyx $=$ 0.79 In $+$ 15.64 ($r = 0.72$, $n = 160$, $P < 0.01$), i.e. hypoxanthine tends to accumulate at a rate 1.27 times slower than inosine and 4.52 times slower than adenosine. This slower accumulation of inosine, and particularly hypoxanthine in brain, contrasts with the equally fast or faster accumulation of inosine and hypoxanthine in other tissues (Rubio *et al.* 1973; Thomas *et al.* 1975; Bockman *et al.* 1976; Mentzer *et al.* 1975). This could be interpreted to mean that in the brain adenosine and inosine have restricted access to their corresponding degradative enzymes. If these enzymes were highly concentrated in the vessel wall then the relative impermeability of the brain capillaries to labelled adenosine and inosine would explain the low production of their degradative products, inosine and hypoxanthine.

Therefore, we decided to apply the histochemical technique described above for the localization of purine-nucleoside phosphorylase in brain tissue. Fig. 9 shows that purine-nucleoside phosphorylase is located in the cytoplasm of capillary endothelial cells. Incubation of brain tissue in a medium containing only ribose-1-phosphate without hypoxanthine yielded negative results (Fig. 10). These findings are in accordance with the concept that in the brain, in contrast to other tissues, adenosine and inosine do not have ready access to their degradative enzymes, possibly because of impermeability of the brain capillary to these nucleosides.

OTHER POSSIBLE FUNCTIONS OF ADENOSINE IN BRAIN

Adenosine is not an inactive substance in brain function; thus, the significance of its production remains to be assessed. Activation by adenosine of the adenylate cyclase (EC 4.6.1.1) system of the brain cortex is well known (Sattin 1971; Schultz & Daly 1973), and recently it has been demonstrated that the excitability of spontaneously firing cortical neurons is depressed by adenosine (Phillis & Kostopoulos 1975). The exact mechanism of this depression is unknown but it is possibly mediated by inhibition of the release of a synaptic transmitter, a Ca^{2+}-dependent process. Adenosine has also been shown to depress the release of transmitter from the motor nerve endings in the rat diaphragm (Ginsborg & Hirst 1972).

ACKNOWLEDGEMENTS

The original research discussed in this chapter was supported by Grant HL-10384 from the Public Health Service and AHA 74962. Dr H. Richard Winn is recipient of a National Institutes of Health Postdoctoral Fellowship NSO5 1F32 NSO5093-01.

References

BERNE, R. M. & RUBIO, R. (1974) Adenine nucleotide metabolism in the heart. *Circ. Res. 35, Suppl. 3*, 109–120

BERNE, R. M., RUBIO, R. & CURNISH, R. R. (1974) Release of adenosine from ischemic brain: effect on cerebral vascular resistance and incorporation into cerebral adenine nucleotides. *Circ. Res. 35*, 262–271

BETZ, E. (1968) The significance of cortical extracellular pH for the regulation of blood flow in the cerebral cortex. *Prog. Brain Res. 30*, 99–102

BILL, A. (1975) Blood circulation and fluid dynamics in the eye. *Physiol. Rev. 55*, 383–417

BOCKMAN, E. L., BERNE, R. M. & RUBIO, R. (1975) Release of adenosine and lack of release of ATP from contracting skeletal muscle. *Pflügers Arch. Eur. J. Physiol. 355*, 229–241

BOCKMAN, E. L., BERNE, R. M. & RUBIO, R. (1976) Adenosine and active hyperemia in dog skeletal muscle. *Am. J. Physiol. 230*, 1531–1537

DAVIES, P. W. & REMOND, A. (1947) Oxygen consumption of the cerebral cortex of the cat during metrazol convulsions. *Res. Publ. Assoc. Res. Nerv. Ment. Dis. 26*, 205–217

ECKENHOFF, J. E., HAJKENSCHIEL, J. H., LANDMESSER, C. M. & HARMEL, M. (1947) Cardiac oxygen metabolism and control of coronary circulation. *Am. J. Physiol. 149*, 634–649

GINSBORG, B. L. & HIRST, G. D. S. (1972) The effect of adenosine on the release of the transmitter from the phrenic nerve of the rat. *J. Physiol. (Lond.) 224*, 629–645

HADDY, F. J. & SCOTT, J. B. (1975) Metabolic factors in peripheral circulatory regulation. *Fed. Proc. 34*, 2006–2011

HARPER, A. M. (1966) Autoregulation of cerebral blood flow: influence of the arterial blood pressure on the blood flow through the cerebral cortex. *J. Neurol. Neurosurg. Psychiatry 29*, 398–403

HARPER, A. M. & GLASS, H. I. (1965) Effect of alterations in the arterial carbon dioxide tension on the blood flow through the cerebral cortex at normal and low arterial blood pressures. *J. Neurol. Neurosurg. Psychiatry 28*, 449–452

HERNANDEZ-PEREZ, M. J. & ANDERSON, D. K. (1976) Autoregulation of cerebral blood flow and its relation to cerebrospinal fluid pH. *Am. J. Physiol. 231*, 929–935

KRNJEVIC, K., RANDIC, M. & SIESJÖ, B. K. (1965) Cortical CO_2 tension and neuronal excitability. *J. Physiol. (Lond.) 176*, 105–122

LARRABEE, M. G. & BRONK, D. W. (1952) Metabolic requirements of sympathetic neurons. *Cold Spring Harbor Symp. Quant. Biol. 17*, 245–266

LENNOX, W. G., GIBBS, F. A. & GIBBS, E. L. (1938) The relationship in man of cerebral activity to blood flow and to blood constituents. *Res. Publ. Assoc. Res. Nerv. Ment. Dis. 18*, 274–297

MCDOWALL, D. G. (1966) Interrelationships between blood oxygen tension and cerebral blood flow, in *Oxygen Measurements in Blood and Tissues* (Payne, J. P. & Hill, D. W., eds.), pp. 205–214, Churchill, London

MCDOWALL, D. G. & HARPER, A. M. (1970) Cerebral blood flow and CSF pH during hyperventilation, in *Progress in Anaesthesiology (Proc. 4th Int. World Congr. Anaesthesiol.)* (Boulton, T. B. *et al.*, eds.), pp. 542–545, ICS. no. 200, Excerpta Medica, Amsterdam

MCILWAIN, H. & JOANNY, P. (1963) Characteristics required in electrical pulses of rectangular time-voltage relationships for metabolic change and ion movements in mammalian cerebral tissues. *J. Neurochem. 10*, 313–323

MENTZER, R. M., RUBIO, R. & BERNE, R. M. (1975) Release of adenosine by hypoxic canine lung tissue and its possible role in pulmonary circulation. *Am. J. Physiol. 229*, 1625–1631

PHILLIS, J. W. & KOSTOPOULOS, G. K. (1975) Adenosine as a putative transmitter in the cerebral cortex. Studies with potentiators and antagonists. *Life Sci. 17*, 1085–1094

RAPELA, C. E. & GREEN, H. D. (1964) Autoregulation of canine cerebral blood flow. *Circ. Res. 15* (Suppl. I), 205–211

RUBIO, R. (1974) Purine nucleoside phosphorylase, in *Electron Microscopy of Enzymes: Principles and Methods* (Hayat, M. A., ed.), pp. 54–67, Van Nostrand & Reinhold, New York

RUBIO, R. & BERNE, R. M. (1975) Relationships of adenosine concentration, lactate levels and oxygen supply in rat brain, in *Blood Flow and Metabolism in the Brain* (Harper, M. *et al.*, eds.), pp. 3.23–3.27, Churchill Livingstone, Edinburgh

RUBIO, R., WIEDMEIER, T. & BERNE, R. M. (1972) Nucleoside phosphorylase: localization and role in the myocardial distribution of purines. *Am. J. Physiol. 222*, 550–555

RUBIO, R., BERNE, R. M. & DOBSON, J. G. (1973) Sites of adenosine production in cardiac and skeletal muscle. *Am. J. Physiol. 225*, 938–953

RUBIO, R., BERNE, R. M., BOCKMAN, E. L. & CURNISH, R. R. (1975) Relationship between adenosine concentration and oxygen supply in rat brain. *Am. J. Physiol. 228*, 1896–1902

SATTIN, A. (1971) Increase in the content of adenosine 3′,5′-monophosphate in mouse brain during seizures and prevention of the increase by methylxanthines. *J. Neurochem. 18*, 1087–1096

SCHMIDT, C. F., KETY, S. S. & PENNES, H. H. (1945) The gaseous metabolism of the brain of the monkey. *Am. J. Physiol. 143*, 33–52

SCHULTZ, J. & DALY, J. W. (1973) Cyclic adenosine 3′5′-monophosphate in guinea pig cerebral cortical slices. *J. Biol. Chem. 248*, 843–852

SHIPLEY, R. E. & STUDY, R. S. (1951) Changes in renal blood flow, extraction of inulin, glomerular filtration rate tissue pressure and urine flow with acute alterations of renal artery pressure. *Am. J. Physiol. 167*, 676–688

THOMAS, R. A., RUBIO, R. & BERNE, R. M. (1975) Comparison of the adenine nucleotide metabolism of dog atrial and ventricular myocardium. *J. Mol. Cell Cardiol. 7*, 115–123

WAHL, M. & KUSCHINSKY, W. (1975) Effects of adenosine and theophylline at pial vessels, in *Blood Flow and Metabolism in the Brain* (Harper, M. *et al.*, eds.), pp. 3.28–3.29, Churchill Livingstone, Edinburgh

WIEDMEIER, V. T., RUBIO, R. & BERNE, R. M. (1972) Incorporation and turnover of adenosine–U-^{14}C in perfused guinea pig myocardium. *Am. J. Physiol. 223*, 51–54

Discussion

Rosendorff: What is the evidence that adenosine or perhaps its precursor, ATP, conforms to the usually accepted criteria for neurohumoral transmission?

Rubio: Adenosine is released as a function of neuronal activity. In rat brains we stimulated the cortex electrically at increasing rates and obtained an increase in adenosine tissue levels proportional to the frequency of stimulation. We have no evidence that adenosine plays a role in synaptic transmission, but when Phillis & Kostopoulos (1975) applied adenosine by iontophoresis to certain neuronal groups the release of transmitter was significantly depressed.

Ginsborg & Hirst (1972) looked at the effect of adenosine on the release of acetylcholine in motor nerve endings and they too demonstrated depression of release of the transmitter by adenosine. The problem so far is that the amounts of adenosine needed to affect the processes are higher than those normally recorded. Adenosine certainly affects these processes, but in order to be sure that it plays a role in modulating synaptic transmission, we would have to determine the concentration of this compound at the level of the synapse. It is difficult to say whether ATP is the compound released. It is possible that one only measures adenosine as a result of ATP breakdown.

Rosendorff: But do you think that adenosine is simply one of the transducing mechanisms between changes in cerebral metabolism and changes in vascular smooth muscle activity? Or are there specialized purinergic nerves going to brain vessels that release adenosine or ATP as their transmitter?

My second question relates to ATP. In other smooth muscle tissue, particularly the gut, it has been suggested that ATP may be just as important as adenosine in its transmitter function. The distinction between the two has been characterized only recently by the evolution of specific blocking agents for ATP and for adenosine. For example, quinidine will block the action of ATP on smooth muscle in the gut whereas methylxanthine will fairly selectively block the action of adenosine. Have you looked at ATP effects or production, or even concentrations in the brain in the same way as you have been measuring adenosine concentrations?

Rubio: Yes, we have measured brain tissue levels of ATP but this value doesn't tell us anything about its release. The release of ATP has been suggested by Forrester (1972; Forrester & Hassen 1973), who used human skeletal muscle as well as isolated frog sartorius muscle and reported that ATP is released when the muscle contracts. However we haven't been able to confirm those findings (Bockman *et al.* 1975; Dobson *et al.* 1971). This does not mean that Forrester is wrong but what happens is that it is very difficult to do the experiments without releasing ATP during the procedure of blood sampling. For instance one problem is that Forrester used EDTA to stop ATPase activity. However, EDTA is known to cause the release of ATP from blood cells.

Purves: Are you suggesting that Forrester's demonstration of a rise over a matter of minutes in venous blood in human muscle is an artifact?

Rubio: We cannot confirm his findings.

Purves: So, from your answer to Professor Rosendorff, you are suggesting that ATP is unlikely to be involved in vasodilatation?

Rubio: That would be my interpretation until evidence is provided to the contrary.

Heuser: Transmitter release is closely linked to calcium uptake. Do you think that one could expect a decrease in local extracellular Ca^{2+} activity under your experimental conditions, which *per se* could be responsible for vasodilatation?

Rubio: In several tissues, particularly mammalian atria, adenosine decreases the influx of calcium. In the depolarized mammalian atria, it is possible to generate the so-called slow action potentials which are known to be strictly calcium-dependent. These electrical responses can be blocked with adenosine, 10^{-6} M (Schrader *et al.* 1975). In the nerve endings Ginsborg & Hirst (1972) showed that the effect of adenosine in decreasing the amount of transmitter release is partially dependent on extracellular calcium. In smooth muscle the action potential is dependent on the external calcium concentration. Thus, one mechanism by which adenosine acts in all these tissues may be by modifying the membrane permeability to calcium.

Meldrum: I assume that the metabolic coupling agent hypothesis should account for the increase in cerebral blood flow during seizures. This increase can be sustained for a period of two hours with a marked reduction of cerebrovascular resistance (Meldrum & Nilsson 1976). One therefore needs to know whether the cerebral vascular response to adenosine shows tachyphylaxis. Relaxation of smooth muscle in the gut through ATP or adenosine certainly shows marked tachyphylaxis. Is this known for the brain?

Rubio: I don't know. In pial vessels with adenosine concentration in the 10^{-6} M range there is sustained vasodilatation and this effect is perfectly reversible.

Meldrum: Some adenosine must be broken down or removed, yet during the two-hour seizure period the adenylate pool remains constant. Sufficient re-synthesis of adenosine nucleotides must be going on throughout the period.

Rubio: Our feeling is that adenosine released is rephosphorylated. The system, because of the blood–brain barrier, is a closed system. For this purpose the brain is in a very privileged situation in contrast to many other organs. In most organs, some of the nucleosides formed are washed out by the circulating blood because the membrane to the capillaries is permeable to these compounds.

Siesjö: As you pointed out, there are obvious differences in some of the results. Further experiments are certainly required. We could confirm your finding that there is a strict correlation between an increase in AMP and an increase in adenosine (Nordström *et al.* 1977). Our experiments were on rats with an exposed dura mater. We induced ischaemia for 10, 20, 30, 40 and 60 s. AMP and adenosine concentrations both increased rapidly. However, our control values for adenosine were about one-fifth to one-tenth of your values.

Furthermore, when AMP increased by 1 μmol/kg adenosine increased by 1.5 μmol/kg, so there was a quantitative difference too.

When a craniotomy is made in the rat, and even if great care is taken, some control animals show increased adenosine concentrations. This increase is always coupled to an increased AMP concentration. We tried to study hypoxia with this model and found it impossible. Thus, there were increases in AMP and in adenosine concentrations, results which are not obtained when the tissue is frozen through an intact skull bone (e.g. Norberg & Siesjö 1975). From these results and other experiments we conclude that craniotomy to some extent disturbs the microcirculation in the tissue. When the flow increases it is perhaps two or three times normal instead of the fivefold increase needed to maintain cerebral energy state.

It should also be added that we have been unable to find any changes in adenosine when we increase the CO_2 concentration.

As a final comment, let me emphasize that we are fully aware that whole tissue analysis may be entirely inadequate. If adenosine is released by membrane-bound 5′-nucleotidase (EC 3.1.3.5), translocating adenosine to the extracellular fluid, then if the vessels are exquisitely sensitive to adenosine we might be dealing with concentration changes that we can't detect. This would also be the case if adenosine or ATP were confined to secretory granules or vesicles that empty their contents into the extracellular fluid. However, if we keep hypoxia going for a 30-minute period, with an arterial Po_2 of 25 to 30 mmHg, we are unable to find an increase in adenosine concentration in cisternal CSF. That may indicate that there is no increase in the extracellular adenosine concentration either.

Moskowitz: Schubert *et al.* (1976) looked at this problem in a slightly different way. They injected radiolabelled adenosine into specific regions of brain and spinal cord. After the adenosine was taken up by cell bodies, this nucleoside, or its trichloroacetic acid-soluble derivatives, is transported to dendrites and axons, released from nerve terminals and transferred to postsynaptic cells; synaptic stimulation can further increase the release of these molecules. Moreover, radiolabelled compounds accumulate within pericapillary foot processes and within vascular endothelial cells. Hence, under physiological conditions, adenosine and its derivatives can be identified in close approximation to the walls of cerebral vessels (Schubert & Kreutzberg 1976).

Purves: Dr Rubio, what is the evidence for the translocation of adenosine in interstitial fluid?

Rubio: We have no evidence for that in brain tissue. However, we know that adenosine is taken up rapidly by many cells. Red cell ghosts also take up adenosine readily. We used these cells because we wanted a simple two-compartment system that we could analyse and use for studying adenosine transport. Even when we raised the concentration of adenosine outside the cells to 1 mM we could barely detect adenosine inside the cells (Schrader *et al.* 1972). We interpreted this as meaning that free adenosine doesn't exist inside the cell, probably because the adenosine kinase is responsible for the rapid adenosine rephosphorylation. We repeated these experiments with dispersed cardiac cells and obtained similar results (Mustafa *et al.* 1975). With dispersed liver cells the results were identical. Other people using other cells such as leucocytes have found exactly the same so we feel that possibly the neurons may not be the exception.

Purves: But isn't that rather an important gap in your argument? It seems that we are still uncertain of the exact sensitivity of vessels to changes in interstitial concentrations of adenosine. Just as for calcium and potassium, in some way we have to match the changes in concentration in interstitial fluid with the known sensitivity of vessels.

Rubio: One of the questions that we have discussed is that we would like to measure perivascular adenosine concentrations with adenosine-sensitive electrodes.

Siesjö: It should be emphasized that there is a constant turnover of the adenine nucleotide pool. As you indicated, AMP is constantly being broken down to IMP, adenosine, inosine and hypoxanthine. These compounds are diffusible in the tissues. That makes it absolutely necessary, especially if there is perturbation of the energy state, for the adenine nucleotides to be constantly resynthesized. Under normal circumstances, *de novo* synthesis in the brain is a very slow process. It seems that the tissue has to use salvage pathways for resynthesis and one such pathway utilizes adenosine in a reaction catalysed by adenosine kinase. In other words, if adenosine is taken up by the tissue that may have nothing to do with regulation of circulation but might simply indicate turnover of the pool.

Owman: In the type of craniotomy experiments that Professor Siesjö mentioned, the brain is extremely sensitive to even small increases in heat produced by the drilling in conjunction with craniotomy, and a local brain oedema easily develops if the area of trephination is not properly irrigated (Edvinsson & West 1972). This damage lasts several hours after the operation. Such simple traumatic factors are usually not taken into consideration in the sophisticated measurements of changes in the microcirculation within exposed areas of the brain.

Rubio: One has to make compromises in designing experiments of this sort. In the particular case of intact skull we had no means of rapidly sampling the tissue. The brain is a *prima donna*—we cannot touch it without introducing a modification. We must obviously try to control all the variables that one can introduce and at the same time be able to sample the tissue satisfactorily. We have discussed the possibility of using a freeze-blowing procedure for brain. Another procedure would be to use microwave irradiation, thus preserving the anatomical structure and making it possible to analyse particular neuronal nuclei (Medina *et al.* 1975). One problem with such a procedure is that there would be such small amounts of tissue that one would have to redesign the procedures for enzymic analysis of adenosine.

References

BOCKMAN, E. L., BERNE, R. M. & RUBIO, R. (1975) Release of adenosine and lack of release of ATP from contracting skeletal muscle. *Pflügers Arch. Eur. J. Physiol. 355*, 229

DOBSON, J. G. JR., RUBIO, R. & BERNE, R. M. (1971) Role of adenine nucleotides, adenosine and inorganic phosphate in the regulation of skeletal muscle blood flow. *Circ. Res. 29*, 375

EDVINSSON, L. & WEST, K. A. (1972) Experimental cerebral heat lesions produced by trephine craniotomy in rabbits. *Acta Pathol. Microbiol. Scand. 80A*, 134–138

FORRESTER, T. (1972) An estimate of adenosine triphosphate release into the venous effluent from exercising human forearm muscle. *J. Physiol. (Lond.) 224*, 611

FORRESTER, T. & HASSEN, M. O. (1973) Appearance of adenosine triphosphate in the perfusate from active frog skeletal muscle. *J. Physiol. (Lond.) 232*, 86P

GINSBORG, B. L. & HIRST, G. D. S. (1972) The effect of adenosine on the release of the transmitter from the phrenic nerve of the rat. *J. Physiol. (Lond.) 224*, 629

MEDINA, M. A., JONES, D. J., STAVINOHA, W. B. & ROSS, D. H. (1975) The levels of labile intermediary metabolites in mouse brain following rapid tissue fixation with microwave irradiation. *J. Neurochem. 24*, 223

MELDRUM, B. S. & NILSSON, B. (1976) Cerebral blood flow and metabolic rate early and late in prolonged epileptic seizures induced in rats by bicuculline. *Brain 99*, 523–542

MUSTAFA, S. J., RUBIO, R. & BERNE, R. M. (1975) Uptake of adenosine by dispersed chick embryonic cardiac cells. *Am. J. Physiol. 228*, 62

NORBERG, K. & SIESJÖ, B. K. (1975) Cerebral metabolism in hypoxic hypoxia. I. Pattern of activation of glycolysis: a re-evaluation. *Brain Res. 86*, 31–44

NORDSTRÖM, C.-H., REHNCRONA, S., SIESJÖ, B. K. & WESTERBERG, E. (1977) Adenosine in rat cerebral cortex: its determination, normal values, and correlation to AMP and cyclic AMP during shortlasting ischemia. *Acta Physiol. Scand. 101*, 63–71

PHILLIS, J. W. & KOSTOPOULOS, G. K. (1975) Adenosine as a putative transmitter in the cerebral cortex studies with potentiators and antagonist. *Life Sci. 17*, 1085

SCHRADER, J., BERNE, R. M. & RUBIO, R. (1972) Uptake and metabolism of adenosine by human erythrocyte ghosts. *Am. J. Physiol. 223*, 159

SCHRADER, J., RUBIO, R. & BERNE, R. M. (1975) Inhibition of slow action potentials of guinea pig atrial muscle by adenosine: A possible effect on Ca^{2+} influx. *J. Mol. Cell. Cardiol. 7*, 427

SCHUBERT, P. & KREUTZBERG, G. (1976) Communication between neuron and the vessels, in *The Cerebral Vessel Wall* (Cervós-Navarro, J. & Matakas, F., eds.), Raven Press, New York

SCHUBERT, P., LEE, K., WEST, M., DEADWYLER, S. & LYNCH, G. (1976) Stimulation-dependent release of 3H-adenosine derivatives from central axon terminals to target neurons. *Nature (Lond.) 260*, 541–542

Final general discussion

Siesjö: I should like to bring up for discussion some problems related to effects of circulating catecholamines on CBF and $CMRo_2$. My reason for doing this is some very preliminary results obtained in our laboratory by Dr Leif Berntman. Previous results from the laboratory (Carlsson *et al.* 1975, 1977; Berntman *et al.* 1977) have shown that both withdrawal of nitrous oxide supply from immobilized and artificially ventilated animals and arterial hypoxia can cause marked increases in CBF and $CMRo_2$ that are blocked or reduced in magnitude by adrenalectomy and by propranolol. Since these results suggest an effect of circulating catecholamines Dr Berntman infused noradrenaline i.v. in rats maintained on 70% N_2O (5 $\mu g\ kg^{-1}\ min^{-1}$) and started measurements of CBF (modified Kety and Schmidt technique) after 10 min of infusion. In the two experiments carried out before we left Lund, cortical CBF showed a three- to fourfold increase while $CMRo_2$ was 130–150% of control.

(*Note added in proof:* Subsequent experiments have shown that the infusion gives rise to increases in Pco_2 and body temperature. When the results are corrected for these increases, six experiments show that CBF is at least doubled, while there is an increase in $CMRo_2$ of about 30%.)

These results were obtained in spite of the fact that no deliberate attempt was made to 'open' the blood–brain barrier to amines, and there was no indication that the barrier was leaky to protein. It would seem profitable to discuss three points. First, could it be expected that the small penetration of amines that occurs normally could have physiological effects? Second, are there reasons to expect species differences in response to noradrenaline infusion? Third, is it possible that deep anaesthesia, as used by others, could blunt the effect of circulating catecholamines on the brain?

Sokoloff: How much does the blood pressure rise in the animals infused with noradrenaline?

Siesjö: About 10 mmHg, on average.

Sokoloff: That finding is not consistent with our results in man. We infused about 4 μg/min continuously for about 30 min and adjusted the infusion rate to increase blood pressure about 20 mmHg. Cerebral oxygen consumption did not change. Cerebral blood flow decreased slightly, but that was probably attributable to a fall in P_{CO_2} in the arterial blood because of hyperventilation.

Siesjö: We have quoted your results extensively but there may be species differences.

Owman: Although the intracerebral arterioles are essentially impermeable to noradrenaline, the pial vessels seem to behave as peripheral vessels in the sense that there is no diffusion barrier to this and other monoamines. If the perfusion time is long enough, noradrenaline will therefore simply diffuse from the pial circulation into the subarachnoid space (cf. Samorajski & Marks 1962). By circumventing the blood–brain barrier under such conditions, even systemic administration of the amine will produce various cerebrovascular effects, either directly or via the metabolism. The difference between the two sets of experiments may be due to the difference in brain sizes. The diffusion distance for noradrenaline coming into the subarachnoid space would be relatively longer in the human brain than in the rat, and during the corresponding time sufficiently deep diffusion from the subarachnoid space will produce more dramatic effects in rats.

Plum: Could you be getting a non-specific arousal effect from stopping nitrous oxide, similar to the effect obtained on blood flow and metabolism during the period of anxiety in the non-starved animal?

Siesjö: Yes, this is possible. We think that after withdrawal of anaesthesia catecholamines may be mobilized from the adrenals, and that causes an increase in CBF and CMR_{O_2}. However, there is a difference between the two sets of experiments. During 'immobilization stress' blood flow and CBF go up to 200% of the control value (30 min). Here, there is a proportionally larger increase in CBF than in CMR_{O_2}. That is, the results are similar to those obtained after injection of amphetamine (Berntman *et al.* 1978). Cerebral blood flow increases and cerebral venous oxygen content is higher than normal.

Reis: Another possibility is that you are stimulating peripheral receptors and getting reflex changes in the brain.

Raichle: What is the evidence that surface vessels on brain are more permeable to amines than deep penetrating vessels?

Owman: There is evidence of this from chemical determinations of noradrenaline in the subarachnoid space, and autoradiography (Samorajski & Marks 1962) shows that pial vessels are permeable to labelled noradrenaline.

There is histochemical evidence that in fairly high doses fluorescing amines penetrate the walls of the pial arteries, whereas they do not penetrate the intracerebral arteries (Bertler *et al.* 1966). Samorajski & Marks (1962) injected radioactive noradrenaline systemically and killed the animals at various times afterwards. Initially noradrenaline was seen only in the lumen of the cerebral vessels. Later there was a deposit also on the surface without anything in the wall proper. The most reasonable explanation was that somehow the intravascular noradrenaline left the vessels and came back through the subarachnoid space in which radioactive deposits were also demonstrable.

Rapoport: I agree with Dr Raichle that there is no definite evidence, at least with respect to the passage of intravascular horseradish peroxidase, that surface vessels generally have different permeability characteristics from central vessels. Westergaard & Brightman (1973) reported that some isolated arterioles, even at the cortical surface, have increased vesicular transport, but as concentrations of large proteins in the cerebrospinal fluid are so trivial, I don't think that this could be quantitatively important.

Table 7 of my paper (this volume, p. 248) shows that the brain normally can take up ^3H label during intravenous infusion of [^3H]noradrenaline. The ^3H space, 10 min and 60 min after continuous infusion of tracer, was 12% and 44%, respectively, as compared to a 3% blood space. The total quantity of tracer taken up by whole brain was 0.06% of the total dose, but we are not quite sure whether it was all noradrenaline. Are you sure that it is unchanged noradrenaline that you are following with the fluorescent technique?

Owman: The fluorescent material was unchanged amine, since the metabolites are not fluorogenic. The radioactive deposits may have included *O*-methylated and deaminated metabolites along with noradrenaline, which was labelled at the 7-carbon.

Rosendorff: The barrier to access of biogenic amines into the brain is not necessarily the same sort of barrier as exists for water or for protein. It is probably multifactorial. We know that noradrenaline is taken up by nerve terminals and by vascular smooth muscle cells. If we accept that the receptors are concentrated on the adventitial side of the vascular smooth muscle, which they almost certainly are, then any intraluminal noradrenaline has to get through a whole thickness of the media. There is a very efficient smooth muscle uptake mechanism before the molecule ever gets to the receptor. There are also of course the enzymes monoamine oxidase and catechol-*O*-methyltransferase to overcome *en route*. The relative impermeability of the blood–brain barrier to noradrenaline may have nothing to do with capillary tight junctions or any property of capillary endothelial cells. On the other hand, it is not difficult to imagine ingress of noradrenaline, and many other substances, into the brain if the capillary endothelial barrier is breached by an osmotic or any other type of insult.

Rapoport: Nevertheless, if any trapping occurred, there would be more label within the brain parenchyma than in the blood.

Rosendorff: We don't know which of these barrier mechanisms is rate-limiting, or even the relative importance of each in the special situation of cerebral vessels.

I was fascinated to hear Professor Siesjö describe experiments in which noradrenaline produced a fourfold increase in cerebral blood flow. This is an astonishing result which contrasts with the published effects, most of which are very subtle.

May I re-emphasize the importance of looking not at single doses of these vasoactive agents but at dose-response relationships? A good illustration of this principle is some work from our laboratory. McCalden & Eidelman (1976) measured cerebral blood flow in the pentobarbitone-anaesthetized baboon by the intracarotid ^{133}Xe clearance technique. Fig. 1 shows the effect of noradrenaline on grey matter blood flow. In the 'normal' animals, the 8 μg/min infusion increases flow by a small (less than 10 ml 100 g^{-1} min^{-1}) but statistically significant amount. As the dose goes up, the vasodilatation gets smaller at 16 μg/min, and then disappears at 32 μg/min.

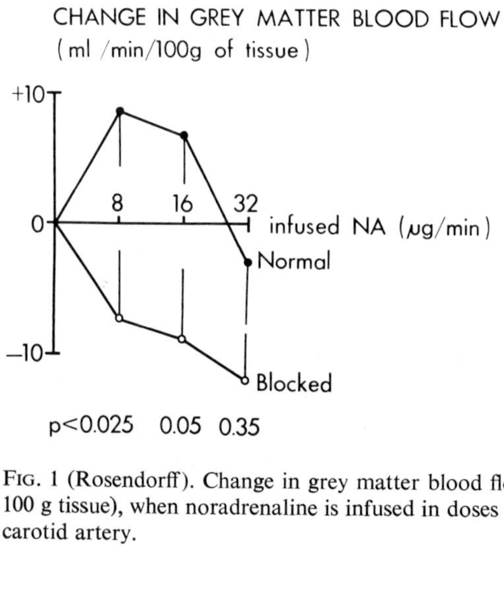

FIG. 1 (Rosendorff). Change in grey matter blood flow in the baboon, measured in ml/(min 100 g tissue), when noradrenaline is infused in doses of 8, 16 and 32 μg/min into the internal carotid artery.

Siesjö: What is the period of infusion?

Rosendorff: There is a continuous infusion. I think that we achieve a steady-state situation for at least the 20 minutes of the xenon clearance curve.

Now, when McCalden & Eidelman block catechol-*O*-methyltransferase with an agent such as 3,4-dihydroxy-2 methylpropiophenone (U-0521), the vasodilator effect of the same dose is converted to a vasoconstrictor effect. All of this suggests to us that lower threshold β receptors mediate the vasodilatation induced by lower doses of noradrenaline. As the dose increases, α receptor vasoconstriction becomes dominant. In the catechol-*O*-methyltransferase-blocked animal, noradrenaline has easier access to receptors, most of which are in the subadventitial region of the media. Therefore the local concentration of noradrenaline in that region is higher, producing an α receptor-mediated vasoconstriction response.

McDowall: What were the blood pressure changes in the two groups?

Rosendorff: None. The different doses were infused into the internal carotid arteries and the spill-over into the systemic circulation was apparently so small as to produce no change in systemic blood pressure.

Sokoloff: What were the changes in blood flow that you were looking at?

Rosendorff: The average grey matter flow is around 80 ml 100 g^{-1} min^{-1}, so this would be about 15%. That is much smaller than the sort of change that Professor Siesjö is talking about. The point is that the 8 μg dose alone would have given a very distorted idea of the whole picture. Secondly, there are several barriers to the ingress of noradrenaline to receptor sites and this is only one of them. If we had combined an uptake-2 blocker with a monoamine oxidase inhibitor and a catechol-*O*-methyltransferase blocker, perhaps we would have got an even more profound vasoconstrictor effect than is shown here.

Plum: Are those cumulative doses?

Rosendorff: No; these were successive experiments with different infusion concentrations for at least 30-min periods. The blood flow is measured in the control and in the uptake-2-blocked animals at the different doses. It doesn't matter how long the infusion lasts as long as we get a reasonably steady state when we are measuring flow.

Raichle: We keep coming back to the idea that levels of noradrenaline in brain tissue may influence overall brain metabolism in some way. Many people have made lesions in the central noradrenergic system and measured levels of noradrenaline in brain tissue. What sort of evidence do we have, from the behaviour of these animals or anything assessed in them, that suggests that profound changes in flow or metabolism have taken place in parallel with changes in brain noradrenaline? I am not talking about pharmacological experiments where one is infusing the drug or breaking the barrier but about animals with chronic lesions whose tissues have low noradrenaline levels.

Reis: There is a controversy about the effect of lesions in the locus coeruleus. The changes are extremely subtle.

Raichle: That would hardly correlate with the change of fourfold in the blood flow and metabolism.

Siesjö: It does with carbon dioxide, which increases CBF four- to fivefold.

Raichle: The inference here is that changes in centrally released noradrenaline cause profound metabolic changes. I hardly see this as a normal state.

Siesjö: It is definitely not a normal state.

Raichle: I am just trying to find a less invasive way of looking at it.

Plum: Sympathectomized rats look perfectly normal, don't they? It is my understanding that if animals in which the locus coeruleus has been acutely destroyed survive, they return to a state in which it is hard to distinguish them from their littermates.

Sokoloff: Is it possible that you were producing seizures in these animals that were masked by the neuromuscular blocking agent, Professor Siesjö?

Siesjö: We don't know. The EEG wasn't measured in these animals. In experiments on immobilization 'stress' there was no seizure pattern in the EEG, and $CMRo_2$ was up to almost 200% of control.

Purves: I am astonished that, apart from the early experiments you were talking about, nobody has found the same thing.

Siesjö: I want to stress two things. First, we work on rats and the rat may be peculiar. Second, the only anaesthetic given is 70% N_2O.

Reis: When autoregulatory curves are being mapped in animals the blood pressure is often raised by the infusion of noradrenaline, and autoregulation is maintained, even when blood pressure may go above 140 or 150 mmHg.

Siesjö: I thought that autoregulation was tested with much shorter infusion periods.

McDowall: I have done many experiments in baboons with infusions of noradrenaline for 20 min to test autoregulation. These animals showed a slight increase in flow, for there was hardly ever perfect autoregulation. We have used an autoregulation index, in an attempt to quantify degrees of impairment of autoregulation (Okuda *et al.* 1976). Using this index we find that under light halothane/nitrous oxide anaesthesia, 60–80% of complete autoregulation is present.

Purves: I thought the whole point was that the increase in arterial pressure was quite trivial?

Siesjö: Maybe the only explanation is that we are dealing with a small brain, as Professor Owman said.

Moskowitz: It might be worth while to emphasize that it is not only difficult to get noradrenaline across the blood–brain barrier into the central nervous system, but it is also extremely difficult to get it out in its unmetabolized state. This is the reason why concentrations of noradrenaline in blood or urine do not reflect the activity of this monoamine in brain.

Reis: Implicit in our concerns about the cerebral circulation and its control is that it is important in delivering metabolites to the brain. But nobody has discussed the possibility that a lot of this regulation may serve in addition a thermoregulatory role. Some of the circulatory effects, particularly on the cortical surface of the pia, may not necessarily be exclusively metabolic but may partake in important thermoregulatory exchanges in brain, possibly in response to slight changes in brain temperature in response to metabolism.

Purves: Do you think this is peculiar to the brain? That function is normally assumed in other vascular beds.

Reis: Hayward (1973) measured intracerebral temperature and showed that there were very wide changes in responses to thermal stimulation. The cerebral circulation might have more to do than just deliver metabolites.

Siesjö: If body and brain temperature is increased by 1 °C cerebral metabolic rate and blood flow are increased by 5%. This means that the changes are much smaller than those seen in blood flow during increased activity.

Reis: That is in relation to an external change. I am talking about dealing somehow with local metabolism of the brain. Heat is cleared so effectively because of vasodilatation.

McDowall: We have a few unpublished measurements of heat clearance on the surface of the brain with Althesin, a drug which reduces cerebral oxygen uptake by half. With the brain surface covered by the thermistor probe, the temperature is within 0.4 °C of the blood temperature. Even with the large metabolic change produced by Althesin, the temperature changes we saw were only within 0.1 °C. But of course flow changes very rapidly also.

Reis: That is the point. If this is an effective heat regulatory mechanism heat will be maintained and the blood flow will change.

References

BERNTMAN, L., CARLSSON, C. & SIESJÖ, B. K. (1977) Cerebral blood flow and cerebral metabolic rate in arterial hypoxia and in mobilization stress, in *Cerebral Function, Metabolism and Circulation* (Ingvar, D. H. & Lassen, N. A., eds.), pp. 4.6–4.7, Munksgaard, Copenhagen

BERNTMAN, L., CARLSSON, C., HÄGERDAL, M. & SIESJÖ, B. K. (1978) Circulatory and metabolic effects in the brain induced by amphetamine sulphate. *Acta Physiol. Scand.* Submitted for publication

BERTLER, Å., FALCK, B., OWMAN, CH. & ROSENGREN, E. (1966) The localization of monoaminergic blood-brain barrier mechanisms. *Pharmacol. Rev. 18*, 369–385

CARLSSON, C., HÄGERDAL, M. & SIESJÖ, B. K. (1975) Increase in cerebral oxygen uptake and blood flow in immobilization stress. *Acta Physiol. Scand. 95*, 206–208

CARLSSON, C., HÄGERDAL, M., KAASIK, A. E. & SIESJÖ, B. K. (1977) A catecholamine-mediated increase in cerebral oxygen uptake during immobilisation stress in rats. *Brain Res. 119*, 223–231

HAYWARD, J. N. (1973) Anatomy of heat exchange, in *Pharmacology of Thermoregulation* (Schoenbaum, E. & Lomax, P., eds.), pp. 22–41, Karger, Basel

MCCALDEN, T. A. & EIDELMAN, B. H. (1976) Cerebrovascular response to infused noradrenaline and its modification by a catecholamine metabolism blocker. *Neurology 26*, 987–991

OKUDA, Y., MCDOWALL, D. G., ALI, M. M. & LANE, J. R. (1976) Changes in CO_2 responsiveness and in autoregulation of the cerebral circulation during and after halothane-induced hypotension. *J. Neurol. Neurosurg. Psychiatry 39*, 221–230

SAMORAJSKI, T. & MARKS, B. H. (1962) Localization of tritiated norepinephrine in mouse brain. *J. Histochem. Cytochem. 10*, 392–399

WESTERGAARD, E. & BRIGHTMAN, M. W. (1973) Transport of proteins across normal cerebral arterioles. *J. Comp. Neurol. 152*, 17–44

Chairman's closing remarks

M. J. PURVES

Department of Physiology, University of Bristol

It is not really practicable to summarize all the topics which have been discussed over these past few days since, as was intended, they have ranged pretty widely. Rather, I shall take this opportunity simply to emphasize one or two points which have emerged from both the presentations and the discussions, where some order appears to be emerging out of chaos and where the techniques involved now appear to be sufficiently advanced for the problems to be tackled analytically in the near future.

In this symposium we have considered the central question, namely, how cerebral vascular smooth muscle is regulated, under two main headings, in keeping with precedent: first, the way in which the cerebral circulation responds to such systemic disturbances as hypoxia, hypercapnia and changes in arterial perfusion pressure, and secondly, the way in which blood flow changes in response to alterations in cerebral metabolic rate. It is reasonable to assume that both types of response are ultimately designed to ensure that the supply of oxygen and substrate to brain tissue is maintained within limits, where the primary stimulus is a threatened reduction in this supply or an increase in metabolic demand. It is, however, far from clear whether the mechanism of response is the same in the two different conditions.

When there is a systemic disturbance, it could act on cerebral blood vessels via a reflex action involving the system of extrinsic nerves which have been so admirably described by Owman. However, several recent experiments have suggested that these nerves affect smooth muscle at the neuromuscular junction in a way which is rather different from the action of the vasomotor nerves in other vascular beds; and it would seem from Heistad's experiments that the neural pathways are not essential for the majority of vasomotor responses but only become important under rather extreme conditions, for example, very high levels of arterial pressure. The systemic disturbance could affect cerebral blood vessels by altering the ionic environment of vascular smooth muscle, notably with respect to H^+ and K^+. However, the evidence presented by Siesjö, Astrup and Heuser would seem to be against this proposition. The vascular response can be due to activation of the adrenergic, dopaminergic or other intrinsic neural pathways, whose existence, distribution and termination are being investigated with vigour at the moment; and although there is as yet no evidence that fibres from such pathways make direct contact with cerebral vascular smooth muscle in the same way as the extrinsic fibres are known to do, it is certainly premature to write these pathways off as having no regulatory function. We should also bear in mind the remarkable example of a nerve termination on elements of the brain capillary which was shown by Raichle. The vascular response could be due to a direct action of oxygen, CO_2 or changes in transmural pressure, but although there is now ample evidence, discussed by Keatinge, that vascular smooth muscle in vessels outside the cranium can be so affected, it has proved to be exceptionally difficult to disentangle such a direct action from the other mechanisms outlined above *in vivo*.

With respect to changes in blood flow which accompany alterations in cerebral metabolic rate, we now have clear quantitative data from Sokoloff and his colleagues that there is remarkably close coupling between metabolic rate and blood flow in all parts of the brain in resting conditions and when the metabolic rate of discrete parts is raised. It would seem that the techniques employed are capable of giving yet further resolution. In addition, the results of experiments by Silver and Lübbers have indicated that the changes in blood flow occur extremely rapidly after changes in metabolic rate have been experimentally induced and that, from measurements of local oxygen tension, the changes in blood flow are more than adequate to meet the new metabolic demand. These observations raise in acute form the question of which part of the cerebral circulation is affected, either by some putative transmitter which couples metabolism and flow or by the extrinsic chemical or physical disturbances. It does not seem to me that we have the answer yet. However, we know that the calibre of both pial arterioles and veins can be affected by hypoxia, hypercapnia, hypotension and cortical seizures; and we know that the level of perfusion of tolerably identifiable volumes of brain tissue measured by the emission of radioactive indicators can similarly be affected. What we do not know is whether the changes in blood flow, which as usually measured represent changes of flow in intracerebral rather than pial vessels, are primary or whether they are secondary to changes in flow or pressure in 'upstream' blood vessels. Experimental results obtained over the last few years have suggested a system which may be described as follows. An external disturbance causes constriction of the larger conducting and/or pial vessels, either by a direct action on vascular smooth muscle or by a reflex action involving sympathetic nerves. The resulting alteration in vascular resistance could lead to a vasodilatation in that part of the cerebral vasculature which consists of vessels of less than 25 μg which are known to contribute about 50% of the total vascular resistance and which lie out of reach of the sympathetic nervous system. Such vessels could be the smallest arterioles, capillaries or, in particular, the post-capillary vessels which would be particularly susceptible to changes in intracranial pressure. As a result of this vasodilatation which occurs through some autoregulatory mechanism, no obvious changes in blood flow, certainly as measured by a radioactive indicator, would occur, although there might be clear evidence of pial vasoconstriction. Such a system might well explain the extraordinary diversity of experimental results obtained over the past decade or so when the proposed neural pathways had been cut or stimulated, for it would be proposed that in many, perhaps the majority, of these experiments, the combined effect of surgery, prolonged anaesthesia and exposure of the brain could variably affect the ability of small vessels to compensate for changes in the larger ones. Certainly, it has been hinted more than once in this symposium that autoregulation is a labile property of the smaller cerebral vessels and that the compensating ability of the smaller vessels can easily be compromised.

If this scheme turns out to be true, it emphasizes that the reaction of small vessels in the brain is the key to the form of response of the cerebral vasculature to both external disturbances and changes in metabolic rate. In turn this would suggest that probably the most important direction in which research should turn is the further exploitation of the methods for measuring local intracerebral blood flow which have been pioneered by Lübbers and Silver. Similarly, it seems clear that with the miniaturization of measuring techniques, such that some function of local cellular metabolism and local perfusion can be measured continuously and in parallel, the question of how metabolism and flow are coupled should be solved before too long. I think it has been made clear in this symposium that it is much more difficult to establish that a substance—whether H^+, K^+, adenosine or others in a fairly long list—is a transmitter either singly or in combination than has previously been realized, and our present technology will have to be stretched to the limit to do so. Thus it is required, on the one hand, that the changes in concentration of a putative transmitter in interstitial fluid be known with precision and, on the other, that the sensitivity of local blood vessels to that substance be known with equal accuracy. Furthermore, as has been made clear by Lübbers and Silver, it is essential to know both the speed and response of blood vessels and flow and the rate of change of the possible transmitter substance before its candidacy as a transmitter can be considered seriously.

In summary, I feel certain that students of the subject will have been greatly encouraged by the advances in techniques which have been made over the past year or so and which have allowed an increasing maturity of conception about the regulation of cerebral vascular smooth muscle. I foresee that, before too long, it should be possible to say something definite about how cerebral blood vessels go about their principal business, namely providing adequate oxygen and substrate to cerebral tissue. I would like to think that the high standards both of presentation and of informed discussion which have characterized this symposium will have played some part, however small, in this analysis.

Index of contributors

Entries in **bold** *type indicate papers; other entries refer to discussion contributions*

Indexes compiled by William Hill

Subject index